Preparing Personnel to Work with Infants and Young Children and Their Families

PREPARING PERSONNEL TO WORK WITH INFANTS AND YOUNG CHILDREN AND THEIR FAMILIES

A TEAM APPROACH

edited by

Diane Bricker, Ph.D.
University of Oregon

and

Anne Widerstrom, Ph.D.
San Francisco State University

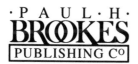

·P A U L·H·
BROOKES
PUBLISHING Cº

Baltimore • London • Toronto • Sydney

Paul H. Brookes Publishing Co.
Post Office Box 10624
Baltimore, Maryland 21285-0624

Typeset by Brushwood Graphics, Baltimore, Maryland.
Manufactured in the United States of America by
BookCrafters, Chelsea, Michigan.

Library of Congress Cataloging-in-Publication Data
Preparing personnel to work with infants and young children and their
    families : a team approach / edited by Diane Bricker and Anne
    Widerstrom.
         p.   cm.
    Includes bibliographical references and index.
    ISBN 1-55766-237-1
    1. Handicapped children—Services for—Study and teaching—United
States.   2. Infants—Services for—Study and teaching—United
States.   3. Child welfare workers—Training of—United States.
4. Health care teams—Training of—United States.   I. Bricker,
Diane D.   II. Widerstrom, Anne H.
HV888.5.p73   1996
362.4'083—dc20   95-39289
                                                            CIP

British Library Cataloguing-in-Publication data are available from
the British Library.

CONTENTS

ABOUT THE AUTHORS

Diane Bricker, Ph.D., Professor, College of Education, and Director, Early Intervention Program, Center on Human Development, University of Oregon, 901 East 18th Street, Eugene, OR 97403

Dr. Bricker is the director of the Early Intervention Program at the Center on Human Development at the University of Oregon. She is a professor of special education: early intervention and speech-language pathology. Dr. Bricker has published widely on personnel preparation and assessment/evaluation in early intervention.

Anne Widerstrom, Ph.D., Professor and Coordinator, Department of Special Education, 4 Tapia Drive, San Francisco State University, San Francisco, CA 94132

Dr. Widerstrom is a professor and coordinator of early childhood special education at San Francisco State University. Her professional experience includes classroom teaching in both general and special education, service as an educational diagnostician, supervision and program coordination, and university teaching. Dr. Widerstrom has published several books and numerous journal articles on early intervention.

Deborah Abelman, Part-Time Lecturer and Doctoral Candidate, Department of Special Education, San Francisco State University, 4 Tapia Drive, San Francisco, CA 94132

Ms. Abelman has taught courses at San Francisco State University and in a rural outreach program. She is a Lekotek leader for a community-based collaborative project funded through the San Francisco Mayor's Office for Children, Youth, and Their Families. She has been a teacher of preschool children with special needs in both public school systems and private nonprofit programs. Ms. Abelman has been a member of the Executive Board of the Division for Early Childhood of the Council for Exceptional Children, and is the president-elect of the California Subdivision of the Division for Early Childhood. She is a doctoral candidate in the Joint Doctoral Program in Special Education at the University of California at Berkeley with San Francisco State University.

Donald B. Bailey, Jr., Ph.D., Director, Frank Porter Graham Child Development Center, University of North Carolina at Chapel Hill, CB No. 8180, Chapel Hill, NC 27599

Dr. Bailey is the director of the Frank Porter Graham Child Development Center, a multidisciplinary research center at the University of North Carolina at Chapel Hill. He is also a professor in medical allied health professions and a research professor of education at the University of North Carolina at Chapel Hill. His research interests include early intervention, families of children with disabilities, the interdisciplinary team process, personnel preparation, and fragile X syndrome.

Deirdre Barnwell, Doctoral Candidate, Department of Special Education, University of Maryland, 1308 Benjamin Building, College Park, MD 20742

Ms. Barnwell has over 10 years of academic and practical experience in early childhood and special education. She has worked in a variety of special education and early childhood settings with families from many diverse cultural and economic backgrounds and with children who present a broad range of disabling conditions. Ms. Barnwell developed a community-wide early intervention program for children with and without disabilities while she was a volunteer for the Peace Corps in Honduras, Central America. Ms. Barnwell has extensive experience training and supervising early intervention personnel, which includes the development of training products and materials and ongoing program evaluation. She is a full-time doctoral candidate and faculty research assistant at the University of Maryland at College Park where she is involved in a variety of scholarly activities and supervising graduate students providing support to families of infants and toddlers with disabilities.

Paula J. Beckman, Ph.D., Professor, Department of Special Education, University of Maryland, 1308 Benjamin Building, College Park, MD 20742

Dr. Beckman is a professor in the Department of Special Education at the University of Maryland at College Park. She received her doctorate degree in 1980 from the University of North Carolina. Dr. Beckman began working with families of infants and toddlers with disabilities in 1974. With over 20 years in the early intervention field, Dr. Beckman has been involved in direct services and personnel preparation and has conducted numerous studies concerned with families of young children with disabilities. In addition to her other responsibilities, she directs a project designed to provide support to families of infants and toddlers with disabilities and a personnel preparation grant for students specializing in work with families.

Lynn Brown, M.S., Department of Special Education, University of Maryland, 1308 Benjamin Building, College Park, MD 20742

Ms. Brown has provided support and assistance to parents of children with disabilities both on an individual and a group basis for many years. In the course of her 20 years in the field, Ms. Brown has worked in both home- and center-based programs and has extensive experience providing preservice and in-service preparation for students in special education. At the University of Maryland, Ms. Brown has been involved in facilitating support groups for families of infants and toddlers with disabilities and providing individual support to families as part of Project Assist. She has also supervised many students in preservice programs who were learning to work with families and participated extensively in statewide in-service training efforts.

Janice Posatery Burke, M.A., O.T.R./L., F.A.O.T.A., Assistant Professor, Department of Occupational Therapy, Thomas Jefferson University, Philadelphia, PA 19107

Ms. Burke is an assistant professor in the Department of Occupational Therapy at Thomas Jefferson University in Pennsylvania. She has served as project director for federally funded graduate programs for occupational and physical therapists in early intervention and special education settings at Thomas Jefferson University, as well as training director for a university affiliated program in California. Her innovative training programs and expertise in theory and research have been recognized with numerous awards and honors.

Camille Catlett, M.A., Coordinator, Southeastern Institute for Faculty Training (SIFT), at the Frank Porter Graham Child Development Center, University of North Carolina at Chapel Hill, Chapel Hill, NC 27599.

Ms. Catlett is the coordinator of the Southeastern Institute for Faculty Training (SIFT) at the Frank Porter Graham Child Development Center at the University of North Carolina at Chapel Hill. Previously she was the director of two federally funded training projects at the American Speech-Language-Hearing Association (ASHA): ASHA's Infant Project (an interdisciplinary trainer-of-trainers project) and Building Blocks. Prior to arriving at ASHA in 1987 as the director of Grants Development and Administration, Ms. Catlett coordinated the special projects grant competition for the U.S. Administration on Developmental Disabilities. She has presented workshops throughout the United States on early intervention, teams and teamwork, family-centered practices, and grantsmanship, and has published articles in each of these areas.

Pamela J. Compart, M.D., Clinical Assistant Professor, Department of Pediatrics, Division of Behavioral and Developmental Pediatrics, University of Maryland, School of Medicine, 630 West Fayette Street, Room 1-120, Baltimore, MD 21230

Dr. Compart is a clinical assistant professor in the Department of Pediatrics, Division of Behavioral and Developmental Pediatrics at the University of Maryland. As a developmental pediatrician, Dr. Compart's clinical area of interest is the multidisciplinary evaluation of young children with a variety of developmental disorders. Her research interest is in medical education. Dr. Compart is a member of the American Academy of Pediatrics, the Society for Developmental and Behavioral Pediatrics, and the Maryland Chapter of the American Academy of Pediatrics Committee on Children with Disabilities.

Ann W. Cox, Ph.D., R.N., Director of Preservice Training, Virginia Institute for Developmental Disabilities, Virginia Commonwealth University, and Assistant Professor, Schools of Nursing and Education, Virginia Commonwealth University, Box 843020, Richmond, VA 23284

Dr. Cox is the director of Interdisciplinary Preservice Training at the Virginia Institute for Developmental Disabilities, a university affiliated program, and holds faculty appointments in the Schools of Nursing and Education at Virginia Commonwealth University. She is the director of an interdisciplinary related services personnel preparation program funded by the U.S. Department of Education that prepares graduate students in nursing, occupational therapy, physical therapy, psychology, and social work for careers in early intervention. Her professional interests include interdisciplinary education, school health, and early intervention. Dr. Cox has authored many training manuals, book chapters, and monographs. She serves as co-chair of the Personnel Development and Training Committee of the Virginia Interagency Coordinating Council.

Nancy Frank, M.S.W., Clinical Social Worker, Department of Special Education, University of Maryland, 1308 Benjamin Building, College Park, MD 20742

Ms. Frank is a clinical social worker and has worked for the past 10 years with parents and children. She has been working for the past 6 years with parents of infants and toddlers with disabilities and has led support groups and provided individual counseling and support services. In addition to her experience working with families and children, Ms. Frank has experience in conducting individual and family therapy groups and assisting families as a case manager.

Barbara Hanft, M.A., O.T.R., F.A.O.T.A., Developmental Consultant, 1022 Woodside Parkway, Silver Spring, MD 20910

Ms. Hanft has more than 20 years of experience as a clinician and counselor and works as a developmental consultant to early childhood agencies and programs. Recognized as a Fellow of the American Occupational Therapy Association for her leadership and advocacy in pediatrics, Ms. Hanft lobbied Congress and the U.S. Departments of Health and Education to enact laws and pass regulations affecting children with disabilities and their families. She has published widely in early intervention and special education and occupational therapy.

Alison Houck, Doctoral Candidate in School Psychology, University of North Carolina at Chapel Hill, Chapel Hill, NC 27599

Ms. Houck is a doctoral candidate in school psychology at the University of North Carolina at Chapel Hill. For 2 years Ms. Houck worked as a graduate assistant for the Southeastern Institute for Faculty Training (SIFT) at the Frank Porter Graham Child Development Center at the University of North Carolina at Chapel Hill. She is working on her dissertation investigating interdisciplinary collaboration among higher education faculty members involved in early intervention. Ms. Houck is on internship at the Kennedy Krieger Institute and The Johns Hopkins School of Medicine in Baltimore, Maryland.

Betsy LaCroix, M.S., O.T.R., Occupational Therapist and Doctoral Candidate, University of Washington, Seattle, WA 98112

Ms. LaCroix is an occupational therapist and doctoral student residing in Seattle, Washington. She received her master's degree in occupational therapy from Colorado State University, began her doctoral studies in early intervention at the University of Oregon, and is continuing her doctoral studies in special education and occupational therapy at the University of Washington. She has worked in schools and early intervention programs and is providing occupational therapy services to young children and their families at Holly Ridge Center in Bremerton, Washington.

Angela Losardo, Ph.D., Assistant Professor of Communication Disorders, Appalachian State University, Department of Language, Reading and Exceptionalities, Boone, NC 28608

Dr. Losardo is an assistant professor of communication disorders and also teaches in the Birth to Kindergarten Program at Appalachian State University. Her principal research interests focus on language and communication of young children, cross-cultural assessment/evaluation procedures, curricular approaches to early intervention, and preparation of personnel to work in early intervention. She is co-directing a model demonstration program exploring the process variables involved in the integration of general and special education curricula in preschool settings.

Jeanette A. McCollum, Ph.D., Professor of Special Education, University of Illinois, 288 Education Building, 1310 South 6th Street, Champaign-Urbana, IL 61820

Dr. McCollum is a professor of special education at the University of Illinois at Champaign-Urbana. Her recent professional career has been devoted to policy and training issues related to early intervention personnel. She has worked at the state and national level, as well as at the University of Illinois, to ensure that personnel working with young children and their families are of the highest quality. Dr. McCollum's other research interests include parent–infant interaction and its role in early development of children with disabilities, as well as personnel skills for supporting and facilitating interaction.

Irene R. McEwen, Ph.D., P.T., P.C.S., Associate Professor of Physical Therapy, University of Oklahoma Health Sciences Center, Post Office Box 26901, Oklahoma City, OK 73190

Dr. McEwen is an associate professor of physical therapy at the University of Oklahoma Health Sciences Center in Oklahoma City. She is the director of a related services personnel preparation project, which is supported by a U.S. Department of Education grant, to prepare occupational therapists and physical therapists at the postprofessional master's degree level to work in early intervention and public school programs. She has been a member and chair of the Pediatric Specialty Council for the American Board of Physical Therapy Specialties and is the associate editor for *Case Reports for Physical Therapy*. Her research focuses on assistive positioning for children with severe neuromotor impairments and evaluation of early intervention programs.

Barbara A. Mowder, Ph.D., Director, School Psychology Program, Department of Psychology, Pace University, Pace Plaza, New York, NY 10038

Dr. Mowder is the director of the School Psychology Program at Pace University in New York City. She has written extensively in the area of school psychology and early childhood special education. In particular, she co-authored *At-Risk and Handicapped Newborns and Infants: Development, Assessment, and Intervention* with Dr. Anne Widerstrom and Dr. Susan Sandall. Her research is in the areas of training school psychologists in the needs of young children with disabilities and their families, parent development and parenting education, and child characteristics as they relate to parenting dynamics.

Sandra Newcomb, M.A., Faculty Research Assistant, Department of Special Education, University of Maryland, 1308 Benjamin Building, College Park, MD 20742

Ms. Newcomb has a master's degree in special education and is a faculty research assistant in the Department of Special Education at the University of Maryland at College Park. She has extensive experience providing support to families of infants and toddlers both in individual settings and in parent support groups. She also has experience providing home-based early intervention services for children from birth to 3 years old. Her experience also includes preservice and in-service personnel preparation and supervision. She is the coordinator of a family specialization training grant that prepares graduate students in early childhood special education to work with families who have young children with disabilities.

Marie Kanne Poulsen, Ph.D., Director of Psychology, University of Southern California University Affiliated Program, Children's Hospital Los Angeles, Mail Stop 53, Post Office Box 54700, Los Angeles, CA 90054

Dr. Poulsen is the director of psychology at the University of Southern California University Affiliated Program, Children's Hospital Los Angeles, and is the director of the Region IX Infant Mental Health Leadership Training Project. She is an associate clinical professor of pediatrics at the University of Southern California School of Medicine and has contributed to the development of effective family-centered policies, programs, and services for infants and young children and families. She has written more than 50 publications concerning developmental and mental health issues and service delivery to infants, toddlers, and young children and their families.

M'Lisa L. Shelden, M.Ed., P.T., P.C.S., Adjunct Assistant Professor of Physical Therapy, University of Oklahoma Health Sciences Center, Post Office Box 26901, Oklahoma City, OK 73190

Ms. Shelden is an adjunct assistant professor of physical therapy at the University of Oklahoma Health Sciences Center in Oklahoma City. In addition to teaching pediatric content in the professional and postprofessional education programs, she is a coordinator of physical therapy for SoonerStart, Oklahoma's early childhood intervention program. She is a primary developer of Oklahoma's Statewide Training and Regional Support (STARS) program of professional development for early intervention personnel and teaches both technical and team-oriented courses. She is the chairperson of the Practice Committee of the American Physical Therapy Association's Section on Pediatrics. Ms. Shelden is completing her dissertation for her doctoral degree in special education. Her research is examining the effects of positioning on fine motor accuracy in children with cerebral palsy.

Jane Squires, Ph.D., Assistant Professor, Early Intervention Program, Center on Human Development, College of Education, 5253 University of Oregon, Eugene, OR 97403

Dr. Squires is an assistant professor in special education/early intervention at the University of Oregon. She directs a master's-level rural personnel preparation program and teaches classes in the early intervention area at the University of Oregon. Dr. Squires has also directed several research studies and outreach projects in the area of developmental screening and the involvement of parents in the monitoring of their child's development. She is a co-author of the *Ages & Stages Questionnaires: A Parent-Completed, Child-Monitoring System.*

Vicki D. Stayton, Ph.D., Professor, Department of Teacher Education, Western Kentucky University, 104 Tate C. Page Hall, Bowling Green, KY 42101

Dr. Stayton coordinates the Office of Interdisciplinary Early Childhood Studies, which houses several state- and federally funded projects specific to early childhood. Project activities include development of performance assessment tasks for the state certification process, implementation of an interdisciplinary early intervention personnel preparation program across four disciplines, and provision of technical assistance services for early intervention personnel. Dr. Stayton also coordinates the master's degree program in interdisciplinary early childhood education and is the chairperson of Kentucky's Part H Interagency Coordinating Council. Her research interests include personnel preparation issues and family-centered services.

Jennifer Stepanek, B.A., Department of Special Education, University of Maryland, 1308 Benjamin Building, College Park, MD 20742

Ms. Stepanek is the mother of four children who have had life-threatening health care needs. She is involved in both preservice and in-service personnel preparation in special education at the University of Maryland at College Park. In her role at the University of Maryland, she provides support to families that have young children with disabilities in both group and individual settings. She also serves as the family/professional resource specialist at the Association for the Care of Children's Health in Bethesda, Maryland. She has experience as a service coordinator for families of infants and toddlers. She has made numerous presentations on the subject of ways to support families who are grieving the loss of a child.

Elizabeth Straka, Ph.D., CCC-SLP, Interdisciplinary Preservice Specialization Project Coordinator, University Affiliated Program for Persons with Developmental Disabilities (UAP), and Adjunct Assistant Professor of Communication Sciences and Disorders, University of Georgia, Dawson Hall, Athens, GA 30602

Dr. Straka is the coordinator of a federally funded personnel preparation project that prepares students pursuing master's degrees in the School of Social Work or the Department of Child and Family Development to serve infants and toddlers who have delays or are at risk for developmental delays and their families. Collaboration with the Department of Communication Sciences and Disorders includes teaching child language courses and graduate student supervision within inclusive settings. She has 9 years' experience with children who have disabilities, the last 4 years of which involved providing in-service transdisciplinary assessment and intervention training. Dr. Straka's primary research interests are related to personnel preparation, collaborative team building, evaluation of preschool environments, and child language assessment and training. She is active in the development of state policy related to early childhood special education, particularly that relating to personnel preparation.

Nancy Striffler, M.S., Senior Policy Associate, Georgetown University Medical Center, Child Development Center, 3307 M Street NW, Washington, DC 20007

Ms. Striffler completed her undergraduate work in speech pathology at Temple University and her master's degree in speech and audiology at the University of Michigan. Ms. Striffler initially worked as a speech-language pathologist and clinical supervisor in both community programs and university settings. She continues to hold state licensure and certification by the American Speech-Language-Hearing Association. Ms. Striffler began her affiliation with Georgetown University Medical Center, Child Development Center (CDC), as a staff speech pathologist in 1973. Since 1980, she has served as the director of the Division of Communication Disorders and the associate director for Interdisciplinary Leadership Training for the CDC. In her role as the senior policy associate, Ms. Striffler provides training, technical assistance, and consultation to states, jurisdictions, and communities to assist in the development of family-centered, community-based services for children with special needs. Interagency collaboration, integrated systems design, and personnel issues have been areas of focus for her technical assistance and consultation activities.

Kathleen Swenson-Miller, M.S., O.T.R./L., Faculty Member, Fieldwork Coordinator, Department of Occupational Therapy, Thomas Jefferson University, Philadelphia, PA 19107

Ms. Swenson-Miller is a faculty member and the fieldwork coordinator for the Department of Occupational Therapy at Thomas Jefferson University in Philadelphia. She has worked extensively with families and children with special needs as a clinician, consultant, administrator, educator, and policy maker. She has served on the Developmental Disabilities Special Interest Committee and the faculty of the Family-Centered Care project for the American Occupational Therapy Association.

Renee C. Wachtel, M.D., Director, Developmental Pediatrics, and Associate Professor of Pediatrics, University of Maryland School of Medicine, 630 West Fayette Street, Baltimore, MD 21230

Dr. Wachtel is a developmental pediatrician who works with many families who have children with disabilities in hospital- and community-based programs. She trains pediatricians and other physicians, nurses, educators, and therapists in the medical care of children with developmental disabilities. She is also very actively involved in the State of Maryland's Infant and Toddler Program, serving on both the state and local Interagency Coordinating Council. In addition, she conducts research in premature infant development and pediatric human immunodeficiency virus infection.

Pamela J. Winton, Ph.D., Director, Southeastern Institute for Faculty Training (SIFT)—Outreach, and Research Fellow and Investigator, Frank Porter Graham Child Development Center, University of North Carolina at Chapel Hill, CB No. 8185, 521 South Greensboro Street, Chapel Hill, NC 27599

Dr. Winton is a research fellow and investigator at the Frank Porter Graham Child Development Center at the University of North Carolina at Chapel Hill. Since 1981, she has been involved in training, curriculum development, and research in the area of family–professional and interprofessional collaboration within the context of early intervention. She has published extensively on this topic, in addition to providing statewide, nationwide, and international training. The training curricula she has developed in collaboration with her colleagues are widely used in preservice and in-service settings. She is the director of the Southeastern Institute for Faculty Training–Outreach, which is a federally funded initiative that extends the interprofessional training model described in her chapter to states outside of the Southeast. Dr. Winton has been a local advocate for children and families in Durham, North Carolina, and is the president of the board of the Durham chapter of The Arc.

PREFACE

BEFORE PLUNGING INTO THE DEVELOPMENT of an edited book, one is wise to give consideration to the project. If we wavered before plunging, it was not for long because of the encouragement that we received. No one cautioned us to reconsider or go slowly. The universal response was to do it and do it now! There was a clear consensus that the literature in fields associated with young children who are at risk and/or have disabilities lacks substantive work on personnel preparation and particularly the preparation of professionals to participate on community-based teams. This book was designed specifically to address this deficit.

The book's content is intended for the variety of professionals engaged in varying levels of preparation in the fields of early intervention, early childhood special education, and allied health. A team approach provides the framework and guidance for the training described in this book and is based on the assumption that no single perspective, orientation, or discipline is adequate to develop and implement effective intervention programs for the range and diversity of problems presented by children and families eligible for public services during the infant, toddler, and preschool years. Most programs that provide services to infants and young children who are at risk and/or have disabilities use a variety of personnel to deliver services. The premise of this book is that the quality and effectiveness of services are enhanced when program personnel function as a team. By this we mean that personnel generally share common philosophies, goals, procedures, and desired outcomes and that individuals coordinate and complement their varying activities by working together as much as possible in the same setting at the same time. We believe that for personnel to function in isolation and without regard for other program elements and goals is simply not acceptable.

PURPOSE

Using a team approach as a foundation and context for service delivery to children from birth to 6 years old and their families, this book is designed to offer the following:

1. A rubric for guiding the development of personnel preparation and a discussion of associated issues
2. A review of training programs across selected disciplines

3. Information for the development of preparation programs for specific disciplines that incorporate a team approach
4. Information that may improve the functioning of teams providing services to young children and their families

CONTENT

This book is divided into three sections. Section I contains three chapters that are designed to provide a foundation and context for the discipline-specific chapters contained in Section II. The 10 chapters in Section II are a sampling of the numerous disciplines that could have been featured in this volume. Space limitations required us to be selective, and so we have attempted to provide a representative cross-section of disciplines participating in early intervention. Each of these chapters follows a similar format: introduction, review of pertinent literature, explanation of disciplinary training practices, analysis of issues associated with team approaches, and outline of potential solutions for barriers to effective collaboration. Section III contains three chapters that address across-discipline issues and one summary chapter that synthesizes the major themes discussed across disciplines.

Audience

This book targets four overlapping groups of readers. The first group is preservice faculty and instructors at institutions of higher education and community colleges. The second group consists of individuals enrolled in graduate training programs who envision becoming involved in preservice and/or in-service training upon graduation. The third group is program developers and administrators who have reason to acquire information on preservice and in-service training focused on infants and young children and their families. The fourth group consists of professionals who deliver services to children and their families and who wish to initiate a team approach or enhance the functioning of their team.

Terminology

Clarity in terminology is essential for successful teams and for effective written communication. To maximize the readability of this book, we have requested that contributors use the term *early intervention* to refer to the age range and services for children from birth to 6 years of age. This has been done unless the author notes otherwise. Thus, the contributors' discussion of *early intervention* encompasses services provided to infants, toddlers, and preschool-age children.

Previous written discussion in the literature on multi-, inter-, and transdisciplinary approaches has brought little clarity to the meaning of these terms. In addition, we have rarely found a team that follows a single model, but rather most teams use a variety of strategies. We, therefore, asked contributors to avoid the multi-, inter-, and trans- terminology whenever possible and to discuss instead the strategies and behaviors that make teams successful.

As we have suggested, we received much encouragement for the development of this volume. The contributors were willing participants who have met tight timelines with, we believe, quality chapters. The need to push the field toward the development of effective team practice is surely upon us. Our hope is that this volume will be the spark that mobilizes personnel to incorporate, study, and improve effective team practice.

To all those who know there is a better way

I

A Team Approach for Early Intervention Personnel

1

AN OVERVIEW OF
INTERDISCIPLINARY TRAINING

Donald B. Bailey, Jr.

I was working as a special education teacher in a resource room for 4- and 5-year-old children with disabilities in the mid-1970s. During the previous year, my co-teacher and I identified children at high risk, decided who was eligible for our class, determined the amount of help each child needed, planned instructional programs, told the general teachers what was going to happen, and provided resource services. All of this was done independently, with little supervision from the special education director and no input from other professionals. In the fall of 1974, however, we saw a dramatic change in the way business was conducted. We were told that eligibility and placement decisions must be made by a team of professionals; furthermore, the team had to agree on the instructional and therapeutic objectives for the child and work together in order to achieve the goals that were established.

I distinctly remember the first meeting. It was an awkward event. We all sat around the table wondering who was in charge and how this new organizational arrangement would work. The meeting was not very well organized, and we struggled to fit our own agendas into the meeting. Although all of us were strongly committed to promoting the development and education of children with disabilities, I am sure that we all were a bit skeptical about whether this approach was really worth the effort it surely would take. I also had misgivings about losing what autonomy I had, not wanting my professional activities to be determined in part by a group of professionals I did not know and who might not share my view of appropriate practice.

MORE THAN 20 YEARS LATER, the interdisciplinary approach remains one of the foundational components of services for children with disabilities. However, the implementation of interdisciplinary practices has been fraught with challenges, and scholars, practitioners, and parents acknowledge that, in most settings, interdisciplinary practices fall short of what was envisioned. Research during this time has reinforced the complex nature of teams and the ecologies within which teams work, and it is now clear that promoting interdisciplinary practices will require effort along a number of critical fronts. One of the most important of these activities is the training of professionals in the skills and philosophical orientation needed to make interdisciplinary practices work.

This chapter has three objectives. The first is to provide a brief overview of the history and rationale for the interdisciplinary perspective. The second objective is to draw on personal experiences and the research literature to highlight what is known about the interdisciplinary process and the implications of that knowledge for personnel preparation. The third objective is to provide an introductory discussion of the goals of interdisciplinary training and models that could be used to achieve those goals.

HISTORY AND RATIONALE FOR THE INTERDISCIPLINARY PERSPECTIVE

The notion of a work team has been of historical importance in sports and military settings and has rapidly grown in acceptance in the business world since the mid-1960s (Sundstrom, DeMeuse, & Futrell, 1990). Although special educators and others committed to improving the lives of people with disabilities and chronic illness have long articulated the importance of a team approach, it was not until the passage of PL 94-142, the Education for All Handicapped Children Act of 1975, that the interdisciplinary team became a required component of special education and related services. In 1996, acknowledgment of the importance of the interdisciplinary perspective is routinely found in almost any publication about services for people with disabilities as well as services for people with other health or mental health concerns (e.g., Findholt & Emmett, 1990; Greening, 1992; Kumpfer, Turner, Hopkins, & Librett, 1993; Saltz, 1992; Saunders, Miller, & Cates, 1989).

The team approach has a particularly strong historical basis in early intervention. Allen, Holm, and Schiefelbusch (1978) presented a detailed rationale for a team approach to early intervention, and this theme has continued to be emphasized in virtually all of the early intervention literature. PL 99-457, the Education of the Handicapped Act Amendments of 1986 (reauthorized as PL 102-119, the Individuals with Disabilities Education Act Amendments of 1991), reinforced the team concept in early intervention and placed a significant emphasis on the role of parents as participating members of the team.

Throughout this literature, four major themes underlie the rationale for a team approach to intervention. It is argued that 1) the complex nature of many disabilities requires high levels of specialization, but the rapidly expanding knowledge base means that no one person or discipline has access to all of the information needed; 2) services need to be integrated; 3) a process is needed to build shared ownership and commitment to goals and services; and 4) decisions made by a group generally are superior to decisions made by an individual.

Complex Nature of Disabilities and the Need for Specialized Knowledge

Children with disabilities represent a highly diverse group with respect to etiology, expression, and treatment. The causes of disabilities are considerable in number and include genetic (e.g., Down syndrome, fragile X syndrome), prenatal (e.g., spina bifida, fetal alcohol syndrome), perinatal (e.g., asphyxiation, low birth weight, other birth trauma), and postnatal (e.g., infections, accidents) etiologies. Children may be mildly affected, with only slight delays in development, or they may have profound delays and multiple impairments. They may have problems with their vision or hearing, brain damage that affects motor development, or severe behavior and/or emotional disabilities. The increased survival rates of children with very low birth weights or other medical problems means that these children may have chronic illnesses or disabilities that require ongoing medical treatment. This incredible diversity requires a high degree of specialization; however, a rapidly expanding knowledge base makes it impossible for any one person or discipline to have or maintain sufficient knowledge about the full range of disabilities or about various educational and therapeutic treatment options. Thus, one argument for the interdisciplinary team is that multiple specialists are needed to address the complex needs posed by children with disabilities.

The Need to Integrate Services

If increased specialization were all that was needed, a *multidisciplinary team* would suffice. The multidisciplinary team model involves professionals from several disciplines who remain independent of each other. The family may have access to a full set of specialists, but there is little attempt to integrate or coordinate activities. The complex nature of disabilities, however, makes it essential that team members meet to share and discuss information, generate ideas about treatment alternatives, and develop an appropriate and functional set of goals and services. The *interdisciplinary team* model provides such a structure, as team members meet and work together to develop a joint plan of action. Although each team member does his or her own assessment and develops an initial set of recommendations, this information is shared along with data generated by other team members and integrated in a comprehensive plan. As Fordyce (1981) suggested, the interdisciplinary team approach differs from the multidisciplinary approach in that the result "can only be accomplished by a truly interactive effort and contributions from the disciplines involved" (p. 51).

A further extension of the collaborative concept is the *transdisciplinary team* model. This model requires a much more complete integration of activities by team members at all levels and is characterized by joint sharing of responsibilities, mutual training of team members, sharing of expertise, and "role release," in which roles and responsibilities of one discipline become embedded in those of another (Lyon & Lyon, 1980; Woodruff & McGonigel, 1988). For example, the physical therapist and the speech-language pathologist might work with the child care teacher to integrate positioning techniques, movement activities, and communication goals into the everyday play activities of a child with cerebral palsy. Linder (1993) described a transdisciplinary model of play-based assessment in which team members conduct assessments jointly using a common assessment tool, further reducing the boundaries between disciplines and encouraging a holistic view of the child.

Shared Ownership and Commitment

A third rationale for the team approach is a recognition that the full implementation of a plan of action (as operationalized in the individualized family service plan [IFSP] or the individualized education program) requires a commitment from all team members to work toward common goals in the agreed-upon fashion. Shared commitment to goals is important because it is unlikely that any one professional will have enough time with the child to achieve the goals for which he or she is individually responsible. For example, the speech-language pathologist alone could be responsible for enhancing communication goals. In reality, however, the child's communication goals will probably not be met unless parents, teachers, peers, and other therapists all are aware of the goals and prompt and reinforce each goal as often as possible.

Commitment is not something that can be legislated or mandated. Commitment comes from a shared vision of desired outcomes for children with disabilities and their families and from a sense of ownership that comes through full participation in the planning process. This can occur only when team members meet together to jointly plan, discuss differences in an open and honest fashion, and work with families to set a team agenda. A multidisciplinary approach results in many team members engaged in their own activities but not working together in a coordinated fashion. Interdisciplinary and transdisciplinary approaches were designed to help ensure that all team members work toward the same goals, building on and reinforcing goals and activities suggested by other team members.

Superiority of Group Decisions

Building on the first three points, a final rationale for the team approach is that a group is more likely to make an appropriate decision about a course of action than any one individual. An individual is likely to be biased by his or her own training and experiences, as well as by limited interactions with the child with a disability and the child's family. Furthermore, an individual usually cannot objectively evaluate the pros and cons of the goals and activities he or she generates. A team can pool information, resources, and experiences to provide a context in which multiple suggestions can be generated, discussed, and evaluated in a collegial yet critical fashion so that decisions can be made on the basis of maximum information and input.

A limited amount of research provides empirical support for the assertion that group decision making can be superior. Wagner (1977) reported that team-generated treatment plans were more "holistic" than plans developed by individual professionals. Pfeiffer and Naglieri (1983) found that there was less variability in placement decisions for teams rather than individuals, suggesting that teams may make fewer placement errors than individuals. In a similar vein, Kuhlman, Bernstein, Kloss, Sincaban, and Harris (1991) found that team consensus ratings of client functioning were substantially more reliable than ratings done by individual team members. Hochstadt and Harwicke (1985) reported that victims of child abuse and/or neglect were more likely to obtain services if they had a team rather than an individual evaluation, and Feiger and Schmitt (1979) found that patients in a medical setting in which there was high team participation had better health outcomes than patients in units in which there was little or no team participation. Stefanich, Wills, and Buss (1991) reported that students who attended middle schools where teachers had a substantial degree of training in interdisciplinary team teaching had higher self-concepts than students who attended schools with low levels of interdisciplinary training; Stefanich et al. suggested that this was likely a result of the increased sense of community fostered by an interdisciplinary approach.

These findings are limited in scope, and little research has provided concrete evidence of the superiority of the team approach, due in part to the complexity of the issue and the challenge of finding a set of outcome measures by which the effectiveness of team approaches can be evaluated. Nonetheless, most authors conclude that if one can assume that the team is composed of competent members who are committed to working together for the good of the child or family requesting services, the resulting decisions are likely to be better than those made by a single individual. As Grofman, Owen, and Feld (1982) suggested, "more heads are better than fewer, as long as they are good heads" (p. 687).

RESEARCH ON TEAMS: IMPLICATIONS FOR PERSONNEL PREPARATION

The interdisciplinary team, with its legal and rational underpinnings, is now a standard part of special education and related services for children with disabilities and their families. What is known about group process and the ecology of teams that is relevant to the central thrust of this text, namely, the preparation of professionals from multiple disciplines to work effectively as a team in early intervention? For more than 15 years, I have had the opportunity to be involved in a number of projects in which some aspect of this question has been addressed. Below is a summary of this work, embedding it in the larger literature on teams and discussing the implications of various findings for personnel preparation.

Describing Individual Participation on Teams

In the 1970s and early 1980s, much of the research on teams focused on the group process, the participation by various team members, and the perceptions participants have of other team members. This research showed that team meetings often lacked substance and true collaboration (Fordyce, 1982; Lowe & Herranen, 1982; Ysseldyke, Algozzine, & Mitchell, 1982), the level of participation varied in part as a function of the disciplinary background and status of team members (Gilliam & Coleman, 1981; Yoshida, Fenton, Maxwell, & Kaufman, 1978), and parents often played minimal roles in the meeting (Goldstein & Turnbull, 1982). In 1981, I was working with a state residential institution for people with severe disabilities to provide training for its staff and wanted to do some evaluation of that work. When the director of the institution was asked to identify the desired outcomes of that training, he said that one of the most important goals was to improve the way team members worked together in planning and implementing services. This led to the exploration of strategies for operationalizing collaboration and subsequently to the study of the interdisciplinary process.

It was decided that although collaboration was a complex construct, the behavior of individuals on the team was fundamental. A scale, validated by experts, was developed to rate individual participation in team meetings. The scale was organized into five dimensions, with multiple items reflecting each aspect of participation:

1. *Preconference preparation*—preparing reports, submitting reports, reviewing the reports of others
2. *Providing information*—providing information, delivering information, using technical terms

3. *Participating in the group process*—seeking information, suggesting goals or strategies, providing feedback, having group discussion, having flexibility, accepting responsibility, suggesting interdisciplinary goals
4. *Distractions*—arriving and departing, distracting behavior
5. *Nonverbal behavior*—physical position within the group, body language

The scale was used to rate the participation of 227 individuals across 23 different team meetings (Bailey, Helsel-DeWert, Thiele, & Ware, 1983; Bailey, Thiele, Ware, & Helsel-DeWert, 1985). These studies provided evidence for the psychometric integrity of the scale. Participation varied as a function of discipline, with professional staff participating more than professional assistants. The lowest ratings were found in the domain of *participating in the group process*, with especially low ratings on seeking information from others, suggesting goals or strategies, providing feedback on suggestions made by other team members, and suggesting interdisciplinary goals. It was also found that self-ratings of participation did not highly correlate with observed ratings.

With respect to personnel preparation, these studies demonstrated that specific behaviors of team members deemed important by the literature and rated as important by professionals were not consistently demonstrated in team meetings. Especially low were those items related to central components of the team process, namely the discussion among team members regarding goals and strategies, the extent to which this discussion is substantive in nature, and the collaborative versus independent nature of goals and strategies. This suggests that professionals need training in effective communication skills and that specific behaviors are important in promoting successful team meetings. It is likely that these skills are the same as those that have been identified as important for communicating effectively with parents, including listening reflectively, questioning effectively, reflecting feelings, reflecting content, and integrating information (Winton, 1988; Winton & Bailey, 1993). In addition, the finding that observed participation is only marginally related to self-reported participation suggests that team members lack sufficient knowledge to evaluate the quality of their behavior in team meetings. Thus, training may need to include specific feedback on behavioral performance.

A Multidimensional Model of Team and Group Process

Although individual participation is central to the team process, group dynamics are likely to reflect more than the sum of the behaviors of individual team members. Drawing on systems theory and a model developed by Tseng and McDermott (1979) to describe families, a "triaxial model" was developed for conceptualizing the interdisciplinary team and group process (Bailey, 1984). The model assumes that teams are complex entities, with three primary dimensions (or axes as portrayed in a visual model). The first dimension, *team development*, is based on the assumption that teams grow, develop, and change over time. For example, a team could move from a multidisciplinary approach to an interdisciplinary approach. Several authors have suggested that teams pass through various stages as they work together over time, beginning with the process of becoming acquainted, passing through periods of trial and error as well as conflicts over how the team should be organized, and eventually reaching a state of equilibrium or maintenance (Lacoursiera, 1980; Lowe & Herranen, 1982; Tuckman & Jensen, 1977). The second dimension, *team subsystems*, assumes that some problems in teams emerge as a function of problems with individuals (e.g., a dominant team member, a social isolate, one member who has conflicts with other members) or with subgroups within the team (e.g., one faction consistently has conflicts with another faction over philosophical or procedural issues). The third dimension, *whole team functioning*, suggests that some problems within teams involve the whole team, such as when a team is overstructured, disorganized, or has ambiguous roles for team members.

Sundstrom et al. (1990) have extended this concept by using an ecological approach to describe the effectiveness of work teams. They argued that teams are heavily influenced by the organizational context in which they work. This would include the collective values of the organization; the nature of the team's task; the clarity of the team's mission; the extent to which the team is allowed to operate in an autonomous fashion; whether teams and team members get feedback on performance; the extent to which rewards and other consequences are contingent on individual versus group behavior; the training, consultation, and support available for teams; and the extent to which the physical environment promotes positive and productive interactions among team members. The real or perceived boundaries that define and link teams and the developmental processes through which teams proceed also determine the ultimate effectiveness of teams. Sundstrom et al. defined effectiveness as a team that performs its intended goals and maintains viability as an entity over an extended period of time.

Teams consist of individuals who try to work together as a group. Groups have their own unique properties; individual behavior can differ from group behavior, and behavior in one group will likely be different from behavior in another group. Furthermore, a team does not operate in a vacuum, but rather in the context of an organization that may or may not support its work. For personnel preparation, several implications are important. Professionals need to be aware of group dynamics and group processes. They need to know how groups can influence individual behavior, and conversely how individuals can affect groups. They must also realize that forces outside the team can serve to shape team functioning in ways that may not be immediately obvious. Furthermore, each group is unique. Training at the preservice level is necessary to prepare professionals to participate in team processes but probably will not be sufficient to support and maintain effective teams. Building effective teams will also require in-service training and ongoing administrative support, especially given the turnover that exists among staff in school and early intervention programs (Palsha, Bailey, Vandiviere, & Munn, 1990).

Preservice Preparation of Professionals for Work on Early Intervention Teams

In 1987, Courtnage and Smith-Davis reported the results of a national survey of training programs for special education teachers to determine the nature and extent of interdisciplinary team training. Only about 50% of the programs in the survey offered training on working with teams, and little was provided by universities in the way of in-service education. The authors argued that the effectiveness of teams could not be fairly evaluated if team members were not adequately prepared to perform their roles.

In 1988, the Carolina Institute for Research on Infant Personnel Preparation, an early childhood research institute at the University of North Carolina funded by the U.S. Department of Education, conducted a series of national surveys of college and university programs to determine the extent to which professionals from 10 disciplines—audiology, medicine, nursing, nutrition, occupational therapy, physical therapy, psychology, social work, special education, and speech-language pathology—were adequately prepared to work with infants and toddlers with disabilities and their families. This research is described in detail in a number of discipline-specific papers (Bailey, Palsha, & Huntington, 1990; Bishop, Rounds, & Weil, in press; Cochrane, Farley, & Wilhelm, 1990; Crais & Leonard, 1990; Holditch-Davis, 1989; Humphry & Link, 1990; Kaufman, 1989; Roush, Harrison, Palsha, & Davidson, 1992; Simeonsson & Brandon, 1988; Teplin, Kuhn, & Palsha, 1993) and summarized in an integrative review (Bailey, Simeonsson, Yoder, & Huntington, 1990).

These surveys revealed considerable variability across and within disciplines on the extent to which entry-level professionals were prepared to work with infants and toddlers with disabilities and their families. Most students received information on typical and atypical infant development, but considerably less information on strategies for infant assessment and infant intervention. Across almost every discipline, little emphasis was placed on working with families or on the interdisciplinary team process. For example, graduate programs reported an average of 11 clock hours of information on team processes, with a low of 2 hours (physical therapy) and a high of 20 hours (nursing). Likewise, programs other than those in social work or nursing reported an average of only 8½ clock hours of information on working with families. With the exception of specialized programs (e.g., early childhood special education), students had few opportunities to work with infants with disabilities and virtually no experiences in working with families or working in the context of interdisciplinary teams. Little change was projected in training programs, primarily due to competing priority areas; perceived and real requirements of state agencies; professional organizations and universities; and lack of faculty with expertise in infancy, families, and teams.

Ideally, all of the major disciplines would have special tracks to provide students with the expertise needed to work with young children and families. The research described above and other similar studies suggest that such a goal is unrealistic in the near future, with the exception of special education, which has a rapidly expanding base of early childhood training programs. However, four policy recommendations for preservice programs seem to be important (Bailey, Simeonsson, et al., 1990).

1. All students should receive an introduction to legislative mandates pertaining to young children and their families and an overview of available programs and services. It has been found that many students have graduated from college and university programs unaware of early intervention legislation or the opportunities for practicing their discipline with young children with disabilities and their families.

2. All students should have at least some exposure to real programs and services for young children and their families. Observing and doing internships

or practicum placements in early intervention programs, especially those with a family-centered, interdisciplinary focus, should provide opportunities for students to obtain a vision of how professionals in their own discipline can and do work with young children and may encourage students to choose early intervention as a career path.

3. Programs should expand the training provided to students on working with families. Data from both preservice and in-service programs document the critical need for expanded family training. Although working with families historically has been the job of the social worker or the nurse, it is recognized that a family-centered approach is necessary for each team member, as each has a responsibility for supporting, enabling, and empowering families.

4. Programs should expand the training provided to students on working in teams with professionals from other disciplines. This training should include both didactic information and practical experiences in working with students and experienced professionals from other disciplines.

These recommendations emerged from the finding that few students left their training programs with the technical skills needed to work with families or on teams (Bailey, Simeonsson, et al., 1990). Furthermore, these roles were not a core part of their professional identity. Placing a value on these skills during a preservice program and providing appropriate peer models would reinforce the essential, rather than peripheral, importance of team-centered and family-centered practices. Parenthetically, it should be recognized that enhancing the family and team aspects of preservice training need not be tied specifically to early intervention, as these skills are likely to be important throughout the age span.

Research on Practicing Professionals

Changes in preservice education are essential for teaching initial skills and fostering a professional identity that centers around teams and families. Given the large number of practicing professionals, however, more knowledge is needed about the complex challenges of working with families and teams in early intervention. Previous work had focused on the skills and behaviors of various team members. However, the importance of perceptions and values became increasingly more apparent as people began working with professionals from multiple disciplines to promote changes in professional practices. Roberts (1989), for example, argued that one of the main challenges to collaboration between social workers and physicians was the conflicting priorities or values held by members of each discipline, as well as values that guide professional thought and decision-making processes. A number of authors have argued that much of early intervention, family therapy, and other human services endeavors are value-laden activities, thus providing a context with considerable potential for disagreement, especially if values are not shared among professionals or between professionals and clients (Aponte, 1985; Dokecki, 1983; Kaiser & Hemmeter, 1989).

To investigate the role that disciplinary training contributed to the various challenges to interdisciplinary collaboration, we conducted two studies of practicing professionals. The first study examined the extent to which 142 early intervention professionals from various disciplines felt competent in working with families, valued family-centered roles, or were concerned about the movement toward family-centered practices (Bailey, Palsha, & Simeonsson, 1991). This study reported that social workers and nurses felt more confident in their skills in working with families than did special educators or allied health professionals (e.g., physical therapists, occupational therapists, speech-language pathologists). When asked to identify the most important roles related to work in early intervention, nurses and social workers were more likely to endorse family-related roles (e.g., assessing family needs, communicating with parents), whereas special educators and allied health professionals were more likely to endorse roles in working with children (e.g., assessing developmental status, designing interventions for children). No differences were found among disciplines in the concerns held by professionals about moving toward a family-centered approach. All professionals expressed concern about how family-centered practices would affect them personally and what impact these practices would have on the children and families they served. One of the highest areas of concern was how the intervention team would work together to implement a family-centered approach. In general, professionals seemed to suggest that they felt comfortable in their traditional disciplinary roles; however, working with families in the context of new federal legislation and the IFSP was a new direction for them. Professionals realized that the whole team would likely be involved in this new approach, but how that would be operationalized, who would take primary responsibility for family work, and the changes in roles of all team members (e.g., from being directive with families to being more responsive to family concerns and desires) were of considerable concern.

In the second study, we conducted a national survey of special educators, occupational therapists, speech-language pathologists, and physical therapists to determine their perceptions of typical and ideal service delivery models in early intervention (McWilliam & Bailey, 1994). We were especially interested in the extent to which professionals from each discipline endorsed "integrated" services (defined as a service delivery model in which therapy and instruction occur in the context of ongoing activities and routines with peers, based heavily on child initiations, addressing functional goals) with the specialist serving primarily as a consultant to the general education teacher. Special educators were found to be more likely to use and endorse integrated practices than were any of the allied health professionals.

These studies indicate that members of interdisciplinary teams have differing values and priorities for early intervention and for the way services are provided. The disturbing pattern of differences in values and priorities regarding family-centered and integrated service delivery models held by educators and allied health professionals could serve as a powerful detriment to the interdisciplinary process. The implication for personnel preparation is that training professionals needs to address more than communication skills and knowledge about group process in order for professionals to participate in the interdisciplinary process. At some point, the field will have to accept the diversity in perspectives that is evident across disciplines. To the extent that professionals differ in fundamental values about families and the way services should be provided, interdisciplinary collaboration will be compromised. Building a shared value base that is endorsed across professions and infusing that value base into preservice and inservice personnel preparation efforts represent critical challenges for the future (Bailey, in press).

Documenting Decision Making within Teams

In another study we extended the work on teams by examining one aspect of the decision-making process within team meetings (Bailey, Buysse, Simeonsson, Smith, & Keyes, 1995). Prior research had suggested that some team members hold more or less power than others (Fiorelli, 1988; Gilliam & Coleman, 1981; Yoshida et al., 1978) and that "team members see themselves primarily as representatives of their own discipline rather than as members of a team" (Sands, Stafford, & McClelland, 1990, p. 55). In this study, 72 professionals working in nine developmental evaluation centers were asked to rate 129 young children with disabilities on an index of functional abilities. The ratings were made independently by each team member, and then the teams met to form a consensus rating. The differences between individual and team consensus ratings were then examined. It was found that in domains in which a professional from a particular discipline was the primary expert (e.g., the physical therapist for ratings of tone, the psychologist for ratings of intellectual functioning), team consensus ratings were more likely to defer to the ratings of the discipline with traditional expertise. Allied health professionals (e.g., physical therapists, occupational therapists, speech-language pathologists) were least likely to change their individual ratings as a function of the team meeting. Expertise, of course, is important and thus, it is logical that the expert would exert a strong influence on team ratings. The areas for which allied health professionals were designated as experts are highly specialized aspects of functioning (e.g., tonicity, arm and hand functioning, communication patterns), but other team members also have perspectives on these areas and their input is likely to be important, especially in documenting functional skills. Further research is needed to examine the processes underlying team and individual decisions, but this study suggests that team decision making is still somewhat compartmentalized and heavily determined by specialized areas of expertise rather than by the team as a whole.

PERSONNEL PREPARATION STRATEGIES: A LOOK TO THE FUTURE

From research, several things have been learned that are relevant to interdisciplinary training. First, interdisciplinary collaboration consists, in part, of individual behaviors that can be described and documented. Those behaviors should be taught and practiced in preservice programs so that entry-level professionals will have the basic skills to perform effectively as team members. Second, it is clear that although work in early intervention involves a set of specific skills, some of which vary across disciplines (e.g., specialized therapeutic techniques) and some of which are common to all disciplines (e.g., communicating effectively with families), it also involves a set of values and assumptions about the goals of early intervention, the methods by which those goals are achieved, and the nature of the relationship between professionals and the families they serve. Preservice training must help students understand the values inherent in early intervention, identify situations in which their values conflict with those of others, and learn effective strategies for resolving value conflicts. Third, the complex ecologies in which teams work and the changing demands and composition of teams require that in-service training and ongoing support for teaming be available if interdisciplinary collaboration is to be effective. In the remainder of this chapter some future directions for personnel preparation at the preservice and in-service level are discussed.

Preservice Preparation of Professionals for Interdisciplinary Collaboration

Preservice preparation is a critical period in the development of a professional. It is during the college or university years that students learn the basic skills associated with their discipline. During this time, the student also begins to develop a professional identity by reading the discipline's literature, listening to and observing the perspectives of professors and practicing professionals, and engaging in internship or other practicum experiences that serve to bring principles and ideals into reality. Some of these skills can be taught within the limited framework of a particular discipline, while others can only be addressed from an interdisciplinary perspective. Dunn and Janata (1987) described five criteria to identify problems that should be addressed through interdisciplinary or interprofessional training:

1. those that are unusually complex;
2. those that are chronic in our society;
3. those that require substantial societal expense;
4. those for which no single profession can provide a solution;
5. those that, despite efforts by a single profession, flow beyond and into another area of the individual's life or have affected a significant other. (p. 100)

These criteria apply to a number of dimensions of early intervention. Three obvious contexts are 1) supporting families, 2) including children with disabilities in programs for typically developing children, and 3) providing services in an integrated fashion.

For interdisciplinary work to be effective, several goals must be accomplished during preservice training. Students need to learn critical skills associated with effective team participation. Perhaps more important, however, is that the development of a professional identity must include the idea that team membership and collaboration with parents and other professionals is a fundamental aspect of what it means to be a professional, regardless of the specific discipline for which the student is being trained. Finally, the values and assumptions underlying early intervention need to be acknowledged, explicated, and supported by faculty and mentor models throughout the training experience.

How can these goals be achieved? Although some information can be provided through special courses and didactic experiences, these are likely to be only marginally effective unless the experiences become a central part of the training program. The following three suggestions are offered for future directions. First, faculty in the disciplinary training program must share a commitment to the interdisciplinary perspective and to the values inherent in certain domains of service delivery. Although most might articulate support of interdisciplinary collaboration, inclusion, and family-centered practices, our research suggests that these ideals are not widely applied in the context of training. True collaboration will only occur when faculty within and across disciplines develop a shared commitment to full implementation of the goals of collaborative practice. This will require cross-disciplinary discussions and collaboration among training programs in college and university settings.

Second, an infusion model, as opposed to a compartmentalized model, is likely to be required if the goals for collaboration are to be achieved. In a *compartmentalized model*, students might receive information about ideals such as interdisciplinary collaboration, inclusion, and family-centered practices in a special course or a module within a course. In contrast, an *infusion model* is one in which these ideas and concepts are embedded throughout every course and practical experience provided for students. For example, information about families and family-centered practices would not simply be a part of a special course on working with families, but would be included in courses on assessment, basic development, and intervention methods. Each course would reinforce the notion that parents are members of the team and that a primary goal of service delivery is to support families in achieving the goals they have for their children and for themselves. In response to this goal, faculty from the Carolina Institute for Research on Infant Personnel Preparation developed a series of curriculum guides for integrating family-centered content into core courses in occupational therapy, physical therapy, and speech-language pathology (Crais, 1991; Hanft, Humphry, Cahill, & Swenson-Miller, 1992; Sparling, 1992).

Likewise, the integrative nature of development (e.g., the interactions among cognitive, language, social, and motor development) would be emphasized in every course and the importance of multiple disciplinary perspectives would be stressed. I distinctly remember when we first had our daughter evaluated in response to some problems she was having in school. Each discipline evaluated her from a specific disciplinary perspective, assigned a label that was consistent with its disciplinary training, and proposed treatment strategies that involved only that discipline. For example, the speech-language pathologist said that she had a receptive language disorder requiring speech therapy, the occupational therapist said she was tactilely defensive and required sensory integration training from an occupational therapist, and the physician said she had an attention deficit disorder and needed medication. The team members could not step outside of their disciplinary perspectives to view our daughter as a child with many interrelated abilities and challenges. Preservice training must create a context in which professionals are encouraged to look at the whole child and work with other professionals to gain a more complete understanding of that child's strengths and needs.

Third, students must have opportunities to interact with students and professionals from other disciplines as well as with families of children with disabilities. An infusion model and broad-based coursework and experiences are essential, but nothing can replace the learning that occurs when students are forced to convey their opinions and listen to professionals from other disciplines. Several examples of this have been provided in the professional literature. Cole and Campbell (1986) described a set of interdisciplinary training experiences for occupational therapy students that involved collaborative training with students in nursing, social work, medicine, psychology, audiology, and speech pathology. The course included skill building, videotaping, observing a number of team meetings, and practical experiences in establishing teams and developing plans for clients. DeSalvo, Arlinghous, and Row (1985) described a graduate-level course for students from pharmacy dietetics, hospital administration, medicine, and nursing programs. Students were assigned to five-member teams that reviewed case studies and applied decision-making strategies to achieve a consensus on courses of action. Winton (1991) developed and field-tested a course for teaching students from multiple disciplines to work with families in the context of early intervention, drawing heavily on case studies (McWilliam & Bailey, 1993), videotaping, and a discussion-oriented format for training in decision making and collaboration. Casto (1987) described an interprofessional preservice training program that is designed to help professionals address complex societal problems. Courses are offered in the interprofessional support of clients, values and ethical issues across professions, policy analyses and implications, and include a clinical seminar on interprofessional practices. A faculty team approach and case study methodology form the underlying basis for this program.

Regardless of the format, interacting with students and professionals from other disciplines provides a unique experience for students. It forces them to develop skills in sharing and communicating with others and in compromising to reach a solution. It also provides key experiences likely to encourage students to think more about children with disabilities and the interrelated nature of developmental domains.

In-Service Training for Professional Collaboration

In comparison with the relatively sparse literature on preservice interdisciplinary training, much more attention has been paid to in-service training to promote team building. A focus on in-service training is logical because although there is a general set of challenges faced by almost any group, teams are unique individuals working in a unique context. In-service training is likely to be needed, both at the global level to encourage the implementation of new models of service delivery and at the level of the specific team to help groups solve problems in collaboration.

A number of models for building teams have been described in the literature. These models have focused on communication and observation skills (Perlman & Whitworth, 1988), problem-solving strategies (Maher, 1983), organizational readiness (Maher & Hawryluk, 1983), attitudes and philosophies (Kealoha & Haase, 1988), building the sense of worth of each team member (FitzSimons, 1977), self-evaluation of team functioning (Fleming & Fleming, 1983), promoting cohesiveness (Callaway & Esser, 1984), team dynamics (Anderlini, 1983), and consensual decision processes (Gero, 1985). This literature suggests that supporting and building teams can be done in a number of ways.

From our research on professionals and the way they work with families, it has been found that moving to family-centered practices represented a major challenge for individual professionals and teams working in early intervention. In considering training strategies to help promote family-centered practices, it became clear that work with families represents a task that is common to all team members, but with varying levels of skill and shared commitment to this task. In order to promote systems change (as opposed to individual skill building), it was concluded that professionals must take an active role in encouraging change and that teams and consumers must be involved in policy decisions. To address the problem, a team-based model was developed for helping programs and teams become more family-centered in their work (Bailey, McWilliam, &

Winton, 1992; Bailey, McWilliam, Winton, & Simeonsson, 1992). The model contains five components. *Team-based training* is considered fundamental; that is, the training must involve all team members and must constantly address the problem from a whole team perspective. *Family participation* in the process is required. Families are members of the interdisciplinary team and should have input in helping programs and teams determine strategies and approaches for family-centered work. A *decision-oriented format* forms the basic core of the model. Instead of telling the teams what they should be doing, a series of workshops addresses six key questions fundamental to team practices vis-à-vis families.

1. What is our philosophy about working with families?
2. How will we involve families in child assessment?
3. How will we assess family needs and resources?
4. How will we involve families in team meetings and decision making?
5. How will we write family goals?
6. How will we implement the IFSP and provide service coordination?

Participants are involved in a set of *guided decision-making activities,* including some presentations, case study discussions, semistructured small-group discussions, and decision-making activities. *Leadership* is provided by a consultant knowledgeable in family-centered practices who could facilitate rather than direct team decision making.

This model was chosen for several reasons. Because professionals and families will need to work together on a daily basis in implementing specific strategies, it was essential that they all be together to wrestle with these issues. Also, based on the literature on adult learning and the change process, decisions were more likely to be implemented if the participants themselves set directions for change, thus building ownership and commitment to the established goals.

Implementing this model has yielded several interesting findings, highlighting the challenges associated with team-based training (Winton, McWilliam, Harrison, Owens, & Bailey, 1992). One of the first challenges was defining the team; this has been difficult in many settings because the team changes with each family and some team members are considered essential participants, whereas others may be optional and less likely to be included. Getting team members to come and participate in these activities has sometimes been difficult, especially for specialists (e.g., therapists) on contract to early intervention programs. The process is time consuming and almost always disruptive, given that arguments occur over desired practices, significant changes in practice are usually recommended, and changes identified sometimes are difficult to implement. Nonetheless, its implementation has forced teams to wrestle with substantive issues about practices, to set concrete goals, and to identify small but meaningful steps leading toward collaborative goal attainment. Also, the research on family participation in this process has demonstrated that family involvement is viewed positively by both parents and professionals, and their presence significantly affects the decisions that are made (Bailey, Buysse, Smith, & Elam, 1992).

It should be noted that this model focuses on an issue common to all team members, rather than on the team process itself. The five components of the model provide the framework, challenges, and supports for team discussion and decision making, but group process is not directly addressed in the training. Despite this, a common reaction of participants is that the experiences led to improved communication among team members and fostered a stronger sense of "teamness" among team members.

CONCLUDING REMARKS: FUTURE DIRECTIONS

The interdisciplinary team will continue to be emphasized in federal and state legislation, and its virtues will continue to be touted in the literature. Full implementation of the goals and processes desired as a result of collaborative teamwork has yet to be achieved, due in part to lack of training and in part to the ecology within which teams work and the constraints under which they function. Genuine collaboration will occur only when team members share a common vision for children and families and interact in an atmosphere of give and take, trust, and open communication in order to evaluate alternatives and design effective interventions and support services. Interdisciplinary training, in which professionals from multiple disciplines interact over an extended period of time to develop the skills and vision necessary for interdisciplinary collaboration, will need to occur at both the preservice and in-service levels. The remainder of this book is devoted to a more detailed discussion of how this can be achieved and a description of various models and approaches.

REFERENCES

Allen, K.E., Holm, V.A., & Schiefelbusch, R.L. (1978). *Early intervention: A team approach.* Baltimore: University Park Press.

Anderlini, L.S. (1983). An inservice program for improving team participation in educational decision-making. *School Psychology Review, 12,* 160–167.

Aponte, H. (1985). The negotiation of values in therapy. *Family Process, 24,* 323–338.

Bailey, D.B. (1984). A triaxial model of the interdisciplinary team and group process. *Exceptional Children, 51,* 17–25.

Bailey, D.B. (in press). Preparing early intervention professionals for the 21st century. In M. Bambring, H. Rauh, & A. Beelmann (Eds.), *Early childhood intervention: Theory, evaluation, and practice.* Berlin/New York: de Gruyter.

Bailey, D.B., Buysse, V., Simeonsson, R.J., Smith, T., & Keyes, L. (1995). Individual and team consensus ratings of child functioning. *Developmental Medicine and Child Neurology, 37,* 246–259.

Bailey, D.B., Buysse, V., Smith, T., & Elam, J. (1992). The effects and perceptions of family involvement in program decisions about family-centered practices. *Evaluation and Program Planning, 15,* 23–32.

Bailey, D.B., Helsel-DeWert, M., Thiele, J.E., & Ware, W.B. (1983). Measuring individual participation on the interdisciplinary team. *American Journal of Mental Deficiency, 88,* 247–254.

Bailey, D.B., McWilliam, P.J., & Winton, P.J. (1992). Building family-centered practices in early intervention: A team-based model for change. *Infants and Young Children, 5*(1), 73–82.

Bailey, D.B., McWilliam, P.J., Winton, P.J., & Simeonsson, R.J. (1992). *Implementing family-centered services in early intervention: A team-based model for change.* Cambridge, MA: Brookline Books.

Bailey, D.B., Palsha, S.A., & Huntington, G. (1990). Preservice preparation of special educators to work with infants with handicaps and their families: Current status and training needs. *Journal of Early Intervention, 14*(1), 43–54.

Bailey, D.B., Palsha, S.A., & Simeonsson, R.J. (1991). Professional skills, concerns and perceived importance of work with families in early intervention. *Exceptional Children, 58*(2), 156–165.

Bailey, D.B., Simeonsson, R.J., Yoder, D.E., & Huntington, G.A. (1990). Preparing professionals to serve infants and toddlers with handicaps and their families: An integrative analysis across eight disciplines. *Exceptional Children, 57*(1), 26–35.

Bailey, D.B., Thiele, J.E., Ware, W.B., & Helsel-DeWert, M. (1985). Participation of professionals, paraprofessionals, and direct-care staff members in the interdisciplinary team meeting. *American Journal of Mental Deficiency, 89,* 437–440.

Bishop, K., Rounds, K., & Weil, M. (in press). The preparation of social workers for practice with infants and toddlers with handicapping conditions and their families: The implementation of P.L. 99-457. *Journal of Social Work Education.*

Callaway, M.R., & Esser, J.K. (1984). Groupthink: Effects of cohesiveness and problem-solving procedures on group decision making. *Social Behavior and Personality, 12,* 157–164.

Casto, R.M. (1987). Preservice courses for interprofessional practice. *Theory Into Practice, 26,* 103–109.

Cochrane, C.G., Farley, R., & Wilhelm, I.J. (1990). Preparation of physical therapists to work with handicapped infants and their families: Current status and training needs. *Physical Therapy, 70*(6), 372–380.

Cole, K.D., & Campbell, C.J. (1986). Interdisciplinary team training for occupational therapists. *Physical and Occupational Therapy in Geriatrics, 4,* 68–74.

Courtnage, L., & Smith-Davis, J. (1987). Interdisciplinary team training: A national survey of special education teacher training programs. *Exceptional Children, 53,* 451–458.

Crais, E.R. (1991). *A practical guide to embedding family-centered content into existing speech-language pathology coursework.* Chapel Hill: Frank Porter Graham Child Development Center, University of North Carolina.

Crais, E.R., & Leonard, C.R. (1990). P.L. 99-457: Are speech-language pathologists prepared for the challenge? *Asha, 32,* 57–61.

DeSalvo, R.J., Arlinghous, E.J., & Row, K.W. (1985). An interdisciplinary-interuniversity health care team management decision-making case study course. *American Journal of Pharmaceutical Education, 49,* 168–172.

Dokecki, P.R. (1983). The place of values in the world of psychology and public policy. *Peabody Journal of Education, 60*(3), 108–125.

Dunn, V.B., & Janata, M.M. (1987). Interprofessional assumptions and the OSU Commission. *Theory Into Practice, 26,* 99–102.

Education for All Handicapped Children Act of 1975, PL 94-142. (August 23, 1977). Title 20, U.S.C. 1400 et seq: *U.S. Statutes at Large, 89,* 773–796.

Education of the Handicapped Act Amendments of 1986, PL 99-457. (October 8, 1986). Title 20, U.S.C. 1400 et seq: *U.S. Statutes at Large, 100,* 1145–1177.

Feiger, S.M., & Schmitt, M.H. (1979). Collegiality in interdisciplinary health teams: Its measurement and its effects. *Social Science and Medicine, 13,* 217–229.

Findholt, N.E., & Emmett, C.B. (1990). Impact of interdisciplinary team review on psychotropic drug use with persons who have mental retardation. *Mental Retardation, 28,* 41–46.

Fiorelli, J.S. (1988). Power in work groups: Team member's perspectives. *Human Relations, 41,* 1–12.

FitzSimons, R.M. (1977). Fostering productive interdisciplinary staff conferences. *Academic Therapy, 12,* 281–287.

Fleming, D.C., & Fleming, E.R. (1983). Consultation with multidisciplinary teams: A program of development and improvement of team functioning. *Journal of School Psychology, 21,* 367–376.

Fordyce, W.E. (1981). On interdisciplinary peers. *Archives of Physical Medicine, 62*(2), 51–53.

Fordyce, W.E. (1982). Interdisciplinary process: Implications for rehabilitation psychology. *Rehabilitation Psychology, 27,* 5–11.

Gero, A. (1985). Conflict avoidance in consensual decision processes. *Small Group Behavior, 16,* 487–499.

Gilliam, J.E., & Coleman, M.C. (1981). Who influences IEP committee decisions? *Exceptional Children, 47,* 642–644.

Goldstein, S., & Turnbull, A.P. (1982). Strategies to increase parent participation in IEP conferences. *Exceptional Children, 48,* 360–361.

Greening, K. (1992). The "Bear Essentials" program: Helping young children and their families cope when a parent has cancer. *Journal of Psychosocial Oncology, 10,* 47–61.

Grofman, B., Owen, G., & Feld, S.L. (1982). Average competence, variability in individual competence, and accuracy of statistically pooled group decisions. *Psychological Reports, 50,* 683–688.

Hanft, B., Humphry, R., Cahill, M., & Swenson-Miller, K. (1992). *Working with families: A curriculum guide for pediatric occupational therapists.* Chapel Hill: Frank Porter Graham Child Development Center, University of North Carolina.

Hochstadt, N.J., & Harwicke, N.J. (1985). How effective is the multidisciplinary approach? A follow-up study. *Child Abuse and Neglect, 9,* 365–372.

Holditch-Davis, D. (1989). In light of Public Law 99-457: How well are novice nurses prepared? *In Touch, 7*(2), 5.

Humphry, R., & Link, S. (1990). Entry level preparation of occupational therapists to work in early intervention programs. *American Journal of Occupational Therapy, 44*(9), 828–833.

Individuals with Disabilities Education Act Amendments of 1991, PL 102-119. (October 7, 1991). Title 20, U.S.C. 1400 et seq: *U.S. Statutes at Large, 105,* 587–608.

Kaiser, A.P., & Hemmeter, M.L. (1989). Value-based approaches to family intervention. *Topics in Early Childhood Special Education, 8*(4), 72–86.

Kaufman, M. (1989). Are dietitians prepared to work with handicapped infants? P.L. 99-457 offers new opportunities. *Journal of American Dietetic Association, 89*(11), 1602–1605.

Kealoha, M.C., & Haase, C.C. (1988). Training models for new and established teams. In D.C. Bross, R.D. Krugman, M.R. Lenherr, D.A. Rosenberg, & B.D. Schmitt (Eds.), *The new child protection team handbook* (pp. 499–534). New York: Garland.

Kuhlman, T., Bernstein, M., Kloss, J., Sincaban, V., & Harris, L. (1991). A team format for the global assessment scale: Reliability and validity on an inpatient unit. *Journal of Personality Assessment, 56,* 335–347.

Kumpfer, K.L., Turner, C., Hopkins, R., & Librett, J. (1993). Leadership and team effectiveness in community coalitions for the prevention of alcohol and other drug abuse. *Health Education Research, 8,* 359–374.

Lacoursiera, R.B. (1980). *The life cycle of groups: Group development stage theory.* New York: Human Sciences Press.

Linder, T.W. (1993). *Transdisciplinary play-based assessment: A functional approach to working with young children* (Rev. ed.). Baltimore: Paul H. Brookes Publishing Co.

Lowe, J.I., & Herranen, M. (1982). Understanding teamwork: Another look at the concepts. *Social Work and Health Care, 7*(2), 1–11.

Lyon, S., & Lyon, G. (1980). Team functioning and staff development: A role release approach to providing integrated educational services for severely handicapped students. *Journal of The Association for the Severely Handicapped, 5*(3), 250–263.

Maher, C.A. (1983). Development and implementation of effective individualized education programs: Evaluation of two team approaches. *Journal of School Psychology, 21,* 143–152.

Maher, C.A., & Hawryluk, M.K. (1983). Framework and guidelines for utilization of teams in schools. *School Psychology Review, 12,* 180–185.

McWilliam, P.J., & Bailey, D.B. (Eds.). (1993). *Working together with children and families: Case studies in early intervention.* Baltimore: Paul H. Brookes Publishing Co.

McWilliam, R.A., & Bailey, D.B. (1994). Predictors of service-delivery models in center-based early intervention. *Exceptional Children, 61,* 56–71.

Palsha, S.A., Bailey, D.B., Vandiviere, P., & Munn, D. (1990). A study of employee stability and turnover in home-based early intervention. *Journal of Early Intervention, 14,* 342–351.

Perlman, M., & Whitworth, J.M. (1988). Group process and interprofessional communication: The human aspects of teamwork. In D.C. Bross, R.D. Krugman, M.R. Lenherr,

D.A. Rosenberg, & B.D. Schmitt (Eds.), *The new child protection team handbook* (pp. 299–320). New York: Garland.

Pfeiffer, S.I., & Naglieri, J.A. (1983). An investigation of multidisciplinary team decision-making. *Journal of Learning Disabilities, 16*, 588–590.

Roberts, C.S. (1989). Conflicting professional values in social work and medicine. *Health and Social Work, 14*, 211–218.

Roush, J., Harrison, M., Palsha, S., & Davidson, D. (1992). Educational preparation of early intervention specialists: A national survey. *American Annals of the Deaf, 137*(5), 425–430.

Saltz, C.C. (1992). The interdisciplinary team in geriatric rehabilitation. *Journal of Gerontological Social Work, 18*, 133–142.

Sands, R.G., Stafford, J., & McClelland, M. (1990). 'I beg to differ': Conflict in the interdisciplinary team. *Social Work in Health Care, 14*(3), 55–72.

Saunders, R.B., Miller, M., & Cates, K.M. (1989). Pediatric family care: An interdisciplinary team approach. *Children's Health Care, 18*, 53–58.

Simeonsson, R.J., & Brandon, L. (1988). Psychology and P.L. 99-457. *Newsletter of the Society of Pediatric Psychology, 12*(4), 11–12.

Sparling, J. (1992). *A practical guide to embedding family-centered content into existing physical therapy coursework.* Chapel Hill: Frank Porter Graham Child Development Center, University of North Carolina.

Stefanich, G.P., Wills, F.A., & Buss, R.R. (1991). The use of interdisciplinary teaming and its influence on student self-concept in middle schools. *Journal of Early Adolescence, 11*, 404–419.

Sundstrom, E., DeMeuse, K.P., & Futrell, D. (1990). Work teams: Applications and effectiveness. *American Psychologist, 45*, 120–133.

Teplin, S., Kuhn, T., & Palsha, S. (1993). Preparing residents for P.L. 99-457: A survey of pediatric training programs. *American Journal of Diseases of Children, 147*, 175–179.

Tseng, W., & McDermott, J.F. (1979). Triaxial family classification. *Journal of the American Academy of Child Psychiatry, 18*, 22–43.

Tuckman, B.W., & Jensen, M.A.C. (1977). Stages of small group development revisited. *Group and Organization Studies, 2*, 419–427.

Wagner, R.J. (1977). Rehabilitation team practice. *Rehabilitation Counseling Bulletin, 20*, 206–217.

Winton, P.J. (1988). Effective communication between parents and professionals. In D. Bailey & R. Simeonsson (Eds.), *Family assessment in early intervention* (pp. 207–228). Columbus, OH: Charles E. Merrill.

Winton, P.J. (1991). *Working with families in early intervention: Interdisciplinary perspectives.* Chapel Hill: Frank Porter Graham Child Development Center, University of North Carolina.

Winton, P.J., & Bailey, D.B. (1993). Communicating with families: Examining practices and facilitating change. In J. Paul & R. Simeonsson (Eds.), *Children with special needs: Family, culture, and society* (pp. 210–230). Orlando, FL: Harcourt Brace Jovanovich.

Winton, P.J., McWilliam, P.J., Harrison, T., Owens, A.M., & Bailey, D.B. (1992). Lessons learned from implementing a team-based model for change. *Infants and Young Children, 5*(1), 49–57.

Woodruff, G., & McGonigel, M.J. (1988). Early intervention team approaches: The transdisciplinary model. In J.B. Jordan, J.J. Gallagher, P.L. Hutinger, & M.B. Karnes (Eds.), *Early childhood special education: Birth to three* (pp. 163–182). Reston, VA: Council for Exceptional Children and the Division for Early Childhood.

Yoshida, R.K., Fenton, D.S., Maxwell, J.P., & Kaufman, M.J. (1978). Group decision making in the planning team process: Myth or reality? *Journal of School Psychology, 16*, 237–244.

Ysseldyke, J.E., Algozzine, B., & Mitchell, S. (1982). Special education team decision making: An analysis of current practice. *Personnel and Guidance Journal, 60*, 308–313.

2

TEAM TRAINING ISSUES

Anne Widerstrom and Deborah Abelman

Imagine these two very different scenarios. First is a group of students gathered around a study table in a university library discussing a journal article on conductive education they have been assigned to read for their class in physical disabilities. The article will be the subject of lecture and discussion during the next several class meetings and will be one of several the students will be assigned to read during the semester about intervention methods for children with cerebral palsy. At the end of the semester there will be some questions on the final exam to test the students' understanding of theories underlying the different intervention approaches. The discussion is lively as the students ask each other questions and take notes to be used in tomorrow's class at which time they will learn more about the theory of conductive education from their university professor.

Second, imagine a program for infants where five staff members are receiving specialized training in positioning a child with cerebral palsy who has just entered the program. The instructor is the physical therapist who works in the program 3 days a week. She is sharing her knowledge with other team members because it is immediately pertinent for the team to be able to handle and position the newest program participant. The training takes place at the end of the program day and includes the child's mother, who is considered a member of the transdisciplinary team.

PERSONNEL PREPARATION IN THE FIELD of early intervention has followed two very different paths. The first path, preservice training, is meant to provide a thorough, in-depth grounding in the theory, knowledge, and skills necessary for successful professional service. It is a lengthy and expensive process, which yields an academic degree and/or professional certification or licensure and usually takes place in a college or university setting. The second path, in-service training (or staff development) and technical assistance, is meant to provide a short-term, inexpensive means for upgrading or updating the skills of professionals who have received preservice training and are working in the field. In-service training can occur in a variety of community-based or academic settings, while technical assistance usually occurs at the site of the early intervention program where services are being delivered. It is important to note that in-service training and technical assistance cannot be substituted for preservice training in meeting long-term personnel needs, but are meant to supplement the basic academic preparation (Bailey, Palsha, & Huntington, 1990; McCollum & Bailey, 1991; McCollum & Yates, 1994; Trohanis, 1994).

The issue of preservice versus in-service training is one of several to be discussed in this chapter. Related to this issue is the role personnel preparation programs play in the translation of theory-based research into current practice in early intervention (Odom, 1987). The relative roles of preservice and in-service training are of current interest in part due to the second issue to be reviewed—namely, the predicted nationwide shortage of early intervention personnel by the year 2000, and related to that, the issue of funding shortages that affects the early intervention field in the same way that other human services fields in the United States are being affected. Another issue is the preparation of nontraditional students who are entering training programs in increasing numbers: older students, students from culturally diverse backgrounds, and students from low-income backgrounds. Yet another issue is the children birth through 5 years old toward which training is directed. Specifically, should there be two different foci to the training, with infants and toddlers seen as separate and different from preschoolers, as reflected in Parts B and H of PL 101-476, the Individuals with Disabilities Education Act (IDEA) of 1990? Or, should training reflect most state certification requirements for early childhood special education and include children birth through 8 years old (Bruder, Klosowski, & Daguio, 1991)? A final issue is preservice training levels in the several disciplines represented on the early intervention team. From the associate degree through doctoral training, questions may be raised concerning certification, licensing and accreditation standards, development of training competencies, and issues of leadership. The purpose of this chapter is to address these issues related to personnel preparation in early intervention.

In this chapter, the term *early intervention* has been deliberately chosen to mean services for children birth through 5 years of age with or at risk for disabilities. There are four reasons for this. First, the early intervention field has developed as a birth-through-5 specialty, despite the fact that the field has been divided by federal legislation into two distinct groups—infants and toddlers (Part H) and preschool children (Part B). As a result of this division and Part H legislation, many authors use *early intervention* to refer to infants and toddlers and *early childhood special education* to refer to preschoolers. The authors of this chapter believe the division into two service delivery categories is confusing and awkward and does not serve the best interests of the early intervention field.

Second, there are more similarities than differences among programs for infants and toddlers and programs for preschoolers. Preschool staffing patterns, for example, are more like those found in infant programs than they are like those found in elementary schools. Curriculum, philosophy, and learning goals and objectives are other areas of strong similarity between infant–toddler and preschool programs.

Third, the authors of this chapter believe it would be a mistake to group preschool programs with elementary school programs simply because elementary programs have primarily an educational rather than an interdisciplinary focus and require the development of an individualized education program rather than an individualized family service plan (IFSP). Some of the most exemplary practices in the field have not come from kindergarten and elementary school but rather have originated in infant–toddler programs and moved to preschool programs (e.g., active role of family, IFSP, interdisciplinary team).

Finally, the field will be stronger in proposing policy changes and more unified in demanding resources if there is one label, *early intervention*, as reflected in the field's primary journal, the *Journal of Early Intervention*. In order to differentiate birth-to-2 programs from programs for 3- through 5-year-olds, it seems logical to speak of infant intervention and preschool intervention or infant–toddler programs and preschool programs.

PRESERVICE AND IN-SERVICE TRAINING

Trohanis (1994) has summarized the factors that continuously influence the quantity and quality of community services available for young children with disabilities and their families. These factors include federal and state laws and regulations, innovations from new research and practice, parent–professional collaboration, interagency coordination, and team service delivery. The field of early intervention is a fast-changing one, creating the need for ongoing, systematic professional training (McCollum & Bailey, 1991). In theory, the roles of preservice and in-service preparation are clear. In practice, there are problems with both approaches. In-service training has been characterized as disjointed, superficial, and ineffective (Meisels, 1989; Trohanis, 1994), while preservice training opportunities are often geographically limited and expensive and, thus, are unavailable to many potential service providers (McCollum & Yates, 1994; Widerstrom, Domyslawski, & McNulty, 1986) (see Chapter 13).

Substitution of In-Service for Preservice Training

As a result of the increase in numbers of children and families served because of federal and state legislation enacted since the mid-1980s, staff shortages exist in all the disciplines associated with early intervention (Hebbeler, 1994). With adequate federal and state support over the long term, preservice programs can be developed to address the shortages. To meet immediate needs, however, several authors have advocated for the development of effective in-service and/or technical assistance programs to provide training until more preservice programs are in place (Bruder & Nikitas, 1992; McCollum & Yates, 1994). For example, McCollum and Yates (1994) described the Partnership Project, a technical assistance project funded by the Office of Special Education Programs (OSEP) to support the implementation of new early intervention personnel standards in Illinois. The project provided funding for collaboration among university, state department of education, and university-affiliated program personnel to carry out three functions: 1) to formulate and implement a new portfolio-based credentialing process, 2) to support field-based training throughout the state for early interventionists to meet the new credential requirements, and 3) to support efforts to increase the number of colleges and universities in Illinois that offer preservice early intervention training. In the portfolio process, a committee of peers consisting of service providers, parents, and preservice and in-service faculty reviews the individual portfolios of early interventionists seeking to be credentialed. Credit for a variety of activities is accepted, including coursework, previous work experience in early intervention, mentoring other professionals, and attending in-service training sessions (McCollum & Yates, 1994).

Another project funded by OSEP has been described by Bruder and Nikitas (1992). Early interventionists from a variety of disciplines and backgrounds attended 4- to 10-week training institutes and then participated in a year of follow-up activities. The content of training focused on topics mandated by PL 99-457, the Education of the Handicapped Act Amendments of 1986 (since updated by PL 102-119, the Individuals with Disabilities Education Act Amendments of 1991), and the process was based on principles of adult learning, including individualized learning based on needs assessment, joint formulation of learning goals, and mutual planning by students and instructors (Bruder & Nikitas, 1992).

Innovative programs like the ones described by Bruder and Nikitas (1992) and McCollum and Yates (1994) have addressed some of the traditional criticisms of in-service training by basing training on established principles of adult learning, providing peer review, and including procedures for follow-up training. In the Illinois Partnership Project, some in-service resources were used to train college and university faculty in early intervention, ultimately increasing the amount of preservice training available in the state. Unfortunately, such exemplary in-service training programs are presently the exception rather than the rule. Many states still rely on fragmented, one-shot in-service training sessions with little input from trainees and little follow up (Trohanis, 1994). It appears unlikely that much positive change in practice results from these one-shot efforts.

A more serious problem occurs, however, when in-service training programs are seen as substitutes for preservice training. There are several reasons in-service training is recommended as a substitute for preservice training. The first, serious personnel shortages, has already been mentioned. An often-proposed solution to the problem of shortages is to use in-service training to upgrade the skills of service providers. A second factor involves the preference of some service providers and administrators for short-term training at their worksites rather than time-consuming coursework offered at university campuses. A third factor is the concern of professionals working in state departments of education, social services, or health services that state personnel standards are not being met due to a lack of preservice training programs. These factors combine to exert pressure for more short-term training measures. Unfortunately, the resources put into these efforts are in many instances subtracted from state dollars that might instead go to fund preservice programs (Gallagher, Shields, & Staples, 1990).

At the same time that an argument is made for continued substantial funding to develop and sustain preservice programs to fill long-term national training needs, there remains an ongoing, lifelong need for professionals to be kept apprised of issues related to their work in early intervention. Therefore, both preservice and in-service training have necessary and unique roles in comprehensive statewide efforts. Preservice training at the undergraduate or graduate level should provide at least basic knowledge about current theory and practice, supervised experience in applying theory to practice, and a repertoire of effective skills for working with children from age birth to 5 who have or who are at risk for disabilities. At the in-service level, professionals should expect a coherent series of activities and experiences sufficient in length and depth to upgrade existing skills, update current knowledge, and provide opportunities for the development of special expertise in specific areas (e.g., fund-raising, technology, public policy, administration).

TRANSLATION OF THEORY-BASED RESEARCH INTO PRACTICE

Odom (1987) wrote that basic research has the primary purpose of building theory, whereas everyday decision making has the purpose of solving problems and guiding actions. Knowledge of theory is an important goal of personnel preparation in early intervention, as is the ability to make informed, effective decisions regarding intervention with children and their families. Although theory and practice may be seen as opposites from which a choice must be made, they are actually integral to each other. Practice generates theory, which in turn guides practice (Berger, 1980).

Professionals who work with young children have a need for research-derived theory that can be incorporated into their practice. Making the link between ongoing research, the development of theory and applications to practice is considered to be a function of the university-based program (Widerstrom et al., 1986). It is the responsibility of the preservice training institution to ensure that practice is guided by theory. Universities are uniquely suited to carry out this task because they have the requisite personnel, resources, and physical space to conduct theory-based research, and they have faculty and staff who can provide the preservice training and supervision (Odom, 1987).

Once preservice training has been completed and the professional has been certified or licensed, further training usually takes the form of in-service training. However, in-service training that attempts to present theoretical knowledge in the absence of adequate application experiences for the learner or that relies on short training experiences that lack any grounding in research or theory will most likely prove ineffective (Widerstrom et al., 1986). Throughout their careers, professionals need practical knowledge thoroughly grounded in both research and theory. In the process of translating research-based theory into practice, cooperation between providers of preservice and in-service training would be ideal. Those engaged in research may not be able to provide practical applications as readily as those engaged primarily in field-based staff development and technical assistance activities. In-service trainers typically do not have the time or resources to conduct research.

EMPLOYMENT AND PROJECTED PERSONNEL SHORTAGES

Although it is generally agreed that shortages in personnel exist in all disciplines associated with early intervention (American Occupational Therapy Association [AOTA], 1990; American Physical Therapy Association, n.d.; Gallagher & Staples, 1990; Hebbeler, 1994; Olsen, 1991; Shewan, 1988; Silver, 1991; Yoder, Coleman, & Gallagher, 1990), specific data are elusive. Many factors affect accurate measurement of personnel shortages, including varying definitional categories across disciplines and also across states, funding considerations for infant programs under Part H and preschool programs under Part B, and different staffing patterns for infant and preschool programs. Nevertheless, data are available from the U.S. Department of Education (1993) and the U.S. Department of Health and Human Services (1992) that suggest that chronic shortages of early intervention personnel are likely to occur as the 21st century approaches. These shortages are projected based on the national trends discussed below.

First, the U.S. population includes an increasing number of older adults, which puts pressure on all human services, resulting in competition for staff between programs for older people and infant–toddler and preschool programs. Second, opportunities for employment for women have expanded since the mid-1970s to include many traditionally male-dominated fields such as law, medicine, and commerce. Although human services positions in social work, education, therapy, and nursing have been filled in the past primarily by women with fewer career options, other fields now compete for women's talents, reducing the pool of potential professionals in early intervention (Hebbeler, 1994). Unfortunately, human services jobs traditionally pay considerably less than jobs in other fields, which increases the difficulty of recruiting new service providers. For example, to be certified by the American Speech-Language-Hearing Association (ASHA) as a speech-language pathologist, a person must have his or her master's degree and extensive field supervision prior to licensing. Nevertheless, the average annual salary for an ASHA member in 1990 was $31,580, well below that of other non–human services professionals with similar educational requirements (Hebbeler, 1994).

Employed Personnel

In order to examine employment in the 1990s and projected personnel shortages in early intervention, it is necessary to distinguish between the different staffing patterns usually found in infant–toddler and preschool programs because the staffing patterns reflect two distinct components of IDEA. Part H for infants and toddlers requires states to establish a coordinated, interagency services delivery system for young children and their families. A range of child and family needs or priorities may be addressed by the interdisciplinary team (Turnbull, 1990). The interdisciplinary focus of Part H is reflected in the fact that more than half of the states in the United States have designated health or social services departments to be the lead agencies to oversee the program (Hebbeler, 1994).

In contrast, preschool programs for children with disabilities under Part B are mandated to provide special education and related services and are under the direction of state departments of education (Turnbull, 1990). The emphasis here is on meeting the child's *educational* needs, and teachers play a primary role on the team. Because of the difference in program focus and because infants require a larger adult–child ratio than preschoolers, infant–toddler programs usually require more staff than preschool programs (Hebbeler, 1994).

Table 1 presents the most current figures on the numbers of professional personnel employed in infant–toddler programs; however, it is difficult to draw firm conclusions about shortages because there is variation in service delivery patterns from state to state and from one discipline to another. As shown in Table 1, data collected by OSEP in 1991 and published in 1993 reveal that nearly 30,000 full-time professionals were employed in infant–toddler programs and nearly 18,000 in preschool special education programs (U.S. Department of Education, 1993). The total for preschool programs included only teachers and teacher assistants. Unfortunately, data are not available for the number of related services personnel who serve preschool programs because these data are collected from public schools as one combined total for children 3–21 years of age (Hebbeler, 1994). The total for infant–toddler programs included only 47 of the 57 states and jurisdictions in the United States, and thus probably underestimates the number of professionals employed nationwide as of 1991. In addition, of the 29,610 total reported for infant–toddler programs in Table 1, more than one half were employed in the state of New York. New York reported employing 15,000 people in infant–toddler programs. It is therefore difficult to generalize the infant–toddler data to a national level.

Table 1 shows that the two largest groups of infant–toddler service providers, 35.2% of the total, were special educators and paraprofessionals. A variety of other professional staff members, including nurses, speech-language pathologists, social workers, occupational therapists, physical therapists, physicians, psychologists, audiologists, and nutritionists, made up the other 64.8% of the total. Hebbeler (1994) noted that many states have indicated difficulty in reporting the number of personnel providing early intervention services because often they are provided by contracted personnel who are hired on a part-time basis. A survey conducted by the National Association of State Directors of Special Education (1993) found that more states tend to contract early intervention services from audiologists, occupational therapists, physical therapists, and physicians rather than employing them on a full-time basis.

As Hebbeler (1994) noted, a problem encountered in collecting national data by personnel category is the wide variation in definition found from state to state. This is especially true for the two largest categories, paraprofessionals and special educators, making it difficult to draw conclusions or generalize across categories. For example, not all states use the term *special educator*. Other titles used include *developmental specialist, early interventionist, interdisciplinary early childhood educator, early intervention specialist, child development fam-*

Table 1. Personnel employed or contracted by infant–toddler intervention programs in 47 states and jurisdictions in December 1991

Categories of personnel	Number	Percent
Paraprofessionals	5,950	20.0
Special educators	4,509	15.2
Other professional staff	3,487	11.8
Nurses	3,248	11.0
Speech-language pathologists	3,239	10.9
Social workers	2,593	8.8
Occupational therapists	1,734	5.9
Physical therapists	1,616	5.5
Physicians	1,332	4.5
Psychologists	1,059	3.6
Audiologists	530	1.8
Nutritionists	313	1.1
Total	**29,610**	

From the U.S. Department of Education (1993).

Note: Percentage of the total full-time equivalents employed and contracted across all categories.

ily specialist, infant specialist, and *early childhood special educator.* It is not clear how many of these individuals are being counted as special educators to indicate personnel shortages.

Similarly, there are differences in the way states define paraprofessionals. In some states the term is used for individuals with a high school diploma; in others it may describe a person with a 2- or 4-year college degree but who lacks the qualifications for licensure in a particular discipline. The term *paraprofessional,* because it implies less than equal status on the team, is losing favor. In the meantime, however, the lack of uniformity in definition requires that data on personnel shortages be cautiously interpreted (Hebbeler, 1994; Striffler, 1993).

Personnel Shortages

Despite limited national data on personnel shortages, data from specific states or regions are sufficient to suggest that some serious personnel shortages have existed for years and are likely to continue throughout the 1990s (AOTA, 1990; Gallagher & Staples, 1990; Hanson & Lovett, 1992; Hebbeler, 1994; Meisels, 1989; Olsen, 1991; Shephard, 1991; Silver, 1991). According to data reported to OSEP in 1991, nearly 7,000 additional service providers were needed to staff infant–toddler programs (U.S. Department of Education, 1993). As shown in Table 2, the three groups in shortest supply for infant–toddler programs were, in order of scarcity, speech-language pathologists, paraprofessionals, and special educators. This number probably underrepresents the actual shortage because not all states were implementing Part H in 1991 (Hebbeler, 1994). Table 2 summarizes data reported to OSEP from the 41 states and jurisdictions that were implementing Part H in 1991.

A review of Table 2 reveals that, in addition to speech-language pathologists, paraprofessionals, and special educators, all other categories of personnel were in short supply in infant–toddler programs. The need for more physical and occupa-

Table 2. Personnel needed in infant–toddler intervention programs in 41 states and jurisdictions from December 1991

Categories of personnel	Number	Percent
Speech-language pathologists	1,576	23.8
Paraprofessionals	964	14.5
Special educators	787	11.9
Physical therapists	636	9.6
Nurses	616	9.3
Occupational therapists	557	8.4
Other professional staff	541	8.2
Social workers	457	6.9
Psychologists	185	2.8
Physicians	129	1.9
Nutritionists	112	1.7
Audiologists	74	1.1
Total	**6,634**	

From the U.S. Department of Education (1993).

Note: Percentage of the total full-time equivalents employed and contracted across all categories.

tional therapists, nurses, and social workers was similar, ranging from 457 social workers to 636 physical therapists. There was a lesser need reported for psychologists, physicians, nutritionists, and audiologists, ranging from 74 audiologists to 185 psychologists.

Due to reporting practices, it is more difficult to determine the extent of personnel shortages in preschool programs. Because preschool data for related services personnel are not reported separately from elementary and secondary data, it is unclear in what disciplines personnel shortages exist and how large they are. OSEP estimated the shortage of preschool special education teachers to be 2,300 nationally in 1991–1992 (U.S. Department of Education, 1993), but no estimates were found for related services personnel working in preschool programs.

The shortage of physical therapists, occupational therapists, and nurses in early intervention is associated with the aging population in the nation. People with multiple disabilities and chronic conditions are living longer, as is the general population, which results in the need for more therapists to address problems found in older adults. In addition, early intervention programs are forced to compete for occupational and physical therapists because of 1) advances in medical technology that allow more individuals of all ages, including infants, to live with serious medical conditions and to need rehabilitation; and 2) the development of new fields (e.g., sports medicine) that employ therapists at relatively higher pay rates than early intervention programs (Hebbeler, 1994).

Because early intervention is a relatively low-paying field, the need to compete with higher-paying fields for service providers will likely have an impact on how quickly shortages can be eliminated. In addition, Shewan (1988) noted that many unfilled positions are in rural areas, in positions associated with low salaries, and in positions with poor working conditions.

As Hebbeler (1994) noted in her summary of personnel shortage data, the extent of the shortages may be masked by a high reliance on contracted services that are usually purchased on a part-time basis and are more expensive than services delivered by full-time salaried staff. This trend exists in both infant–toddler and preschool programs and leads to the spending of scarce resources for high-cost personnel because full-time staff positions go unfilled.

Certification Standards and Personnel Shortages

To further complicate the discussion of personnel shortages, many professionals meet certification requirements for early intervention positions but lack training and experience working with children under 5 years old. For example, some states accept certification with school-age children with disabilities for teachers working in preschool classrooms. Conversely, other professionals may have a great deal of knowledge and experience but lack appropriate certification (Bailey, Simeonsson, Yoder, & Huntington, 1990). Because early intervention is a young, emerging profession, not all states have fully developed standards for qualifying people to work in the profession (Bailey, Simeonsson, et al., 1990; Bennett, Watson, & Raab, 1991; Bruder et al., 1991; Hanson & Brekken, 1991; McCollum & Bailey, 1991; McCollum, McLean, McCartan, & Kaiser, 1989; Stayton & Miller, 1993). In fact, as of the fall of 1994, only 35 of the 50 states required some form of certification for educators employed in infant–toddler programs, and two other states had optional certification (National Early Childhood Technical Assistance

System, 1994). Clearly, if infant, toddler, and preschool programs for children with disabilities employed only people who were qualified and certified, both current and projected shortages would be much higher. Issues related to personnel standards and certification and/or licensing requirements are discussed below.

REDUCTIONS IN FUNDING

Reductions in funding have affected both training institutions and programs for young children and their families since the 1980s. The reductions have meant cutbacks in personnel that may affect the quantity and quality of services available (Bruder, Lippman, & Bologna, 1994; Meisels, 1989). At colleges and universities with no training programs for early intervention professionals, plans do not exist to create new programs (Gallagher & Staples, 1990). In addition, at universities with existing training programs, the reductions have meant larger classes, less faculty time for supervision, and larger student-advising loads. This situation makes it particularly difficult for faculty to engage in the mentoring activities that are important to the successful education of nontraditional students (Widerstrom, 1995). Because in many instances state and federal training funds are scarce, preservice programs are placed in the unhappy position of competing with state-funded in-service programs for resources. It is unfortunate, for example, that the greatest portion of Part H (PL 99-457) funds allocated to states was earmarked for planning rather than for training or direct services.

In addition, students themselves face funding shortages for financing their training and, as a result, many students attend school on a part-time basis. There are problems associated with part-time students who hold jobs in order to finance their education. These problems include lack of time to devote to coursework and field experiences, lack of energy to concentrate fully on training, and often the inability to quit the job in order to complete practicum and internship requirements (Widerstrom, 1995).

Solutions

There are several possible solutions to the shortages of funds and personnel for early intervention. The most obvious is to train more providers for full-time employment, reducing vacancies and reducing reliance on expensive contract services. Most professions involved in serving young children are advocating for an increase in the number of preservice programs that offer training in early intervention, despite the fact that universities seem reluctant to create new programs (Bailey, Palsha, et al., 1990; Bennett et al., 1991; Brandt & Magyary, 1989; Gallagher & Staples, 1990; Godfrey, 1995; Hanson & Lovett, 1992; Rowan, Thorp, & McCollum, 1990; Shephard, 1991). In addition, several authors have recommended using in-service training and technical assistance programs as means for improving the quality of service providers who may lack qualifications or competence (Bruder & Nikitas, 1992; Eggbeer, Latzko, & Pratt, 1993; McCollum & Yates, 1994).

Other solutions may involve increased recruitment and retention efforts to reduce turnover in the field (Widerstrom, 1995; Widerstrom et al., 1986). The effectiveness of these efforts depends on how successful the field is as a whole in raising pay standards for entering professionals. Professional organizations may need to take a more active role in recruiting new personnel (AOTA, 1990; Hebbeler, 1994). In addition, institutions of higher education should be encouraged to expand their preservice transdisciplinary training efforts (Bailey, Palsha, et al., 1990; Bruder et al., 1994). However, it should be emphasized that university faculty face the same below-average pay for professional work found in the rest of the early intervention field; if increased numbers of faculty are to be recruited to staff higher education training programs, pay inequities will have to be addressed.

A final solution may be to reduce the number of highly trained specialists who serve as team members and replace some of them with professionals with less specialized training (Striffler, 1993). The career ladder advocated by some (Hanson & Brekken, 1991; Kemple, Hartle, Correa, & Fox, 1994) could be a part of this proposed solution. Career ladders, with hierarchies of levels of training and employment, may appeal to young people wishing to commit to a career that offers advancements in responsibility as well as increases in pay (Hanson & Brekken, 1991).

RECRUITMENT AND TRAINING OF NONTRADITIONAL SERVICE PROVIDERS

As early intervention services become more family centered, parents of children with disabilities have more opportunities to express their preferences for how the services should be delivered. In response to parents' complaints about difficulties in finding and having access to services, better coordination between agencies is now occurring, which is reducing redundant, overlapping services and making a variety of services—health, social, and educational—available at a single site. At the same time, many parents are requesting service providers from their own communities who speak their language, share their values, and understand their customs. Yet, according to a study of early intervention service providers conducted in California, the majority of early interventionists are Caucasian women (Hanson & Lovett, 1992), a trend that is probably duplicated nationally.

In her study of multicultural competencies needed to work with families from diverse backgrounds, Christensen (1992) found that professionals (primarily of Caucasian, middle-class background) rated the ability to acknowledge one's own cultural heritage, beliefs, and biases as having a low level of importance. Interestingly, clarification of one's own value system appears to be an essential prerequisite for cross-cultural competence (Lynch & Hanson, 1992). As Christensen (1992) wrote, "Each individual has a unique cultural background with differing values, beliefs, and biases, and this cultural background can have a powerful effect on the relationship between professionals and the families they serve" (p. 55).

In most discussions of multiculturalism, the issues usually focus on racial, cultural, linguistic, and ethnic diversity. Little, if any, attention is paid to those issues pertaining to religious minorities. Yet, the concerns they have are often similar to those of people from racial and/or cultural minorities. It is possible that these concerns may be overlooked by professionals in part due to a belief that one's culture and religious beliefs are the same. But for African American

Jewish people, for instance, the issues that they face as a religious minority are different from those they face as a cultural minority. The Caucasian, middle-class professionals who participated in Christensen's (1992) study reported that they received minimal training in working with families from a variety of religious backgrounds; furthermore, they did not believe they needed additional training in this area. Yet, religion may affect much of everyday life for a family. "There appears to be a need to reexamine the importance of religion to ascertain how it shapes a specific culture and, more importantly, how it affects individual families" (Christensen, 1992, p. 56).

In order to increase diversity within the ranks of professionals serving young children, it is necessary to recruit a more diversified student population. According to the National Black Child Development Institute (1994), only half as many African American (14%) as Caucasian (31%) teachers in child care hold a bachelor's degree. According to membership data for the Division for Early Childhood of the Council for Exceptional Children (DEC), a primary professional organization for early intervention service providers, only 2% of the membership is African American and 7½% is non-Caucasian (Council for Exceptional Children, personal communication, September 30, 1994).

The factors discussed previously have contributed to a trend in institutions of higher education to recruit and train students from a variety of backgrounds to serve in diverse communities (Widerstrom, 1995). This trend is apparent in early intervention as well as in other areas and has found formal support in federal funding through OSEP. Institutions that enroll significant numbers of students from ethnic groups may compete for special funds to train members of racial and cultural groups in special education. As a result, 82 personnel preparation grants were awarded to minority institutions between 1992 and 1996 (OSEP, personal communication, August 1995). The primary purpose of these grants is to provide minority student financial support. It is an important factor in recruitment, as "it is difficult for many African Americans [and other ethnic groups or low-income students] to obtain the financial resources to attend college, especially a four-year college" (National Black Child Development Institute, 1994, p. 33). Graduate training necessary for a master's or doctoral degree is even more difficult to finance, making federal support of low-income students from ethnic groups especially important.

Another nontraditional student is the older person who may require additional training after working for several years in early intervention or a related field, or who may wish to change fields, entering early intervention for the first time. Many of these students are women who, having raised families, are returning to school to finish their education and to enroll in graduate training. Like students from ethnic backgrounds, many are the first in their family to receive a bachelor's or master's degree (Widerstrom, 1995). There are advantages and disadvantages in training older students. On the positive side, they often bring valuable experience to their studies, both general life experience and prior professional experience. They are typically highly motivated to complete their studies and work in their chosen field. They will, however, probably retire before younger students, limiting the potential number of years of service they can offer, while at the same time they are just as expensive to train; and, therefore, in an overall sense, older students may be less cost effective than younger ones. Until the 1980s this fact was reflected in the policy of many American medical schools that would not admit students over 30 years of age. In 1996, most people would agree that older service providers contribute a great deal to the early intervention field; excluding them is discriminatory and thus illegal.

Training nontraditional students involves accepting special challenges not usually encountered with other types of students. Students from nontraditional backgrounds may have unique needs for support, assistance, and understanding. They respond well to mentoring from faculty members, more experienced students, and their peers (Widerstrom, 1995). Establishing a one-to-one relationship with a supportive mentor that lasts throughout the training experience can make the difference between success and failure for many students. Mentoring and other techniques for supporting nontraditional students tend to require additional faculty time and therefore represent more intensive use of an already scarce resource.

DEFINING EARLY CHILDHOOD

According to the DEC, National Association for the Education of Young Children (NAEYC), and the Association of Teacher Educators (ATE) (1994), *early childhood* is defined as being bounded by birth and age 8. This definition has both a theoretical and pragmatic rationale: Development is seen as occurring on a continuum, with gradual changes in emphases.

> A program serving infants and toddlers will look markedly different from one serving children aged five through eight; yet, each will share underlying organizational principles that put both in stark contrast to programs for older children, such as the role of families, the way in which the child's role as active learner and discoverer is supported, and the way in which information is conveyed to the learner. (DEC, NAEYC, & ATE, 1994, p. 7)

From a pragmatic perspective, there are clear benefits to be derived from linking the entire birth-to-8 age range. In particular, it provides an effective response to the trend toward the downward escalation of academic curriculum and formal instruction in programs for younger children (Bredekamp, 1993). Nevertheless, while the term *early childhood* includes ages birth to 8, the term *early intervention* is restricted to children from birth to 5 years of age. This differentiation reflects both legal and programmatic definitions. The issue for training early interventionists can be summarized in two related questions:

1. Toward what groups of young children and their families should training be directed?
2. What are the training implications for inclusion if general early childhood programs serve children from birth to 8 years of age?

These questions are related to other issues, training levels, personnel standards, and leadership training, all of which are discussed below.

LEVELS OF TRAINING

Included in a discussion of training levels are questions related to developing personnel standards for the several disciplines involved in early intervention, their various certification and licensing requirements at each level, and training for leadership. Personnel standards and licensing requirements are of interest in examining the various disciplines that make up early intervention teams. Of the professionals involved in providing services to young children, speech-language pathologists and social workers have the highest educational requirements, the master's degree, while occupational and physical therapists require a bachelor's degree. Educational requirements for teachers and nurses vary greatly from state to state (Bruder et al., 1991; Hebbeler, 1994; Shewan, 1988). Early childhood special education requires the master's degree in several states, but graduates of those programs nationwide are approximately evenly divided between having bachelor's and master's degrees (Gallagher & Staples, 1990).

In the education field there is general agreement that there should be a hierarchy of personnel holding appropriate degrees (Brandt & Magyary, 1989; Hanson & Brekken, 1991; NAEYC, n.d.). The recommendations of the DEC, NAEYC, and ATE (1994) in their guidelines for licensure suggest that there should be separate licenses for the early childhood educator and the early childhood special educator, but there should be a link between the two so that professionals are capable of both upward and horizontal mobility within the greater early childhood education field.

The *NAEYC Guidelines for the Preparation of Early Childhood Professionals* (n.d.) suggest that the development of qualified personnel is a process that is ongoing. It recommends the following continuum for professional development:

1. **Associate degree:** The ability to plan and implement curricula
2. **Bachelor's degree:** The ability to develop curricula and develop and conduct assessments
3. **Master's degree:** The ability to analyze and refine knowledge and to evaluate and utilize research to improve practice
4. **Doctoral degree:** The ability to conduct research to expand the knowledge base and influence systems change

In 1994, the DEC, NAEYC, and ATE recommended that preservice undergraduate training be required for entry-level competence to serve children from birth to 8 years old. Graduate training should involve specializing in a particular area, such as the birth-to-3 population. This in essence creates a career ladder for early interventionists with a hierarchy of personnel (e.g., assistant, interventionist, specialist) holding appropriate degrees (e.g., high school diploma, bachelor's degree, master's degree). Each level in the hierarchy would have its appropriate certification (DEC, NAEYC, & ATE, 1994).

PERSONNEL STANDARDS

Personnel standards are the basis for developing certification and licensing guidelines, and these guidelines, in turn, are what dictate content for preservice personnel preparation programs. The need for the development of personnel standards for early interventionists received official recognition through PL 99-457 (Bennett et al., 1991). States are required to identify appropriate standards and establish a long-term structure to support the standards (McCollum & Bailey, 1991).

In a discussion of who should be responsible for setting the appropriate standards, Gallagher et al. (1990) suggested that professional organizations may be best suited to develop standards for their own disciplines, thus ensuring the development of national standards. If each state were allowed to set its own standards, it would take longer to develop them, and each discipline would have 50 sets of standards as opposed to a single one. If, however, professional organizations develop the standards, there is the concern that a professional organization might have a monopoly on the professional standards of a particular discipline. As of 1996, for example, the American Speech-Language-Hearing Association controls the professional standards for speech-language pathologists.

In making recommendations for personnel standards, the DEC, NAEYC, and ATE (1994) stated that although infant–toddler programs differ from those for preschoolers, they share at least six underlying principles that may guide the development of personnel standards and hence licensure requirements for personnel working in programs for young children. The first principle is based on the idea that children from birth to 8 years of age develop and learn differently from older children.

The second principle is based on the philosophy that families play a significant role in their children's development. Families are equal members of the decision-making team and their priorities and concerns should be met. Professionals need to develop collaborative relationships with family members.

The third and fourth principles address service delivery, stating that it should be developmentally appropriate and inclusive. Developmentally appropriate practice can be divided into two major components—*age appropriateness* and *individual appropriateness* (Bredekamp, 1993). Age appropriateness refers to programs developed for particular chronological and developmental ages, while individual appropriateness refers to the adaptations within programs for a particular child. "Th[e] practice of inclusion is based on the belief that young children with disabilities are more similar to than different from their peers, and that all young children benefit from learning together as members of a diverse community" (DEC, NAEYC, & ATE, 1994, p. 11).

The fifth principle is based on the concept that professionals must behave in a culturally competent manner. Development and learning occur within and are influenced by the contexts of ethnicity, culture, and religion (DEC, NAEYC, & ATE, 1994). Yet, there is not always a match between the ethnicity, culture, and religious background of families and service providers.

The sixth principle is based on the importance of collaboration with families, colleagues, and professionals in other fields. If families are to be included in the decision-making process and services are to be provided for children in inclusive settings as recommended in the second and third principles, then it should be done in a manner that enhances outcomes for children (DEC, NAEYC, & ATE, 1994).

Professionals who work in related services should develop their own standards that are consistent with recommended practices in early intervention (DEC, NAEYC, & ATE, 1994). For instance, standards for nurses who work in early intervention programs have been formalized by the nursing divisions of the American Association of University Affiliated Programs and the American Association on Mental Retardation (Brandt & Magyary, 1989).

LEADERSHIP TRAINING

The relationship between leadership-training and teacher-training programs should be recognized (Bowen, 1990), because students in leadership training programs will ultimately be responsible for personnel preparation programs. There are several issues related to doctoral leadership training that have implications for personnel preparation. One issue is that there are different categories of educational leadership with different content to be mastered, such as clinical, policy, administrative, research, and university teaching (Thurman et al., 1990). Each may require the development of different approaches to problem solving. For instance, a researcher may use different problem-solving techniques from a clinician. Related to this are the differences in requirements for the doctor of philosophy (Ph.D.) versus the doctor of education (Ed.D.) degrees. The Ph.D. is research oriented, whereas the Ed.D. degree emphasizes administration. It has been suggested that a third degree be developed that emphasizes clinical skills. Some have questioned which degree is the most appropriate for those engaged in early intervention training (Thurman et al., 1990).

Bowen (1990) discussed barriers to leadership training in education. These barriers include a lack of adequate financial support for students, competition with careers in more lucrative fields, the training in isolation from other disciplines, the generally low status of education faculty on university campuses, and the fact that in some cases beginning faculty salaries are lower than the mean salary of classroom teachers.

Bowen (1990) also raised concerns about the quality and strength of doctoral training programs. He cited the lack of procedures for monitoring student progress, the lack of validated guidelines for quality practice (including quality of program faculty and program practices), and the lack of emphasis on problem solving and knowledge generation as areas for consideration. Because training early interventionists can be only as effective as the faculty who develop the programs and carry on the training, the factors Bowen mentioned indirectly affect the quality of early intervention training programs. It is important that the early intervention field ensure the continuation of excellent doctoral training. One successful avenue has been the leadership training grants awarded annually by the U.S. Department of Education, which are intended to provide resources for expanding and updating existing university doctoral programs in special education and related services disciplines.

CONCLUDING REMARKS: FUTURE DIRECTIONS

The issues discussed in this chapter are varied and complex. They present substantial challenges to the field of early intervention and no doubt will be the subject of considerable discussion as the 21st century approaches. It seems obvious that certain changes are necessary in order to achieve an optimal national system of personnel preparation in all the disciplines represented in early intervention.

The following list summarizes the primary points raised in this chapter and offers suggestions for addressing the identified needs:

1. Adequate funding to develop and support additional preservice training programs is essential.
2. In-service programs and technical assistance should be relied upon to upgrade and update personnel's existing skills and knowledge, not to be a substitute for preservice training.
3. Nontraditional students bring new energy and experience to training programs. At the same time, they often need additional resources and support.
4. Service delivery should be within a seamless system for children from birth to 8 years old, with continuity from infant–toddler programs to preschool programs to primary programs. Training should prepare early interventionists to work in inclusive settings (preschool programs) and home environments (infant–toddler programs).
5. Standards and certification should reflect the transdisciplinary nature of early intervention, with coordination among the 50 states and across the various disciplines for the development of training competencies, personnel standards, and licensing standards to provide a hierarchy of high-quality service providers. National coordination of this system is necessary and might be jointly provided by the relevant professional organizations in collaboration with government standards.

REFERENCES

American Occupational Therapy Association (AOTA). (1990). *Shortages in occupational therapy: Fact sheet.* Rockville, MD: Author.

American Physical Therapy Association. (n.d.). *Physical therapy manpower estimates by state.* Alexandria, VA: Author.

Bailey, D.B., Palsha, S.A., & Huntington, G.S. (1990). Preservice preparation of special educators to serve infants with handicaps and their families: Current status and training needs. *Journal of Early Intervention, 14,* 43–54.

Bailey, D.B., Simeonsson, R.J., Yoder, D.E., & Huntington, G.S. (1990). Preparing professionals to serve infants and toddlers with handicaps and their families: An integrative analysis across eight disciplines. *Exceptional Children, 57,* 26–35.

Bennett, T., Watson, A.L., & Raab, M. (1991). Ensuring competence in early intervention personnel through personnel standards and high-quality training. *Infants and Young Children, 3*(3), 49–58.

Berger, K.S. (1980). *The developing person.* New York: Worth.

Bowen, M.L. (1990). *Leadership training in special education: A status analysis.* Washington, DC: Project FORUM, National Association of State Directors of Special Education. (ERIC Document Reproduction Service No. ED 346 660)

Brandt, P.A., & Magyary, D.L. (1989). Preparation of clinical nurse specialists for family-centered early intervention. *Infants and Young Children, 1*(3), 51–62.

Bredekamp, S. (1993). The relationship between early childhood education and early childhood special education: Healthy marriage or family feud? *Topics in Early Childhood Special Education, 13*(3), 258–273.

Bruder, M.B., Klosowski, S., & Daguio, C. (1991). A review of personnel standards for Part H of PL 99-457. *Journal of Early Intervention, 15,* 66–79.

Bruder, M.B., Lippman, C., & Bologna, T.M. (1994). Personnel preparation in early intervention: Building capacity for program expansion within institutions of higher education. *Journal of Early Intervention, 18,* 103–110.

Bruder, M.B., & Nikitas, T. (1992). Changing the professional practice of early interventionists: An inservice model to meet the service needs of P.L. 99-457. *Journal of Early Intervention, 16,* 173–189.

Christensen, C.M. (1992). Multicultural competencies in early intervention: Training professionals for a pluralistic society. *Infants and Young Children, 4*(3), 49–63.

Division for Early Childhood of the Council for Exceptional Children (DEC), National Association for the Education of Young Children (NAEYC), & Association of Teacher Educators (ATE). (1994, October). *Personnel standards for early education and early intervention: Guidelines for licensure in early childhood special education.* Washington, DC: Authors.

Education of the Handicapped Act Amendments of 1986, PL 99-457. (October 8, 1986). Title 20, U.S.C. 1400 et seq: *U.S. Statutes at Large, 100,* 1145–1177.

Eggbeer, L., Latzko, T., & Pratt, B. (1993). Establishing statewide systems of inservice training for infant and family personnel. *Infants and Young Children, 5*(3), 49–56.

Gallagher, J., & Staples, A. (1990). *Available and potential resources for personnel preparation in special education: Dean's survey.* Chapel Hill: Carolina Policy Studies Program, University of North Carolina.

Gallagher, J.J., Shields, M., & Staples, M. (1990, May). *Personnel preparation options: Ideas from a policy options conference.* Chapel Hill: Carolina Policy Studies Program, University of North Carolina.

Godfrey, A.B. (1995). Preservice interdisciplinary preparation of early intervention specialists in a college of nursing: Faculty reflections and recommendations. *Infants and Young Children, 7*(3), 74–82.

Hanson, M.J., & Brekken, L.J. (1991). Early intervention personnel models and standards: An interdisciplinary field-developed approach. *Infants and Young Children, 4*(1), 54–61.

Hanson, M.J., & Lovett, D. (1992). Personnel preparation for early interventionists: A cross-disciplinary survey. *Journal of Early Intervention, 16*(2), 123–135.

Hebbeler, K. (1994). *Shortages in professions working with young children with disabilities and their families.* Chapel Hill, NC: National Early Childhood Technical Assistance System.

Individuals with Disabilities Education Act (IDEA) of 1990, PL 101-476. (October 30, 1990). Title 20, U.S.C. 1400 et seq: *U.S. Statutes at Large, 104* (Part 2), 1103–1151.

Individuals with Disabilities Education Act Amendments of 1991, PL 102-119. (October 7, 1991). Title 20, U.S.C. 1400 et seq: *U.S. Statutes at Large, 105,* 587–608.

Kemple, K.M., Hartle, L.C., Correa, V.I., & Fox. L. (1994). Preparing teachers for inclusive education. *Teacher Education and Special Education, 17*(1), 38–51.

Lynch, E.W., & Hanson, M.J. (Eds.). (1992). *Developing cross-cultural competence: A guide for working with young children and their families.* Baltimore: Paul H. Brookes Publishing Co.

McCollum, J.A., & Bailey, D.B. (1991). Developing comprehensive personnel systems: Issues and alternatives. *Journal of Early Intervention, 15,* 57–65.

McCollum, J.A., McLean, M., McCartan, K., & Kaiser, C. (1989). Recommendations for certification of early childhood special educators. *Journal of Early Intervention, 13,* 195–211.

McCollum, J.A., & Yates, T.J. (1994). Technical assistance for meeting early intervention personnel standards: Statewide processes based on peer review. *Topics in Early Childhood Special Education, 14*(3), 295–310.

Meisels, S. (1989). Meeting the mandate of Public Law 99-457: Early childhood intervention in the nineties. *American Journal of Orthopsychiatry, 59,* 451–460.

National Association for the Education of Young Children (NAEYC). (n.d.). *NAEYC guidelines for the preparation of early childhood professionals.* Washington, DC: Author.

National Association of State Directors of Special Education. (1993). *Preliminary results of NASDSE early intervention personnel survey.* Alexandria, VA: Author.

National Black Child Development Institute. (1994). Constraints and opportunities for African American leadership in early childhood education. *Young Children, 49*(4), 32–36.

National Early Childhood Technical Assistance System. (1994). *Part H personnel profile.* Chapel Hill, NC: Author.

Odom, S.L. (1987). The role of theory in the preparation of professionals in early childhood special education. *Topics in Early Childhood Special Education, 7*(3), 1–11.

Olsen, G.G. (1991, April/May). Therapist shortage threatens access to care. *REHAB Management,* 28–29.

Rowan, L., Thorp, E., & McCollum, J. (1990). An interdisciplinary practicum to foster infant–family and teaming competencies in speech-language pathologists. *Infants and Young Children, 3*(6), 58–66.

Shephard, D. (1991, February 11). Hospital initiatives can boost supply of allied health care personnel. *American Hospital Association News,* 4.

Shewan, C.M. (1988). *ASHA work force study final report.* Rockville, MD: American Speech-Language-Hearing Association.

Silver, S. (1991, January 10). "Allied health: Chronic shortages predicted." *The Washington Post,* p. G7.

Stayton, V.D., & Miller, P.S. (1993). Combining general and special early childhood education standards in personnel preparation programs: Experiences from two states. *Topics in Early Childhood Special Education, 13*(3), 372–387.

Striffler, N. (1993). *Current trends in the use of paraprofessionals in early intervention and preschool services.* Chapel Hill, NC: National Early Childhood Technical Assistance System.

Thurman, S.K., Brown, C., Bryan, M., Henderson, A., Klein, M., Sainato, D., & Wiley, T. (1990). *Some perspectives on preparing personnel to work with at-risk children birth to five.* Washington, DC: U.S. Department of Education, Office of Educational Research and Improvement. (ERIC Document No. ED 343 342)

Trohanis, P.L. (1994). Planning for successful inservice education for local early childhood programs. *Topics in Early Childhood Special Education, 14*(3), 311–332.

Turnbull, H.R. (1990). *Free appropriate public education: The law and children with disabilities* (3rd ed.). Denver, CO: Love Publishing.

U.S. Department of Education. (1993, July 1). [State reports to OSEP of personnel employed or contracted in early intervention as of December 1991.] Unpublished raw data.

U.S. Department of Health and Human Services. (1992). *Health personnel in the United States: Eighth report to Congress, 1991.* Washington, DC: Author.

Widerstrom, A.H. (1995). *Recruitment and retention of nontraditional students for graduate work in early intervention.* Unpublished manuscript.

Widerstrom, A.H., Domyslawski, D., & McNulty, B.A. (1986). Rural outreach training in early childhood special education: A cooperative model. *Journal of the Division for Early Childhood, 10*(1), 84–92.

Yoder, D.E., Coleman, P.P., & Gallagher, J.J. (1990). Personnel needs—Allied health personnel meeting the demands of Part H, P.L. 99-457. Chapel Hill, NC: Carolina Policy Studies Program.

3

TRAINING PRACTICES

Diane Bricker and Betsy LaCroix

In June, Karen received a bachelor's degree in special education and a state endorsement qualifying her as an early intervention teacher. She had three job interviews and was offered three positions. Karen chose the early intervention position in a medium-size town because the program staff appeared knowledgeable, parent friendly, and genuinely interested in assisting young children with disabilities. Karen's first weeks on the job were hectic but exciting. She liked the children who were assigned to her classroom, found their parents to be interested and supportive, and enjoyed working with her instructional aide. During the fourth week, Karen's supervisor asked her to attend a team meeting to discuss the recent evaluation of a child who participated in her class. When Karen arrived at the meeting, she was briefly introduced to the physical therapist, communication specialists, social worker, and developmental pediatrician. Karen, of course, knew the parents, who were also in attendance. Prior to the meeting Karen was not asked to assess the child nor asked to bring any information to the meeting. At the meeting each of the professionals presented his or her evaluation findings separately. Neither the parents nor Karen were asked to contribute any evaluation information or to assist in revising the child's individualized family service plan (IFSP). During the meeting, Karen attempted to maintain her composure and appear to be a competent professional, yet she felt confused and intimidated by the other team members. She noticed the parents appeared unhappy as well.

As Karen walked home from work that evening she pondered the "team" meeting and wondered why she felt so dissatisfied with her performance and the outcome. She arrived at two conclusions. First, while in her university training program she had received only minimal exposure to students, faculty, supervisors, and material from other disciplines (e.g., physical therapy, speech-language pathology). She did not understand the jargon used by the professionals on the team nor did she understand how they assessed young children and designed intervention programs. In fact, Karen concluded she was very poorly prepared to contribute to a meeting such as this one. Second, she did not understand why the members of this team presented separate evaluation findings and developed separate IFSP goals. She also did not understand why neither she nor the parents were asked to participate in the child's evaluation or the development of the IFSP. As she listened to the team's discussion, she found herself disagreeing with them about the child's capabilities and what she thought would be appropriate IFSP goals. Karen concluded from this meeting that "team" means that each professional conducts individual evaluations and selects IFSP goals appropriate to his or her discipline.

Was Karen's first experience with a team unusual or is it representative? Are most students better prepared than Karen to participate on a team? This chapter attempts to answer these and similar questions by examining a range of university training programs focused on preparing early intervention personnel.

THE PASSAGE OF PL 99-457, the Education of the Handicapped Act Amendments of 1986, and subsequent amendments (e.g., PL 102-119, the Individuals with Disabilities Education Act Amendments of 1991) have made clear the federal intent that services for young children with disabilities must be provided by a range of qualified, well-trained professionals (Brown & Rule, 1993; Klein & Campbell, 1990). Federal regulations require states to establish personnel standards that meet certification and licensing stipulations for personnel working with young children with disabilities that are at least equivalent to personnel standards that are in place for school-age children. It is interesting to note that personnel certification and licensing standards can and do differ across disciplines (Bruder, Klosowski, & Daguio, 1991). Disciplines such as occupational therapy, physical therapy, psychology, and speech-language pathology have combined state and national standards leading to uniformity in training goals and outcomes, while education standards are determined individually by each state. This latter practice does little to foster a national set of personnel guidelines, standards, or benchmarks to assist in the development of personnel training efforts by educationally based disciplines. Addressing this problem, the Division for Early Childhood of the Council for Exceptional Children (DEC), National Association for the Education of Young Children (NAEYC), and Association of Teacher Educators (ATE) (1994) have begun to develop and disseminate national guidelines or standards for personnel who will be offering services to young children with disabilities. Although this beginning represents a step forward, a great deal remains to be done in the formulation of state and national guidelines that can direct the preservice and in-service training philosophies and practices to ensure the consistent output and maintenance of quality personnel. This chapter focuses on personnel preparation efforts offered by educationally based disciplines.

When the first formal intervention efforts were initiated with infants and young children with disabilities during the early 1970s, there were no degree programs nor professional licensure available to individuals providing educational services to this population (Bricker & Slentz, 1988). Most educational personnel associated with these early programs had been trained to work with older populations (e.g., school-age children, adults) in settings (e.g., public schools, institutions) that bore little resemblance to the typical home environments of infants and young children. The application of content and strategies derived for older populations proved to be less than effective with infants and young children (Bricker & Carlson, 1981). Over the years, often initially through trial and error, the field of early intervention, which in this chapter includes the birth- to 5-year age range, has accumulated a knowledge and skill base that has been formalized into systematic programs of personnel preparation. According to a survey conducted by the National Early Childhood Technical Assistance System (1993), 33 states have some type of professional licensure or certification available for early intervention. Many professional organizations are considering recommending a special credential or at least special training for professionals working with infants and young children with disabilities (Baer, Blyler, Cloud, & McCamman, 1991; Crais & Leonard, 1990; Effgen, Bjornson, Chiarello, Sinzer, & Phillips, 1991; Hanft & Humphry, 1989; McLinden & Prasse, 1991). In addition, most states appear to have at least one institution of higher education that offers formal coursework in early intervention, degree programs (Office of Special Education Programs [OSEP], 1993), and special certification for early intervention personnel (Bruder et al., 1991).

The dramatic growth in degree granting and licensure programs for early intervention personnel raises a number of important questions: 1) What philosophies or orientations direct these programs? 2) What are course and practica requirements? 3) What competencies are graduates expected to acquire? and 4) What type of credentials are issued?

The purpose of this chapter is to address questions of program philosophy, content, and credentialing associated with the preparation of early intervention personnel. Addressing these questions required collecting descriptive information on early intervention personnel preparation programs in the mid-1990s; therefore, a formal survey of preservice programs located throughout the United States was conducted. Before describing the survey and presenting the results, a review of relevant literature is offered. Finally, this chapter addresses the salient issues raised by the survey data.

PREVIOUS SURVEYS AND RELEVANT LITERATURE

Understanding the contemporary status of early intervention personnel preparation can be enhanced by examining the history of its training efforts. Although oral recollections and observations can be useful, most professionals tend to give written accounts more credence in terms of objectivity and accuracy. Unfortunately, the brief history of personnel preparation in early intervention is not well-documented. An examination of the available literature finds two types of foci: 1) descriptions of specific programs (e.g., McCollum, Rowan, & Thorp, 1994; Mills, Vadasy, & Fewell, 1987) and statewide efforts (Hanson & Lovett, 1992; McCollum, 1987), and 2) descriptions of competencies and content that training programs should address (Bruder, Lippman, & Bologna, 1994; Fenichel & Eggbeer, 1990). With notable exceptions (e.g., Bailey, Palsha, & Huntington, 1990; Bricker & Slentz, 1988; Bruder et al., 1991), the literature contains few empirically based descriptions of national program content, training efforts or certification and/or licensure requirements, and studies focused on the effectiveness of training models or specific training programs. McCollum and McCartan (1988) wrote, "If the question is 'How much of what we do in teacher education in ECSE [early childhood special education] is supported by research?' the answer is 'not much'" (p. 269). Klein and Campbell (1990) reinforced this conclusion, suggesting that "data related to the effectiveness of training personnel to work with handicapped infants, toddlers and preschoolers and their parents is almost nonexistent" (p. 682). Likewise, a combing of the literature in 1996 suggests modest gains in the development of an empirical base focused on the study of training efforts and effects.

Given the importance of personnel preparation, why has so little objective study been undertaken to address this area? There are three important reasons. First, the conduct of methodologically sound research is expensive. With a few notable exceptions (e.g., University of North Carolina's Research Institute, Carolina Policy Studies Program), training monies for early intervention

personnel have been largely directed to preparation and not to the study of training outcomes or the effectiveness of training approaches. Although federally supported training efforts require projects to address evaluation of student outcomes
and program effectiveness, budget limitations severely restrict these evaluation
efforts. In a review of 40 federally funded projects designed to train specialists to
work with infants, Bruder and McLean (1988) noted that "evaluation sections of
the proposals were sparse" (p. 304) and projects appear to be engaging in only cur-
sory evaluation. Comprehensive and meaningful evaluation efforts (e.g., long-
term follow-up of students' performances on the job) likely do not occur in part
because most training grants lack sufficient funds.

Second, individuals responsible for personnel preparation (e.g., faculty, staff)
may be poorly prepared to plan and implement well-designed evaluations of
training efforts and outcomes. Without assistance from evaluation specialists,
chosen measures, procedures, and methodology may lack validity, reliability,
and appropriateness (Lazzari & Bruder, 1988). For example, many homemade
tools may be used to gauge program impact. Unfortunately, these tools often
lack psychometric data that would ensure the user or the consumer of outcomes
of the measure's validity and reliability. Or, conversely, psychometrically sound
measures may be selected, but these measures may be at best tangential to the
training emphasis of the program.

Third, program personnel often receive little external encouragement for
conducting sound evaluation research. Institutions of higher education appear
more driven by documented personnel shortages than by determining whether
training program graduates can contribute to their field in substantial and meaningful ways. State and national licensing and certification agencies and/or organizations require program evaluations, but these groups provide little support for
the study of training models, program effectiveness, or long-term student outcomes. The lack of fiscal support, trained personnel, and external encouragement for the study of early intervention training efforts help to explain its
meager empirical base. Although meager, studies of early intervention training
efforts and comprehensive surveys of practice do exist. A number of surveys
were located that directly or indirectly related to providing a historical context
and comparative base for the descriptive survey of early intervention personnel
preparation programs contained in this chapter.

Courtnage and Smith-Davis (1987) conducted a national survey focused on
examining the extent to which 360 special education teachers were involved in
team training—a topic of specific concern in this book. Courtnage and Smith-
Davis reported that 48% of the surveyed teachers indicated receiving no team
training, and of those who did, only 18% reported taking a specific course or
practicum that focused on team training. Because the subjects of the study were
special education teachers, the results are of questionable applicability when examining training efforts with personnel in early intervention (Bricker & Slentz,
1988; Bruder et al., 1991; McCollum & Bailey, 1991). Nevertheless, the outcomes do provide a potentially useful benchmark against which to examine the
shifting emphasis on team training in special education and in particular early
intervention.

Using resources from an OSEP-funded research institute, Bailey and his
colleagues examined the extent to which students enrolled in preservice undergraduate and master's programs across eight disciplines (nursing, nutrition,

occupational therapy, physical therapy, psychology, social work, special education, and speech-language pathology) were provided training focused on infants with disabilities and their families (Bailey, Simeonsson, Yoder, & Huntington, 1990). A survey was developed to determine the core curriculum that was provided for typical students in each of the eight professions. In this study, a telephone survey was conducted by trained interviewers with representatives from 237 undergraduate and 212 master's programs. The authors reported a number of troubling findings. First, they found considerable variability *between* disciplines in the students' exposure to infant, toddler, and family content. Second, they found similar variability *within* disciplines. Third, they found that little time and attention were devoted overall to content focused on infants and toddlers and their families. Of the time spent, most was directed toward typical and atypical early development, suggesting serious gaps in attention to content and experience addressing infant and family assessment and intervention.

A related study, directed exclusively toward surveying training content in special education programs, yielded similar findings (Bailey et al., 1990). Using results from combined telephone ($n = 20$) and mail ($n = 37$) surveys, Bailey et al. (1990) reported that students enrolled in programs that did not have an infancy or early childhood focus received little information about intervening with infants with disabilities and their families. The authors voiced concern about meeting early intervention personnel shortages, given the small number of infant-focused programs in higher education and the minimal attention given to early intervention by general special education personnel preparation programs. Gallagher and Staples (1990) echoed a similar concern based on their survey of 249 deans of colleges of education. Respondents reported that 162 of the 249 schools had no early intervention programs, and furthermore, 60% of the deans indicated little interest in developing or expanding programs focused on infants and toddlers with disabilities because of limited resources.

Findings from these three surveys focused on Part H programs are of interest but may not be representative of programs in the preschool range. A telephone survey to determine national personnel standards conducted by Bruder et al. (1991) was also restricted to Part H programs. The respondents ($n = 49$) were Part H coordinators; they were asked to indicate which states have licensure or certification for specialists in the 10 disciplines named in PL 99-457 and what types of state standards occur across these 10 disciplines. Interestingly, most states reported having standards in place for children from birth on for all 10 disciplines; however, according to Bruder et al. (1991), the standards are not specific to infants and toddlers.

The study most similar to the survey discussed in this chapter was conducted by Bricker and Slentz (1988). The subject list for this national survey was derived from two sources: 1) the OSEP directory of funded personnel preparation programs, and 2) an early childhood special education personnel preparation conference held in 1984. A list of programs was obtained by combining these two sources, and a 22-item questionnaire was mailed to the 131 training programs that indicated they offered at least some training in early intervention. Survey questions addressed program resources, levels of training, and program content. In addition, respondents were asked to agree or disagree with four position statements about practice in the early intervention field. There was a 50% return rate ($N = 65$). In general, the findings were similar to those reported by Bailey et al.

(1990) in that large variations in number and type of required courses and practicum were found. The variations precluded determining clear standards for coursework, practica, and competencies that operated to direct early intervention personnel preparation efforts in the mid-1980s. A comparison of the specific findings from this study with the present survey findings is of interest and appears in the results and discussion sections that follow.

THE SURVEY

As indicated, the purpose of this chapter is to describe, from a national perspective, personnel programs offering preservice training in the area of early intervention.[1] To accomplish this goal, a survey tool was developed to obtain a range of information from a sample of programs offering preservice training at the graduate and undergraduate levels. These programs were developed to prepare personnel to deliver services, develop programs, and conduct research focused on infants, toddlers, and preschool-age children who are at risk or have disabilities and their families.

Finding a list of preservice training programs was a challenge. A central registry of programs specifically designed to prepare personnel to work with young children with disabilities was not available. The most comprehensive listing we discovered was the directory compiled and disseminated by OSEP. The directory, *Selected Early Childhood Programs* (OSEP, 1993), lists project grants in two program categories: the Early Education Program for Children with Disabilities and the Division of Personnel Preparation (DPP). The DPP category lists and briefly describes all federally supported personnel preparation programs focused on training special education and related services personnel to work with young children who are at risk and/or have disabilities. The list includes grants for 1) infant, toddler, and preschool personnel; 2) leadership personnel; 3) low incidence, minority institutions; 4) related services, rural special projects; 5) special educators, special populations, special projects; and 6) state education agencies. Our sample was drawn from the first two categories.

Because our sample was obtained from the OSEP directory, it may not be representative of all programs that train personnel to work with young children who are at risk or have disabilities and their families. There are preservice programs that train personnel to work with young children with disabilities, which do not receive federal funds and therefore do not appear on the OSEP list. To our knowledge, there is no source to assist in determining the number of non–federally funded programs in the area of early intervention. In addition, as an agency, OSEP may be more closely allied with special education, resulting in a higher proportion of personnel training grants submitted from special education than from other disciplines. The 1992–1993 OSEP-compiled list of 245 personnel preparation projects did include training grants awarded to departments of physical therapy $(n = 6)$, occupational therapy $(n = 7)$, speech-language pathology $(n = 43)$, school psychology $(n = 11)$, early childhood education $(n = 20)$, nursing $(n = 1)$, physical education and adaptive physical education $(n = 3)$, and

---

[1]The authors are not referring only to training special educators but also to other disciplines that provide training focused on young children with disabilities, including occupational therapy, physical therapy, school psychology, early childhood education, psychology, and speech-language pathology.

social work ($n = 1$); special education received 79 training grants. We were unable to classify 74 of the programs based on the information given in the directory. Therefore, these numbers do not represent the total number of grant projects in each discipline category. Given these circumstances, it is not clear how representative of the nation's overall early intervention training efforts this survey is; however, it is representative of OSEP-funded training efforts.

Measure

The survey tool used in this study was developed through several iterations. Initially, content areas were derived by examining previous surveys on personnel preparation and by analyzing major areas of concern discussed in the early intervention literature. Areas in which little objective personnel preparation information existed were also identified. Examining previous surveys yielded a variety of topics, which were classifiable into content areas (e.g., program description). Using the selected topics, a series of questions was developed into a four-page survey form. The tool was reviewed by several professionals considered experts in training personnel to work with young children and their families. Feedback from these professionals resulted in deleting, adding, and modifying items. The revised survey tool was then formally piloted through a telephone interview with four early intervention faculty members from universities in California, Colorado, and Oregon. These faculty members were associated with longstanding early intervention training programs and were experienced and knowledgeable in the area of personnel preparation. Items identified by these four respondents as needing clarification or further definition were modified. The final version of the survey tool contained 27 questions addressing the following areas: program description, program philosophy, training approach or model, program content, professional background of faculty and students, credentials or certification, and issues surrounding personnel preparation. A complete copy of the survey tool is contained in Figure 1.

Procedure

As indicated previously, the OSEP Division of Personnel Preparation–funded training grants for 1992–1993 served as the pool from which the survey sample was randomly selected. A total of 132 training projects is listed in either the leadership ($n = 28$) or infant, toddler, and preschool ($n = 104$) personnel category. From this sample, 40 were randomly selected from the infant, toddler, and preschool projects and 10 from the leadership projects. In addition, 15 alternate projects were selected for replacing the original sample as needed, 10 from the infant, toddler, and preschool category, and 5 from the leadership category. Ten of these alternate programs were used to replace 10 of the original samples. Programs were eliminated from the original sample for the following reasons: 1) the program did not meet the specifications of an early intervention preservice training program (i.e., training did not lead to a degree or certificate), and 2) programs were selected from the same university that had two or more grant-funded projects.

A copy of the survey and a cover letter were sent to each of the originally selected 50 programs. Following receipt of the letter, each program contact person

EARLY INTERVENTION PERSONNEL PREPARATION QUESTIONNAIRE

Time start: _____

Time finish: _____

1. Interviewer: _____ Date: _____

2. Interviewee: _____

3. Department: _____ University: _____

4. Position: _____

5. Discipline or training: _____

6. Type of preservice training program(s) and number of students in each:

   Associate in Arts: _____ Bachelor's: _____ Master's: _____

   Doctoral: _____ Other: _____

7. Does your program have an early intervention focus?

   Yes: _____ No: _____ Some: _____

8. Program title: _____

   Description of program: _____

   _____

   _____

   _____

   _____

9. Does your program have an interdisciplinary or transdisciplinary focus in coursework?

   Yes: _____ No: _____ Some: _____

   Example: _____

   _____

10. Which disciplines (for master's, doctoral, certificate programs) are represented by
    students?

    Early childhood education: _____ Early childhood special education: _____

    Speech-language pathology: _____ Occupational therapy: _____

    Physical therapy: _____ Social work: _____

    School psychology: _____ Nursing: _____

(*continued*)

Figure 1. A questionnaire on preparing personnel in early intervention and early childhood special education.

Figure 1. (*continued*)

Physical education: _____ Other: _____

11. Does your program have an interdisciplinary faculty? Yes: _____ No: _____

Number of faculty: _____ Disciplines represented:

Early childhood education: _____ Early childhood special education: _____

Speech-language pathology: _____ Occupational therapy: _____

Physical therapy: _____ Social work: _____

School psychology: _____ Nursing: _____ Physical education: _____

Other: _____

12. Is your program competency based? Yes: _____ No: _____

Number of competencies to complete degree: _____

(Please send copy of competencies)

13. Length of program: _____

14. Number of credit hours to graduate:

Quarter hours: _____ Semester hours: _____

(Please send list of required courses and course descriptions)

15. Number of practicum hours required to graduate:

Quarter hours: _____ Semester hours: _____

16. Where are the students placed for practicum and field experience?

Infant and toddler program: _____ Preschool program: _____

Community-based program: _____ University-based program: _____

Child care program: _____ Hospital program: _____

Home-based program: _____ Parent program: _____

Site at which currently employed: _____

Other (please describe): _____

17. Other requirements:

Comprehensive examination: _____ Thesis: _____ Project: _____

Other: _____

18. Does your program provide training in team process and team building?

Yes: _____ No: _____ If so, how?

(continued)

Figure 1. *(continued)*

Specific course(s): Yes: _____ No: _____

Part of course(s): Yes: _____ No: _____

Practica: Yes: _____ No: _____

Other _____

19. Is your program accredited? Yes: _____ No: _____

    If yes, by whom? _____

20. Do your students receive state or national licensing, certification, or credentials?

    Yes: _____ No: _____

    Please describe: _____

    _____

21. Very briefly, what do you see as the most significant change in early intervention personnel preparation in the last 5 years?

22. What do you think will be the most significant change in the next 5 years?

23. What do you see as the greatest current challenge in the preparation of early intervention and early childhood special education personnel?

Please agree or disagree with each of the following statements:

24. Individuals who work with infants who are at risk or have disabilities and their families require information and skills different from personnel working with children in the 3- to-5-year age group, and training programs should reflect these differences.

    Agree: _____ Disagree: _____

(continued)

Figure 1. (*continued*)

---

25. The primary focus of intervention with children birth to 3 years old should be the primary caregiver(s) and family members, and training programs should reflect this emphasis.

    Agree: _____ Disagree: _____

26. Because intervening with infants and their families requires professional maturity and judgment, training programs should require extensive practical experience.

    Agree: _____ Disagree: _____

27. Intervening with infants and their families often requires coordination of many disciplines and agencies, and training programs should reflect this need.

    Agree: _____ Disagree: _____

Comments:

Thank you for your participation!

---

was telephoned to schedule an appointment to complete the survey. At least four follow-up telephone calls were made in an attempt to contact program personnel before being replaced with an alternate program. Two of the alternate programs had to be eliminated from the sample because one of the programs did not meet the specifications of an early intervention preservice training program and the other program was no longer in existence. Only one follow-up telephone call was made to the alternate programs because of time constraints. Representatives from a total of 48 programs were interviewed.

The interviews were conducted by telephone for two important reasons. First, the interview process provided an opportunity for each item to be explained in a similar manner to each respondent. Prior to the interviews, terms were defined so each respondent would receive the same definitions and information. Second, as questions arose, they could be answered in a consistent manner to help eliminate individual interpretation of items and question intent.

The length of the interviews ranged from 10 to 45 minutes, with a mean of 25 minutes, and were conducted between March and August 1994 by two interviewers, both graduate students in the University of Oregon early intervention program. Prior to the first interview, the two interviewers worked together to develop a standard interview format and to establish agreement in how they recorded the respondents' replies to the survey questions. The interviewers conducted two joint interviews. Their responses to each survey question were reviewed by a third party to determine the percent of agreement and disagreement. The agreement for these interviews was 93%. Subsequent interviews were conducted individually. All surveys were conducted over the telephone with one exception, which was completed in writing. A copy of the survey was sent to each respondent at least 2 weeks before the interview was conducted.

With the exception of the four position statements on the survey, items were read aloud by the interviewer, who wrote down the respondent's answer or checked the appropriate category. Respondents were asked to agree or disagree with the four position statements and the interviewer marked their choices. These four statements were taken from an earlier survey by Bricker and Slentz (1988). In the initial survey, the statements were presented in writing. Therefore, in order to allow for valid comparison of the results to those previously obtained, respondents were asked to read these items and respond. Two respondents did not have access to the survey tool during the interview. In these cases, the interviewer read each item to the respondents.

Upon completion of the interviews, the respondents' answers were entered into computer files for subsequent analyses. The findings from this survey are presented in the following section.

Results

Several programs included in the survey sample offered more than one preservice degree and/or certification; therefore, respondents provided data on 15 certificate, 8 bachelor's degree, 36 master's degree, and 13 doctoral programs.

The number of students in each program varied from a mean of 6.1 for doctoral programs to 63.6 for bachelor's programs. The mean numbers of students in master's and certificate programs were 31.3 and 22.3, respectively. The number of faculty involved in each program was 5.4 for certificate, 6.9 for bachelor's, 7.0 for master's, and 8.8 for doctoral programs. These numbers included faculty who taught core coursework as well as faculty who taught required coursework for a program or a degree. However, these figures do not include faculty teaching elective courses or adjunct faculty. A number of program respondents indicated the use of community practitioners and parents as instructors in addition to faculty; however, data were collected regarding faculty only. Table 1 lists the percentage of certificate, bachelor's, master's, and doctoral programs that have faculty in the disciplines of early childhood, early childhood special education, special education, occupational therapy, physical therapy, social work, school psychology, nursing, and adaptive physical education.

All respondents for bachelor's and doctoral programs and 93% of certificate and master's program respondents described their programs as having an interdisciplinary and transdisciplinary focus in both coursework and practica. One program reported having a combined interdisciplinary and transdisciplinary focus in practica but not in coursework. Over 90% of respondents indicated that their programs offered training in team-process skills in coursework. The number of programs offering an entire course focused on team process ranged from 44% for master's programs to 63% for bachelor's programs. In addition, 87%–100% of respondents indicated their programs provided training in team process through practica. Most programs offered a variety of practicum opportunities and indicated that the amount of training in team process varied with the practicum placement. Table 2 lists practicum sites and the percentage of programs offering practica in each type of site. The last entry indicates the percentage of programs offering practica at the students' own places of employment. It was not possible to compute the mean number of practicum hours required by programs because of variations in reporting these data (e.g., clock hours versus credit hours, professional hours versus degree hours, practica versus internship,

Table 1. Percent of certificate, bachelor's, master's, and doctoral programs having faculty from specific disciplines or areas

Discipline or area	Type of program			
	Certificate (N = 15)	Bachelor's (N = 8)	Master's (N = 36)	Doctoral (N = 13)
Early childhood education	60	75	47	46
Early childhood special education	73	88	69	69
Special education	20	25	42	39
Speech-language pathology	47	63	64	77
Occupational therapy	20	13	17	15
Physical therapy	20	25	25	0
Social work	20	38	22	15
School psychology	27	63	31	46
Nursing	33	38	31	31
Adaptive physical education	7	0	11	23

core early intervention versus noncore hours, teaching versus field experience, grant-related versus non–grant-related hours).

Respondents were surveyed regarding program competencies and indicated that 79% of certificate, 86% of bachelor's, 74% of master's, and 50% of doctoral programs were competency based, meaning they had a list of specific knowledge and/or skills that participating students were to acquire through coursework and practica.

Respondents were asked about other program requirements, such as research and comprehensive examination requirements. Of the certificate programs, 14% required students to complete a research project in addition to regular coursework, 7% required the completion of comprehensive examinations, 19% required students to write a thesis, and 33% reported that writing a thesis was presented as one option but was not required. Of the master's programs, 17% required students to complete a research project, while 11% presented this as an option, and 42% required that students in the master's programs complete comprehensive examinations, while 17% presented this as an option. Of the doctoral programs, 91% required students to complete comprehensive examinations in addition to writing a dissertation.

Along with the program-specific data collected, respondents were asked to agree or disagree with four position statements regarding the preparation of personnel in early intervention. Agreement and disagreement percentages for each statement are presented in Table 3, in comparison with the 1988 survey conducted by Bricker and Slentz.

Respondents were also asked three open-ended questions regarding changes and challenges in early intervention personnel preparation. These questions were intended to identify the general impressions of the respondents regarding trends in the field as they relate to personnel preparation. The questions were as follows:

1. What do you see as the most significant change in early intervention personnel preparation in the last 5 years?

Table 2. Percent of practicum sites used by certificate, bachelor's, and master's programs

	Type of program		
Type of practicum site	Certificate (N = 15)	Bachelor's (N = 8)	Master's (N = 36)
Infant and toddler	93	88	100
Preschool	87	88	97
Community based	80	88	89
University based	40	50	64
Child care	53	63	56
Hospital based	47	75	67
Home based	80	100	81
Parent program	40	38	44
Employment site	67	75	56

2. What do you think will be the most significant change in the next 5 years?
3. What do you see as the greatest current challenge in the preparation of early intervention personnel?

Responses to each question were noted by the interviewer and they were then coded and categorized. These data are presented in Tables 4, 5, and 6. Responses indicated by two or fewer individuals are not included in these tables.

DISCUSSION

The purpose of the national survey discussed in this chapter was to develop a "sense" of the focus, content, and structure of early intervention personnel preparation programs, which seemed particularly important because no national standards or guidelines for training in this area exist (as of 1996). Creating a survey to acquire information that was neither too specific nor too general was a challenge. Narrowly focused questions often prevented respondents from providing simple, straightforward answers. For example, program credit hour requirements for undergraduate programs can be reported in a variety of ways, depending on whether one is referring to the entire baccalaureate degree or the specialization area of early intervention. For a graduate program, credits may vary depending on whether a student is interested in obtaining a certificate in addition to earning a master's degree. Posing broad-based questions was equally troublesome. For example, the question concerning the interdisciplinary focus of a program tended to consistently elicit a positive response. However, programs varied in the amount of time and energy they directed toward this goal, making the usefulness of the responses questionable. Even with extensive piloting of the survey, we found it difficult to arrive at a set of questions that would yield accurate and meaningful outcomes. Nevertheless, we believe the survey sheds some light on four important areas associated with early intervention personnel preparation: 1) the focus on team training, 2) competency and coursework requirements, 3) philosophical positions affecting training, and 4) challenges and changes facing early intervention training programs.

Table 3. Comparison of 1988 and 1994 survey results addressing comparison of four position statements

| Position statement | Percentage | | | | | |
| | 1988 survey | | | 1994 survey | | |
	Agree	Disagree	Neither	Agree	Disagree	Neither
1. Individuals who work with infants who are at risk or have disabilities and their families require information and skills different from personnel working with children in the 3- to-5-year age group, and training programs should reflect these differences.	89	3	8	83	15	2
2. The primary focus of intervention with children birth to 3 years old should be the primary caregiver(s) and family members, and training programs should reflect this emphasis.	79	14	7	88	5	7
3. Because intervening with infants and their families requires professional maturity and judgment, training programs should require extensive practical experience.	97	3	0	93	5	2
4. Intervening with infants and their families often requires coordination of many disciplines and agencies, and training programs should reflect this need.	100	0	0	98	0	2

Note: The 1988 survey results are from Bricker, D.D., & Slentz, K. (1988). Personnel preparation: Handicapped infants. In M. Wang, H. Walberg, & M. Reynolds (Eds.), *The handbook of special education: Research and practice* (Vol. 3), Copyright 1988, pp. 319–345, with kind permission from Elsevier Science Ltd, The Boulevard, Langford Lane, Kidlington OX5 1GB, UK.

INTERDISCIPLINARY TEAM TRAINING

The findings from this survey of randomly selected personnel preparation programs strongly suggest a heavy emphasis on preparing students to work as members of a team. The evidence comes from three sources. First, most programs, which included all levels (i.e., certificate, bachelor's, master's, and doctoral), reported having faculty from a variety of disciplines. A review of Table 1 shows representation in the surveyed programs of faculty from early childhood education, early childhood special education, special education, speech-language pathology, occupational therapy, physical therapy, social work, school psychology, and nursing. Faculties with such broad-based disciplinary representation surely must help promote an interdisciplinary perspective and orientation.

Table 4.   Recent changes in personnel preparation identified by survey respondents

Identified changes	Number of respondents[a]
Blending of early childhood education and early childhood special education; inclusive, community-based, and natural environments	18
Family-centered practice	15
Interdisciplinary and transdisciplinary team collaboration	10
Increased focus on birth to 3, recognition of continuity from birth to 5	6
Increased use of competencies, quality standards	5
Emphasis on diverse and multicultural populations	5
Child-directed intervention (e.g., activity-based intervention, developmentally appropriate practice)	4
Increase in early childhood focus in special education and related service training programs	4

[a]Respondents could identify more than one change.

Second, all programs at the bachelor's and doctoral levels and nearly all of the certificate and master's programs reported that their coursework and practica have an interdisciplinary team focus. At least 60% of the bachelor's and certificate programs reported having specific courses on team-process skills, while 44% of the master's and 50% of the doctoral programs offered specific courses on team processes.

Third, the variety of practicum placements for students also suggests a strong team focus. Settings vary from hospital-based to child care programs. It is likely that these settings offer students the opportunity to observe and work with professionals from a variety of perspectives and disciplines.

Since the passage of PL 99-457 in 1986, leaders in the field have given consistent voice to the need for early intervention personnel to adopt and employ team approaches to assessment, intervention, and evaluation (Bailey et al., 1990; Campbell, 1990). The data from our survey suggest that the majority of early intervention training programs represented in this sample were addressing this goal. Studies are needed to measure the effectiveness of the team-process skills of the professionals who were the recipients of this training (Johnson, 1995).

Table 5.   Expected changes in personnel preparation identified by survey respondents

Identified changes	Number of respondents[a]
Blending of early childhood education and early childhood special education; inclusive, community-based, and natural environments	20
Interdisciplinary and transdisciplinary team collaboration	5
Increased attention to diverse populations	5
Family-centered practice	5
Need for cost containment	3
Increased service delivery options, nontraditional models	3

[a]Respondents could identify more than one expected change.

Table 6. Current challenges in personnel preparation identified by survey respondents

Identified challenges	Number of respondents[a]
Scope of knowledge and skills needed for extensive range in population and service delivery models	9
Finding inclusive training sites with well-trained personnel	9
Obtaining funding, need to prioritize limited resources	7
Recruiting and/or retaining minority students	4
Assessment and/or intervention with diverse populations	4
Facilitating interaction across disciplines	4
Incorporating families and home-based training	3
Preparing adequate numbers of qualified personnel, making training accessible (e.g., to students in rural areas)	3
Gap between recommended practice and reality, resistance to change	3

[a]Respondents could identify more than one current challenge.

COMPETENCY AND COURSEWORK

Except for the doctoral programs, only 50% of which are reported to be competency based, over three fourths of programs at the other levels indicated they are competency based. We were surprised by the finding that many programs were not competency based and wished we had identified the alternative approaches used by these programs.

Only 16 programs in the sample sent copies of their competencies, and 23 provided information on coursework requirements, creating a smaller subsample from the original and replacement group. The competency and course requirement data came from degree programs at the bachelor's, master's, and doctoral levels.

The coursework and competencies identified by this subsample resemble those described by Bruder and McLean (1988) in their review of 40 federally funded personnel preparation projects for infant specialists. Our results also approximate minimum content areas recommended for certification in early childhood special education (McCollum, McLean, McCartan, & Kaiser, 1989). Individual programs, however, fell short of some of these recommendations. For example, McCollum et al. (1989) recommended that content include life-span development and learning, as well as the integration of all areas of child development. Many of the programs we surveyed listed competencies and coursework that addressed a more narrow scope of development (e.g., birth to 5 years of age *only*; one aspect of development *only*, such as language development).

Many of the programs in the subsample lacked other recommended content (McCollum et al., 1989) as well. Although the majority identified coursework and competencies in foundations of early intervention, few included social and philosophical foundations of education. Other content reported by a small percentage of programs in the subsample included physical and medical management and environmental and behavior management. These content areas may be included in methods courses; therefore, it is difficult to draw conclusions regarding the number of programs that do not address these areas.

Although Bailey et al. (1990) found that programs in a variety of disciplines provide minimal exposure to family issues, the majority of programs in the subsample identified both coursework and competencies related to working with families. The subsample differed from the Bailey et al. (1990) sample that focused on non–early intervention programs, while all the programs in the subsample were early intervention programs. It seems clear that a greater emphasis on family involvement exists within early intervention programs versus those training personnel in other disciplines to work with young children with disabilities and their families.

PHILOSOPHICAL POSITION STATEMENTS

Bricker and Slentz (1988) asked representatives from a previous national survey to agree or disagree with four position statements. For comparison, we asked respondents of the present survey to respond to the same four statements. Table 3 contains the statements and the percentage of agreement between the 1988 and 1994 survey populations. For three of the statements, opinion appears to have shifted little. Of those surveyed, 83% or more agreed that interventionists working with infants require different information and skills from those required for working with 3- to 5-year-olds, interventionists in training should have extensive practicum experience, and intervention requires the coordination of many disciplines and agencies. There was a 9% shift from the 1988 survey (79%) to the present survey (88%) in agreement with the statement that the primary intervention focus for infants should be the primary caregivers and family members. The data from the present survey, if representative of the field, suggest a shift toward more family-focused intervention for infants and toddlers. The lack of change on the other issues may suggest that early intervention has had its basic direction set since at least the mid-1980s and is maintaining its course, at least in those areas addressed by these position statements.

CHALLENGES AND CHANGES

Although survey respondents were asked to identify the most significant change (past and future) and the most significant challenge in the preparation of early intervention personnel, many responded with several salient issues, all of which were recorded and coded. Many of the responses were indicative of changes and challenges in the field of early intervention in general and not necessarily specific to personnel preparation. It was implied by respondents that changes in personnel preparation parallel changes in the field; the link, however, was not always explicit.

Almost 50% of those interviewed identified issues related to the inclusion of young children with disabilities in programs with typically developing children as a significant change since the late-1980s. A similar number were expecting inclusion-related issues to change significantly during the 1990s. This category encompassed responses related to the joint training of personnel in early childhood education and early childhood special education, as well as issues of service delivery to young children with disabilities in more inclusive, community-based, or natural environments, and the resulting implications for training.

Other trends expected to continue include 1) increased focus on family-centered or family-guided practice, 2) increased attention to interdisciplinary or transdisciplinary team collaboration models, and 3) increased emphasis on training personnel to serve culturally and economically diverse populations.

The two most frequently identified challenges faced by those involved in the preparation of personnel to serve young children with disabilities and their families relate to inclusion. Nine respondents indicated one of the greatest challenges is preparing students for the extensive range of children and families being served. This includes children at various levels of development as well as an increasing age range (e.g., birth to 8 years). Another challenge identified was preparing students for the array of service delivery models, including team collaboration in inclusive settings. One specified obstacle to providing adequate training is a lack of inclusive practicum sites with personnel who are qualified to train students in these service delivery models. A few respondents identified a more general gap between recommended practice and current practices in the field and a perceived resistance to change.

CONCLUDING REMARKS: FUTURE DIRECTIONS

The data provided by the survey in this chapter do assist in creating a more complete and accurate picture of certain aspects of early intervention personnel preparation in the United States; however, it is important to keep in mind the limitations of the study. The random sample included only projects that receive federal funding. How representative these programs are of nonfederal projects remains unknown. Our belief is that these programs represent the best training efforts available in the United States because successfully competing for external federal support indicates the program's quality. Even though the survey was piloted, the interviewers encountered respondents who found items unclear and/or difficult to answer; therefore, information provided may not be perfectly matched with the questions asked. We do not know what training programs do; we only know what their representatives say they do. The reported emphasis on preparation of students for teams may have been biased by the field's apparent universal acceptance of this perspective. In other words, early intervention trainers may give lip service to the perspective without providing students adequate opportunities to acquire the information and develop the skills necessary for effective team participation. We hope not; however, only further study will provide the information needed to draw conclusions about the effectiveness of training efforts for future professionals.

Given these cautions, what do the survey findings suggest regarding trends and themes? First, training programs appear to be aiming toward generally accepted standards for the preparation of their students. Those standards appear to include an interdisciplinary perspective and the ability to deliver coordinated, family-focused services. Although programs use traditional strategies such as coursework, practical experience, and competencies to help students achieve these standards, there appears to be significant variability in how training programs select, cover, and sequence their chosen content. This lack of consistency across training programs is not surprising because educationally based disciplines have as yet no national standards or guidelines to direct their training activities.

Second, it appears that, at least conceptually, training faculty are committed to helping students acquire a team perspective. We were pleased and surprised to note the variety of disciplines associated with early intervention training programs at all levels. Participation by faculty representing a range of disciplines should offer students insight, skills, and content that are not possible from exposure to faculty and trainers from only one or two disciplines. Furthermore, faculty from across disciplines who do work together provide a model of successful teamwork for students to observe and emulate.

Third, competency-based approaches have been a long-time trend in special education and that trend appears to be continuing in early intervention. Not only do most programs operate using a competency-based model, but there also seems to be strong agreement about the general nature of the competencies to be targeted as well. Wording may vary but there is consensus about the importance of developing competence in child development (typical and atypical), assessment and evaluation, intervention strategies, family involvement, administration and management, service delivery and coordination, and team functioning.

A fourth consistent theme is the importance assigned to practical experience with children and families. All programs require that students spend time working directly with the target population. Most programs have selected a range of practicum sites that can provide students with a variety of important and diverse experiences. We suspect that the quality of sites varies considerably and that most programs would like to expand their practicum offerings to include community-based programs that are effectively integrating young children with disabilities.

In comparing the 1988 and 1994 survey results, we noted that respondents consistently reported that they believe personnel working with birth- to 2- and 3- to 5-year-old children should have different skills. This consistent theme poses a serious dilemma to educationally based early intervention training programs as well as for personnel being trained by other disciplines. The dilemma is how to balance generalized and specialized training. That is, what skills, content, and competencies cut across the birth-to-5 age range, and when are specific skills and content needed for specific populations? To complicate the problem further, there appears to be a national move toward extending the purview of early intervention from 5-year-old children to 8-year-old children to match the traditional age span of early childhood educators (DEC, 1993). Such an expansion will have a significant impact on training efforts. How such an expansion will be accomplished is a serious question, particularly because training issues covering the birth to 2 and 3–5 age ranges remain, for the most part, unresolved.

A final theme we have identified from our findings is the overriding concern for the practice of inclusion and its implications for training programs. How to effectively include young children with disabilities in community-based programs is a major concern in the early intervention field. We appear to *know* that personnel must be properly prepared if children with disabilities are to be successfully integrated; however, we appear to not *know* how to prepare personnel to meet this goal. Gaining this knowledge is a major challenge for all of us associated with the preparation of early intervention personnel (Kemple, Hartle, Correa, & Fox, 1994).

This chapter, as well as the others in this book, underscores the need for study of early intervention training efforts. There appears to be general acceptance of the tenet that early intervention programs are only as good as the staff they employ. Descriptive surveys, such as the one described in this chapter, can provide useful information about training efforts, but they should be complemented by investigations of the fidelity of training models and approaches and the effectiveness of those approaches, as evidenced by the skills of practicing professionals.

REFERENCES

Baer, M.T., Blyler, E.M., Cloud, H.H., & McCamman, S.P. (1991). Providing early nutrition intervention services: Preparation of dietitians, nutritionists, and other team members. *Infants and Young Children, 3*(4), 56–66.

Bailey, D.B., Palsha, S., & Huntington, G. (1990). Preservice preparation of special educators to serve infants with handicaps and their families: Current status and training needs. *Journal of Early Intervention, 14*(1), 43–54.

Bailey, D.B., Simeonsson, R.J., Yoder, D., & Huntington, G. (1990). Preparing professionals to serve infants and toddlers with handicaps and their families: An integrative analysis across eight disciplines. *Exceptional Children, 57*(1), 26–35.

Bricker, D.D., & Carlson, L. (1981). Issues in early language intervention. In R. Schiefelbusch & D. Bricker (Eds.), *Early language: Acquisition and intervention* (pp. 477–515). Baltimore: University Park Press.

Bricker, D.D., & Slentz, K. (1988). Personnel preparation: Handicapped infants. In M. Wang, H. Walberg, & M. Reynolds (Eds.), *The handbook of special education: Research and practice* (Vol. 3, pp. 319–345). Oxford, England: Pergamon Press.

Brown, W., & Rule, S. (1993). Personnel and disciplines in early intervention. In W. Brown, S.K. Thurman, & L.F. Pearl (Eds.), *Family-centered early intervention with infants and toddlers: Innovative cross-disciplinary approaches* (pp. 245–268). Baltimore: Paul H. Brookes Publishing Co.

Bruder, M., Klosowski, S., & Daguio, C. (1991). A review of personnel standards for Part H of P.L. 99-457. *Journal of Early Intervention, 15*(1), 66–79.

Bruder, M.B., Lippman, C., & Bologna, T. (1994). Personnel preparation in early intervention: Building capacity for program expansion within institutions of higher education. *Journal of Early Intervention, 18*(1), 103–110.

Bruder, M., & McLean, M. (1988). Personnel preparation for infant interventionists: A review of federally funded projects. *Journal for the Division of Early Childhood, 12*(4), 299–305.

Campbell, P.H. (1990). Meeting personnel needs in early intervention. In A.P. Kaiser & C.M. McWhorter (Eds.), *Preparing personnel to work with persons with severe disabilities* (pp. 111–134). Baltimore: Paul H. Brookes Publishing Co.

Courtnage, L., & Smith-Davis, J. (1987). Interdisciplinary team training: A national survey of special education teacher training programs. *Exceptional Children, 53*(3), 451–458.

Crais, E., & Leonard, C. (1990, April). P.L. 99-457: Are speech-language pathologists prepared for the challenge? *Asha, 32*, 57–61.

Division for Early Childhood of the Council for Exceptional Children (DEC). (1993, December). *DEC position on early intervention services for children birth to age eight.* Reston, VA: Author.

Division for Early Childhood of the Council for Exceptional Children (DEC), National Association for the Education of Young Children (NAEYC), & Association of Teacher Educators (ATE). (1994, October). *Personnel standards for early education and early intervention: Guidelines for licensure in early childhood special education.* Washington, DC: Authors.

Education of the Handicapped Act Amendments of 1986, PL 99-457. (October 8, 1986). Title 20, U.S.C. 1400 et seq: *U.S. Statutes at Large, 100,* 1145–1177.

Effgen, S., Bjornson, K., Chiarello, L., Sinzer, L., & Phillips, W. (1991). Competencies for physical therapists in early intervention. *Pediatric Physical Therapy, 3*(2), 77–80.

Fenichel, E., & Eggbeer, L. (1990). *Preparing practitioners to work with infants, toddlers and their families: Issues and recommendations for educators and trainers.* Arlington, VA: National Center for Clinical Infant Programs.

Gallagher, J., & Staples, A. (1990). *Available and potential resources for personnel preparation in special education: Dean's survey.* Chapel Hill, NC: Carolina Policy Studies Program.

Hanft, B.E., & Humphry, R. (1989). Training occupational therapists in early intervention. *Infants and Young Children, 1*(4), 54–65.

Hanson, M., & Lovett, D. (1992). Personnel preparation for early interventionists: A cross-disciplinary survey. *Journal of Early Intervention, 16*(2), 123–135.

Individuals with Disabilities Education Act Amendments of 1991, PL 102-119. (October 7, 1991). Title 20, U.S.C. 1400 et seq: *U.S. Statutes at Large, 105,* 587–608.

Johnson, J. (1995). *Passwords: Participants' reactions to a preservice family and professional collaboration class.* Unpublished doctoral dissertation, University of Oregon, Eugene.

Kemple, K.M., Hartle, L.C., Correa, V.I., & Fox, L. (1994). Preparing teachers for inclusive education. *Teacher Education and Special Education, 17*(1), 38–51.

Klein, N., & Campbell, P. (1990). Preparing personnel to serve at-risk and disabled infants, toddlers, and preschoolers. In S. Meisels & J. Shonkoff (Eds.), *Handbook of early childhood intervention* (pp. 679–699). New York: Cambridge University Press.

Lazzari, A., & Bruder, M. (1988). Teacher evaluation practices in early childhood special education. *Journal of the Division for Early Childhood, 12*(3), 238–244.

McCollum, J.A. (1987). Early interventionists in infancy and early childhood programs: A comparison of preservice training needs. *Topics in Early Childhood Special Education, 7*(3), 24–35.

McCollum, J.A., & Bailey, D. (1991). Developing comprehensive personnel systems: Issues and alternatives. *Journal of Early Intervention, 15*(1), 57–65.

McCollum, J.A., & McCartan, K. (1988). Research in teacher education: Issues and future directions for early childhood special education. In S.L. Odom & M.B. Karnes (Eds.), *Early intervention for infants and children with handicaps: An empirical base* (pp. 269–286). Baltimore: Paul H. Brookes Publishing Co.

McCollum, J.A., McLean, M., McCartan, K., & Kaiser, C. (1989). Recommendations for certification of early childhood special educators. *Journal of Early Intervention, 13*(3), 195–211.

McCollum, J.A., Rowan, L., & Thorp, E. (1994). Philosophy as training in infancy personnel preparation. *Journal of Early Intervention, 18,* 216–226.

McLinden, S., & Prasse, D. (1991). Providing services to infants and toddlers under P.L. 99-457: Training needs of school psychologists. *School Psychology Review, 20,* 37–48.

Mills, P., Vadasy, P., & Fewell, R. (1987). Preparing early childhood special educators for rural settings: An urban university approach. *Topics in Early Childhood Special Education, 7*(3), 59–74.

National Early Childhood Technical Assistance System. (1993, June). *Section 619 profile* (4th ed.). Chapel Hill, NC: Author.

Office of Special Education Programs (OSEP). (1993). *Selected early childhood programs.* Washington, DC: U.S. Department of Education.

II
DISCIPLINARY PERSPECTIVES ON TRAINING

4

PREPARING EARLY CHILDHOOD SPECIAL EDUCATORS

Jeanette A. McCollum
and Vicki D. Stayton

Andrea is a child development specialist for 20 families who have young children with special needs. Because the area she works in is very rural, Andrea provides a combination of center- and home-based services. Most of the therapists and other professionals with whom Andrea works are assigned across the agency's several sites and not just to her program. Some of the children and families also receive some of their services in a clinic located in the next county. Andrea tries to meet regularly with her core team members to coordinate the interventions they provide to these children and families. Sometimes the team plans a home visit so that it combines the goals that each of the members is working on; then, whoever makes the visit will be able to incorporate all of these areas of emphasis. Sometimes one of the other core team members also is able to spend a couple of hours in Andrea's classroom. However, the fact that members of the team are geographically dispersed and some services are contracted to other clinics has made it difficult to share information and provide a cohesive intervention. Andrea has made a practice of sending regular notes to other staff and of always inviting clinic staff to team meetings when "their" families are involved. In addition, she sometimes attends the clinic with the families she serves; often, they ask her to help them understand the information and instructions that they receive. One of Andrea's goals is to help families integrate this information into the routines of their daily lives. This also helps her provide a more integrated program when the children are in the classroom. Because she is familiar with the children's therapy goals and procedures, she can communicate progress and issues to parents and to other members of the team as well.

THIS SCENARIO ILLUSTRATES THE MULTIPLE types and contexts of the interactions that early childhood special educators[1] may have with professionals from other disciplines in providing early intervention services to young children (birth

---

[1]For the purposes of this chapter, the term *early intervention* is used to refer to the range of services delivered to children from birth to 5 years old who have disabilities and their families or to the team of professionals who deliver these services. The term *early childhood special education* is used to refer to the services provided specifically by early childhood special educators and to the discipline itself. The term *interdisciplinary early childhood education* is used to refer to services delivered by personnel trained in a unified program combining early childhood education and early childhood special education. *Infant–toddler* or *preschool* is used where appropriate to distinguish age levels within this broader age period. In cases in which titles of a discipline or a program are specific to the state or university being discussed, those titles are used as they are employed in that state or university.

through 5 years) with disabilities and their families. Two aspects of this illustration may be particularly relevant for considering interdisciplinary training for the discipline of early childhood special education (ECSE): 1) the wide variety of potential roles that the educator may take in relation to individuals from other disciplines, and 2) the different types and depths of information and experience needed to fill these roles. For some roles, a simple awareness of the areas of expertise of other disciplines may be sufficient. For other roles, a deeper understanding of the knowledge base of other disciplines may be necessary in order to assist in blending the experiences each child and family is having into a cohesive whole. In addition, when early childhood special educators work on a tightly knit direct services team with professionals from other disciplines, they need to sufficiently understand the goals and techniques of these disciplines to enhance the interconnections with the goals and techniques of their own discipline. In some cases, these educators may be using activities and procedures recommended by a professional from another discipline, or assisting families to do so. In others, they may be teaching their educational procedures to members of other disciplines. The variations among these roles have critical implications for programs in personnel preparation.

The team roles of educators are influenced to a large extent by the same factors that affect the roles of any professional working with young children with special needs and their families. These include extra-program variables (e.g., geography, population density, personnel availability) as well as intra-program variables (e.g., funding sources) and whether services in the community are structured within a single agency or across several agencies. Within any particular service model, variations occur with regard to where the services are provided; whether the services involve the child, the parent, or both; who is seen as the primary recipient of the services; and whether services are provided on a one-to-one basis or in groups. The other disciplines available and the team model of choice within the agency will also influence how the educator will work with members of other disciplines (McCollum & Hughes, 1988). As noted by McCollum and Maude (1994), when a family-centered philosophy is employed, the roles of the early childhood special educator also will vary in relation to the configuration of services chosen by each family. Flexibility in services provided and in the roles assumed has been identified as an overarching theme of early intervention service provision (Thorp & McCollum, 1994); preparation for flexibility in assuming different aspects of multiple roles, as well as for the roles themselves, must be a central concern in personnel training (Fenichel & Eggbeer, 1991). In addition, the interactions that early childhood special educators have with individuals from other disciplines will reflect the beliefs and values that they hold about their own discipline, other disciplines, and interdisciplinary team functioning. These beliefs and values therefore must become an explicit focus of training for work with young children and their families, regardless of discipline. Nevertheless, of all of the early intervention disciplines, ECSE is the one in which the similarities and differences between the traditional functions of the discipline and those performed in early intervention may be most elusive, particularly at the birth-to-3-year level. Neither the content taught at older age levels nor the instructional methods employed translate easily to the infant–toddler level or even to the preschool level (Bricker & Slentz, 1988). Moreover, the services of the early childhood special educator may be provided not only in settings apart from the public school classroom but also by agencies other than the local school. Although the unique contributions of this discipline to the early intervention team are fairly well agreed upon within the field of ECSE, they are not clearly recognized by other disciplines, by educators who work with older children, or by the early intervention programs that employ these educators; hence, role identity is another factor that may have considerable influence on the early childhood special educator's interactions and relationships with other team members, indicating that it also must receive attention during preservice training.

Underlying the formulation of training for early childhood special educators is an understanding of both the unique contributions that early childhood special educators make to the early intervention team and the important and extensive functions that they perform as generalists on the early intervention team. Distinctions between generalist and specialist roles have long been apparent in the lists of functions ascribed to special educators working with young children. For instance, both types of functions appear in the areas of expertise identified by Bailey, Palsha, and Huntington (1990) as special contributions of the early childhood special educator to services for children from birth to 3 years old, which include integrating goals from multiple developmental domains within the context of activity-based intervention; using a comprehensive and systematic approach in which assessment, intervention, and evaluation are combined into a coordinated whole; and advocating for children and families. This list mirrors five major roles of an early childhood special educator outlined by Bricker (1989): conceptualizer, synthesizer, instructor, evaluator, and counselor. Another generalist role assuming increased importance as more young children receive intervention services in community-based programs is consultation (Coleman, Buysse, Scalise-Smith, & Schulte, 1991).

Although models of teaming vary greatly across early intervention programs, each of the various specialist and generalist roles enumerated above was seen in the earlier scenario describing Andrea's early intervention work. Nevertheless, what distinguishes the generalist roles of ECSE from those of other disciplines are not the roles themselves but rather the variety of generalist roles assumed and the extent to which these roles characterize the daily work of the early childhood special educator. Often, it is the early childhood special educator who is the consistent member of the early intervention team and who functions as the primary interventionist and service coordinator, whether in an infant or toddler setting (McCollum & Hughes, 1988) or in a preschool (Bricker, 1976). Because either generalist or specialist roles may be performed in a variety of team contexts from unidisciplinary to transdisciplinary, the early childhood special educator may be called upon to change the skills employed depending on other team members. Therefore, skills and information to support the educator's generalist roles, as well as skills and knowledge to support the unique specialty-based contributions of this discipline, make important contributions to the early intervention team. Recognition of these roles as they may be applied across multiple team contexts has broad implications for training and warrants an explicit focus on the team process within the context of training.

The remainder of this chapter is devoted to describing the content and process of preservice teacher education directed toward preparing early childhood special educators to work in team contexts, with particular emphasis on components of training that directly address preparation for team roles. A brief overview of the literature related to the content and process of interdisciplinary training of early childhood special educators follows, as do descriptions of two specific personnel preparation programs. The discussion is limited to the concept of team training as it applies to interactions with professional disciplines outside of education and does not include issues of team interaction that arise among early childhood special educators, early childhood educators, and special educators. The discussion also is limited to the training of the professional members of the team.

INTERDISCIPLINARY TRAINING OF
EARLY CHILDHOOD SPECIAL EDUCATORS

Any program preparing early childhood special educators for interdisciplinary work with young children with special needs and their families faces two questions: "What?" and "How?" The first, a question about the content of the program, concerns the areas of competence important for performing the multiple roles that this professional may fill. The second, a question about the program's processes, asks which training procedures are most likely to prepare professionals for complex roles that are grounded in interdependence among multiple individuals at multiple levels of interaction, across multiple settings, and over time (Fenichel & Eggbeer, 1991; Thorp & McCollum, 1994). Although the majority of the literature on preparing early childhood special educators for interdisciplinary roles relates to work with children from age birth to 3 and their families, much of this work applies directly to the preschool level as well (even though a number of specific differences may occur across this age range). These differences in competencies will reflect the changing developmental needs of the child and family during this early period of development, the purposes of intervention during this time period, the nature of the service systems that provide these services, the contexts within which the services are delivered, and the intervention strategies that are employed (Bailey, 1989; Fenichel & Eggbeer, 1991; Thorp & McCollum, 1994). As seamless systems of service are developed across the birth- to 5-year age range, values and practices originally delineated for services at the birth- to 3-year level are making their way upward into the preschool level (McCollum & Maude, 1994). New teacher certifications in ECSE, which reflect a specific focus on young children with special needs from birth to 5 or birth to 8 years of age, will support this trend by encouraging the development of training programs that encompass a broader age span.

For educators, as for other disciplines working with young children, required areas of competence include those unique to the discipline, reflecting the specialist roles performed by members of the discipline, and those held in common across disciplines, reflecting more generalist roles (McCollum & Thorp, 1988). The distinction between within- and across-discipline competencies provides a useful framework for designing training programs. Thorp and McCollum (1994) discussed four broad categories for organizing knowledge and skill competencies for disciplines working with young children with special needs:

1. Child-related (understanding of typical and atypical development, ability to learn from observation)

2. Family-related (awareness of family systems, understanding of sources of vulnerability in families, supporting family competencies)
3. Team-related (common vocabulary, joint-planning and problem-solving strategies, conflict resolution skills)
4. Interagency, advocacy-related (knowledge of state legislation, coordination of programs across agencies)

These authors and others (Fenichel & Eggbeer, 1991) also stressed personal qualities (e.g., flexibility, maturity, independence, willingness to share, tolerance) that may be particularly critical for interventionists working with very young children and their families. The particular relevance of these personal qualities to teamwork is the emphasis on building relationships that are based on shared knowledge and respect. The ability to reflect on oneself as a helper and as a team member is a critical skill across all early intervention disciplines (Fenichel & Eggbeer, 1991).

Attention also has been given to what is unique about the skills and knowledge that the early childhood special educator brings to the early intervention team (Bailey, Palsha, et al., 1990; Geik, Gilkerson, & Sponseller, 1982; Thorp & McCollum, 1994). Using the same four broad categories described above, Thorp and McCollum (1994) identified competencies that are more unique to the specialist roles of the early childhood special educator:

1. Child-related competencies (cognitive, social, and affective development; skills in developmental assessment; design of learning environments; strategies to promote engagement and interaction; skills in data collection and evaluation)
2. Family-related competencies (strategies for including family members as partners in planning and implementing intervention, strategies for promoting interaction between parent and child)
3. Team-related competencies (skill in integrating the knowledge and recommendations of multiple disciplines into the child's and family's daily routines)
4. Agency-related competencies (knowledge of community resources, developing blended service plans)

These and other delineations of areas of competence (e.g., Division for Early Childhood of the Council for Exceptional Children [DEC], Association of Teacher Educators [ATE], & National Association for the Education of Young Children [NAEYC], 1995; McCollum, McLean, McCartan, & Kaiser, 1989) provide significant guidance to training programs in the development of program content by helping to clarify the many generalist and specialist roles of the early childhood special educator across the early childhood years. Moreover, they help to tie these roles to those of educators who work with older children by clarifying commonalities in roles across the age range. Again, however, these areas also demonstrate the salience of the variety of roles engaged in by professionals who work with young children and their families; the younger the child, the closer the ties among developmental systems and the family ecology within which early development occurs, and the greater the interdependence among disciplines. When a child is young, discipline differences tend to be ones of focus, context, or emphasis, rather than representing the performance of mutually exclusive functions.

In contrast to the substantial amount of information related to the competencies needed by early intervention personnel, much less information is available with regard to the training structures and processes that might be used to develop this content in preservice students, or how these processes might best be matched to the specific content to be taught. Fenichel and Eggbeer (1991) identified three process variables critical to the preparation of interventionists who work with very young children:

1. Opportunities are needed for direct observation and interaction with young children and families who represent the heterogeneous array of characteristics of the children and families with whom these interventionists will work.
2. Individualized supervision is needed to allow the trainee to reflect upon all aspects of work with children, families, and colleagues from a range of disciplines.
3. Support from colleagues is needed, both within and across disciplines, that begins early in training and continues throughout the practitioner's professional life.

Bailey and his colleagues (Bailey, Simeonsson, Yoder, & Huntington, 1990a), summarizing results from a national survey and from a multidisciplinary working conference of professionals from eight disciplines, suggested that all students should have clinical experiences working with families, as well as coursework and clinical experiences involving students and professionals from multiple disciplines. Exposure to a variety of program settings also appears crucial to preparing students for the heterogeneity of settings and roles in which they may work with professionals from other disciplines. Part H of the Individuals with Disabilities Education Act (IDEA), gives explicit sanction to utilizing interdisciplinary interaction as an important training process by specifically mentioning the desirability of training that occurs on an interdisciplinary basis (McCollum & Bailey, 1991).

Recommended training practices, like recommended training content, may be difficult to implement. Bailey et al. (1990) found that students in university programs in special education, like those in other programs (Bailey, Simeonsson, Yoder, & Huntington, 1990b), rarely had an opportunity to work on interdisciplinary teams or to have direct experience with young children with special needs or their families (Bailey et al., 1990b; Bruder & McLean, 1988). Further evidence comes from a within-state survey in Illinois (reported in McCollum & Thorp, 1988) in which personnel working in infant–toddler programs were asked to identify what they believed to be the most important training elements missing from their own preservice preparation. A common element was direct experience with infants and families and with students preparing for other disciplines. These patterns also were corroborated in three within-state studies that included programs affiliated with early childhood education as well as with special education (Bevins, 1992; Hanson, 1990; Sexton & Snyder, 1991). Students enrolled in programs more directly focused on young children do appear to have more exposure to content related to a range of roles relevant to early intervention services than do students in less focused programs. Nevertheless, training emphases vary substantially across schools (Bailey, Palsha, et al.,1990; Bailey et al., 1990b), and the emphasis continues to be on the more traditional child-directed roles of the educator, to the relative exclusion of the family, and team roles increasingly found in all early childhood settings. Hence, it appears that neither recommended content nor recommended training practices have found their way into the majority of programs preparing students from any early intervention discipline, including ECSE.

Interaction among students and faculty from multiple disciplines requires that programs step outside of the disciplinary lines in developing new courses or experiences (Bailey, 1989). However, there are significant barriers to the development of interdisciplinary training (Bailey et al., 1990b). Several of these barriers relate directly to the ability of program faculty to prepare students for interdisciplinary team roles or to use interdisciplinary interactions as part of the training process, including the following:

1. Shortage of faculty with expertise with young children or with interdisciplinary and interagency collaboration
2. Already crowded curricula, often tied closely to state or national certification or licensing requirements
3. The lack of available practicum settings that can provide students with experience in interdisciplinary team roles or other components of recognized recommended practice
4. University structures and reward systems that do not support or recognize the value of faculty or programs crossing disciplinary lines

State and university policies and practices are important contexts influencing the design of any training program; for programs that set out to provide training in nontraditional ways, as may be true of interdisciplinary training, these contexts will necessarily influence the design process in critical ways.

Many questions remain with regard to training early childhood special educators who will become interdisciplinary specialists working with young children with disabilities and their families. Nevertheless, there is considerable guidance available from personnel preparation programs that have already experienced the interdisciplinary program design process. Two programs, each directed by one of the two authors of this chapter, are described in more detail in the next section. Emphasis is given to program elements reflective of team training, especially those developed to foster the acquisition of skills and values supportive of a team process. A historical and ecological context for each program is presented in order to illustrate how the structure and practices adopted by each program reflect the conditions present in its ecosystem. The reader also is referred to other chapters in this book for additional models that might be adapted to the preparation of early childhood special educators.

A TALE OF TWO PROGRAMS

In each of the programs described in this section, interdisciplinary content and process are part of a larger program preparing early childhood special educators to work with young children from birth to 5 years of age. In both, graduate students from several departments participate in program activities directed toward gaining expertise with young children who have special needs and their families. Despite these similarities, there are many differences between the two programs that may be helpful in considering how to overcome barriers to providing such training within the unique contexts of different university systems.

Many aspects of the programs described apply across the different disciplines involved. For the purpose of this chapter, the ECSE perspective is emphasized. A similar format will be followed for each program description. First, a context is provided by describing state and university variables that have a bearing on how the program is organized. The ways in which each program evolved within the parameters set by its own context, as well as its goals, content, and training processes, are delineated. The aspects of the program that reflect or facilitate interdisciplinary interaction and support training explicitly directed toward the team process are emphasized. Factors that act as supports and barriers to interdisciplinary training also are described. Finally, similarities and differences in approach between the two programs are summarized in order to assist readers in drawing generalizations that may be relevant to their own individual situations.

University of Illinois at Champaign-Urbana

State and University Context

In Illinois, both preschool and infant–toddler services are under the administrative umbrella of the Illinois State Board of Education. However, the models of service delivery used in these two systems are very different. Preschool services for 3- to 5-year-olds with disabilities and developmental delays have been a part of the public schools since 1975 when Illinois became one of the first states to pass a preschool mandate. Since that time, services have been provided primarily in self-contained classrooms located in the public schools. In some districts, classroom services are provided for 4 days a week, with the fifth day being used for home visiting and team meetings. Family centers established in many schools provide a range of services, such as parent–child play groups, toy-lending libraries, and parenting classes. There also has been a trend toward using more inclusive community settings. Blending of disciplinary roles is increasing, with many programs using transdisciplinary assessment teams and integrating therapies (and therapists) into daily classroom routines. Preschool teachers are certified by the Illinois State Board of Education in either special education (kindergarten–grade 12) or in early childhood education. Special education certification is categorically based and emphasizes training with school-age populations. Early childhood certification, although written to include third grade and under, emphasizes primarily the preschool and primary levels. In addition to holding one of these two types of certification, teachers working with preschoolers with disabilities also must complete four additional academic courses to obtain an Illinois Approval in Early Childhood Special Education.

In contrast to preschool services, infant–toddler services are provided through a heterogeneous mixture of state-funded, not-for-profit, and private providers, using service contexts that include the home, center-based groups for children alone, center-based groups for children and parents, and specialized clinics. The Department of Mental Health and Developmental Disabilities is the largest state funder of infant–toddler services (McCollum, Cook, & Ladmer, 1993). However, many other state agencies also contribute resources to support these services. It is not uncommon for an individual program to combine funding from as many as a dozen different sources to employ or contract individuals representing an array of disciplines. As the infant–toddler system in Illinois moves toward a new configuration envisioned by the state interagency council, services will become system based, rather than program based, with funding flowing through a central billing system to reimburse providers from all disciplines for their respective individual services.

Typical personnel configurations in most local programs mirror those found at the national level by McCollum and Hughes (1988); the child development specialist (the title used for the early childhood special educator on the team) is the most consistent member of the program team across the state's approximately 100 infant–toddler programs, as well as the member most likely to be involved in the widest variety of program functions (McCollum et al., 1993). Qualifications for all disciplines have been outlined by the Personnel Committee of the interagency council and approved on a trial basis for 5 years. These are external to the teacher certification system used for personnel in the public schools. For the child development specialist, these qualifications combine a basic level of preparation (defined as a bachelor's degree in early childhood education, special education, or child development) with an additional specialization in the infant–toddler period. The specialization may be obtained through one of two means—university coursework or a portfolio review (McCollum & Yates, 1994). In developing the guidelines for credentials needed to support this specialization process, which apply across disciplines, attention has been given both to the interdisciplinary coursework and to the practicum placements of students as they work to meet these qualifications. Interdisciplinary experiences available to individuals already in the field as they work through the portfolio review also have been emphasized. Only three universities in Illinois (as of 1996) provide a full course of study allowing ECSE students to focus specifically on the infant–toddler population. Preparation for the add-on state approval in ECSE, enabling teachers to teach preschoolers with disabilities, also is not an integral part of most preservice training programs.

Although the University of Illinois at Champaign-Urbana is the state's largest public university, the training programs for most of the major disciplines that provide early intervention services are located at the Chicago campus, 140 miles to the north. This has placed significant constraints on the development of interdisciplinary training, as the intensive interdisciplinary specialization sequence in which students participate is primarily restricted to students from three disciplines: ECSE, speech and hearing science, and social work. In addition, individual students from the Department of Curriculum and Instruction (early childhood education) and Human Development and Family Resources (child development) have chosen to participate in various aspects of the interdisciplinary training without taking the full specialization sequence.

Supported by a grant from the Bureau of Education for the Handicapped, the graduate program in ECSE at the University of Illinois began in 1975. In 1983, an infant–toddler practicum component was added to the program. Grant support was obtained from the Office of Special Education and Rehabilitative Services in 1986 to offer an interdisciplinary specialization at the birth- to 3-year level, funding graduate students from different departments. The interdisciplinary aspects of the program, with the exception of the interdisciplinary practicum, are required for all students in ECSE; the practicum is required only for students specializing at the infant–toddler level.

Beginnings of Interdisciplinary Training

Although many faculty at the University of Illinois interact across departments, the university is structured along departmental lines, with few formal mechanisms to support team training. Discussions of cross-departmental collaboration were first initiated in 1986 by two faculty members from the Department of ECSE and two from the Department of Speech and Hearing Science around the topic of developing a collaborative practicum. Following 2 years of successful implementation of the new practicum, these faculty, with the addition of another faculty member from the School of Social Work, successfully collaborated in preparing an interdisciplinary grant proposal to provide a cross-department infant–toddler specialization. As outcomes for students were clarified during the first year of this grant, additional formal structures were put in place to support the specialization. The emphasis on preparing students for team-based, family-centered, and child-responsive practice that grew from this project is the foundation of all coursework and field experience in ECSE.

The rationale for developing the interdisciplinary specialization was based on four premises. First, the close interrelationship among developmental areas in very young children makes interrelationships among the goals and procedures of different disciplines inevitable; similarly, the family context of early development has major implications for the professional roles of all disciplines (Thorp & McCollum, 1994). An interrelated service model therefore was viewed not only as the most effective and efficient model, but also as the most child and family friendly because each professional would be more likely to support a broader range of goals important to the child and family. A second premise of the rationale for the development of interdisciplinary training came from participating faculty members' increasing awareness of the commonalities and uniquenesses among early intervention disciplines (Bailey et al., 1990a). Third, through collaboration, faculty had begun to develop and articulate shared beliefs about interdisciplinary training. One belief was that some content important in early intervention (e.g., respect for how disciplines complement one another within the early intervention context) cannot be learned within a single-discipline training framework. To gain a common frame of reference about service delivery and to develop a common set of values about children, families, and services, students need to participate together in learning. Fourth, faculty believed that to develop values and commitment to a team process, students would need not only to directly experience team interaction, but also to reflect extensively on that experience and on themselves as team members. These beliefs were supported by training needs identified by practitioners in Illinois (McCollum & Thorp, 1988), and also by the four guidelines for program development outlined by Fenichel and Eggbeer (1991).

Structure of the Interdisciplinary Specialization

A three-level model (McCollum & Thorp, 1988) was used as the framework for outlining interdisciplinary coursework and field experiences. For each discipline, based on emerging consensus in the literature, consideration was given to Level 1—

the discipline's traditional body of knowledge; Level 2—specialized disciplinary knowledge as it would apply to infants and toddlers; and Level 3—the body of knowledge held in common across students from all disciplines. In each of the participating programs, courses were identified that could meet the needs of each level. In necessary cases, modifications were made to the courses to better meet these needs and additional courses were proposed to fill gaps.

A typical program of study for an interdisciplinary specialization student in ECSE is shown in Table 1, outlined according to this three-level model. The student would complete the requirements of the Department of Special Education as outlined for students in ECSE (Levels 1 and 2), as well as the cross-discipline courses taken in common with other interdisciplinary students (Level 3). In Levels 1 and 2, courses might include students from other disciplines or, in some cases, might be taken from faculty in other departments. However, it is at Level 3 that cross-discipline interaction and interdisciplinary content are emphasized.

Three academic courses comprise the interdisciplinary emphasis for all ECSE students and, for students specializing at the infant–toddler level, the interdisciplinary practicum also is required. Two of the academic courses (interdisciplinary teams and atypical development) were developed specifically for the specialization, whereas the third (families) was redesigned to achieve a greater

Table 1. Structural framework of the University of Illinois interdisciplinary specialization

Program content	Participating disciplines
Level 1—Within-discipline knowledge base	
Child development	Early childhood special education
Language development	Early childhood special education, speech and hearing science
Organizing for early intervention	Early childhood special education
Selected courses in:	
Educational psychology	—
Educational policy	—
Level 2—Within-discipline age level specialization	
Assessment	Early childhood special education
Intervention issues and practices	Early childhood special education
Practicum	Early childhood special education
Level 3—Cross-discipline specialization	
Families of children with special needs	Early childhood special education, speech and hearing science, social work
Development of young children with special needs	Early childhood special education, speech and hearing science, social work, other[a]
Interdisciplinary teaming	Early childhood special education, speech and hearing science, social work, other[a]
Interdisciplinary practicum	Early childhood special education, speech and hearing science, social work, other[a]

[a]Other students, regardless of discipline, taking the specialization sequence.

family-centered perspective. The interdisciplinary practicum, taken by all students enrolled in the infant–toddler specialization, regardless of discipline, was
already in place prior to the rest of the program, but was integrated into this
overall framework. It is in the parents' interaction with infants (PIWI) practicum
that students practice and evaluate their own roles as team members. PIWI is designed to complement experiences already available in the community by providing opportunities for extensive interaction with infants and toddlers and their
families, experience working as equal members of the team, the opportunity for
some degree of independence in developing and evaluating a service program,
and the opportunity to experience elements of emerging recommended practice.
As described elsewhere (McCollum, Rowan, & Thorp, 1994; Rowan, McCollum,
& Thorp, 1993; Rowan, Thorp, & McCollum, 1990), the PIWI practicum is based
on a set of philosophy statements related to children, families, teams, and supervision of students. These philosophy statements have been expanded further
into a set of program standards, used as an integral part of the training that occurs within this practicum by providing the framework around which students
develop and evaluate the services that they deliver. The beliefs and values em-
bodied in these philosophy statements also are infused throughout the rest of the
interdisciplinary coursework.

Although the elements of the philosophy are emphasized throughout the
program, it is in the interdisciplinary team class and in the PIWI practicum that
the process of team building among disciplines is an explicit focus of training.
The primary team competency areas include the following:

1. The knowledge and skills of interpersonal interaction in the group process,
    including effective communication, decision making, and conflict resolution
2. The knowledge of roles and tasks of early intervention disciplines
3. The skills of role release across disciplines

In the interdisciplinary team course, each of these competency areas is addressed
at all levels, from knowledge to skills and values. To accomplish this, a variety of
methods are used including self-evaluation, case studies, and team development
activities. All students majoring in ECSE, including those in the PIWI practicum,
also participate with other ECSE students in weekly practicum seminars in
which they learn a specific model of peer collaboration as they consider issues
that apply to their profession across the birth- to 5-year age span. The PIWI students then apply this model within their PIWI team meetings.

It is in the PIWI practicum that the focus on team process and on team- and
self-analysis is most explicit. This practicum is taken concurrently with coursework, usually during the student's second semester in the program. Teams of
two to four students, representing different disciplines, are responsible for planning, implementing, and evaluating parent–child play groups for two different
sets of six to eight parent–child dyads per week over a full semester (McCollum
et al., 1994; Rowan et al., 1990; Rowan et al., 1993). A team meeting after each
session is used to evaluate not only what was provided to children and families,
but also the team process that was used to do so. Thus, within the context of the
play group and the team meeting, students practice team roles, provide peer feed-

back, and engage in team-evaluation and self-evaluation activities. The two teams of students involved in PIWI during the same semester also meet together weekly as a total team to assist one another in problem solving through the use of scenarios that they bring to the group or videotapes that they have made of their play groups or of their team meetings. The assumption is made that the skills learned through this intensive experience, if supported by self-analysis and reflection at both the team and individual levels, will translate to working with a broader array of disciplines in other team situations.

One primary purpose of the PIWI practicum is to provide students with the opportunity to independently design, implement, and evaluate an early intervention service. Although no cooperating professional is involved, a doctoral student from one of the participating disciplines is assigned to each team to function as team and individual supervisor. The supervisor is present throughout the groups and the team meeting but does not enter the team process unless needed. Using a clinical supervision model to support the students as they learn team processes, the supervisor's goal is to match the level of supervisory involvement with the team's need for support, gradually shifting all responsibility for observation and analysis to the team. Supervisors also provide individual supervision to each team member on a rotating basis. Together, the two supervisors assigned to the PIWI practicum plan and implement the weekly total team meetings. The content of these meetings responds to specific needs that have emerged from the implementation of the groups and also systematically introduces new skills to be incorporated into implementation of the groups (e.g., supporting parent–child interaction, embedding individual objectives through matrix planning). Team analysis and problem solving through the use of case presentation also play a prominent role in these total team meetings.

In summary, several factors characterize the interdisciplinary specialization as experienced by students majoring in ECSE at the University of Illinois. First, the program of study is based on an organizational framework that incorporates competency areas identified as important to the specialist and generalist roles of the early childhood special educator working with very young children and their families. Second, the interdisciplinary specialization was developed to fill gaps identified in each participating department with regard to working with young children, particularly at the birth- to 3-year level. Third, a new practicum site was created jointly by participating faculty to complement field placements available within the community and to address specific areas of competence that required intensive, focused training beyond that available in other placements. Fourth, because few disciplines were available on the Champaign-Urbana campus to participate in interdisciplinary training, the decision was made to focus on the team process through an intensive interdisciplinary practicum and through an interdisciplinary team course; less extensive exposure to more disciplines was obtained through other practicum sites. Finally, it has been essential that participating faculty agree on desired outcomes for students and then devote considerable time to recruitment, advisement, and negotiating for departmental resources. Ongoing collaboration at the faculty level has been key to the management and continuation of the specialization because these faculty provide the link to other faculty and students in their respective departments.

Western Kentucky University at Bowling Green

State and University Context

Kentucky's preschool services are administered by the Kentucky Department of Education (KDE), while infant–toddler services are administered by the Department of Mental Health/Mental Retardation (MH/MR). Beginning in 1984, when kindergarten became a mandated public school program, school districts began to offer services for 5-year-olds with disabilities. Mandated public school services began in 1990 for 3- and 4-year-olds with disabilities and for 4-year-olds identified as at risk by qualifying for the federal free school lunch program. Some school districts voluntarily provide services for all 3- and 4-year-olds regardless of special needs.

Inclusion as a recommended service delivery practice has been stressed in Kentucky's preschool programs since their inception. During the 1980s, school districts were encouraged to participate in a grant-supported program, funded through Part B Preschool Incentive Grant monies, in which kindergarten staff participated in training institutes and periodic consultation on recommended practices for integrating children with disabilities into kindergarten programs. Since 1990, the majority of 4-year-olds with disabilities have been served in center-based programs with other 4-year-olds identified as at risk. Based on the individual needs of 3-year-olds and their families, services may be center based (typically with 4-year-olds) or home based. School districts also have the option of contracting with Head Start or child care centers to provide services for preschoolers with disabilities or those who are at risk. Beginning in 1995, lead teachers in all public school programs serving young children with or without disabilities must be certified through the KDE in interdisciplinary early childhood education, birth to primary (IECE, B–P). Most school districts employ speech and/or communication disorders specialists and school psychologists from whom the preschool staff receive assistance. Preschool staff also work closely with family resource centers, often staffed by a social worker. Services from other related services professionals are typically provided on a contractual basis.

In contrast to preschool services, the majority of infant–toddler services in Kentucky are provided through 14 regionally operated, state-funded MH/MR districts. Although MH/MR has been the major funding source, a variety of other sources include Medicaid, Maternal and Child Health, and United Way. With the passage of state legislation in 1994 and the implementation of the new state system of services for infants and toddlers, a centralized billing system has been instituted that has access to funds primarily from three state agencies—the Departments of MH/MR, Medicaid, and Health. Some programs provide a combination of center- and home-based services, while others provide only one service delivery option; similarly, some programs employ professionals from several disciplines, while in others the majority of services are provided by the child development specialist with other services contracted through separate agencies.

The personnel committee of the Kentucky Early Intervention System Interagency Coordinating Council has delineated both generic and discipline-specific competency areas for early intervention personnel working with children from birth to 3 years old in Kentucky. Developmental interventionists (early childhood special educators) are required to obtain the IECE, B–P Certification. Due to the newness of this certificate, universities are just beginning to establish programs. Moreover, few universities prepare students in other disciplines to work specifically with infants and toddlers and their families.

Western Kentucky University is a regional university with an enrollment of approximately 15,000 students. Many of its students work full time and live some distance from the campus. The IECE graduate program was initiated in 1990, offering a unified certificate in Early Childhood Education and Early Childhood Special Education; it has been partially grant supported since the fall of 1991 through the U.S. Department of Education, Office of Special Education Programs. Students completing the program are eligible to apply for the IECE, B–P Certification, thereby becoming qualified as early childhood/early childhood special educators at both the infant–toddler and preschool levels. This is accomplished by requiring assignments and practicum experiences to be completed with children and families across the age range. Students enter the major in IECE from a range of backgrounds including special education (kindergarten–12th grade), primary level elementary education (kindergarten–fourth grade), child development, speech/communication disorders, psychology, and physical therapy.

In addition to the master's program in IECE, the university offers programs in nursing, school psychology, social work, and speech/communication disorders. Interdisciplinary training activities occur at different levels of intensity with students and faculty from each of the on-campus disciplines.

Beginnings of Interdisciplinary Training

An interdisciplinary focus has been part of the IECE master's program at Western Kentucky University from its beginning. As discussed elsewhere (Stayton & Miller, 1993), a committee representing the disciplines of child development and family studies, early childhood education, early childhood special education, school psychology, special education, speech/communication disorders, and social work was appointed in the fall of 1989 at the request of the head of the Department of Teacher Education to assist in developing a master's program in IECE. The primary goal of forming this committee was to design a program that would facilitate early childhood special educators' understanding of other disciplines and enhance their ability to work collaboratively with professionals from those disciplines. The philosophy statement articulated by this faculty committee is guided by six premises related to program content and process. Through both content and program structure, students were to be prepared to 1) provide services in inclusive settings (Miller, 1992; Odom & McEvoy, 1990), 2) participate as team members (Nash, 1990), and 3) deliver family-centered services (Winton & Bailey, 1990). In addition, the philosophy statement stresses that the program should 1) recognize training needs of nontraditional students, 2) have as its foundation a competency-based curriculum (McCollum et al., 1989; Smith & Powers, 1987), and 3) provide opportunities for students to problem-solve and make decisions about their own learning and experiences (Knowles, 1984).

Through the process of discussing and developing a philosophy statement to undergird the preparation of students in the IECE program, the interdisciplinary faculty committee began to envision an interdisciplinary master's program with an emphasis in early childhood for students from multiple disciplines. Benefits for cross-disciplinary training for all students and faculty involved were clarified.

Roles for which students would be prepared were then delineated and curriculum content developed. External grant funds were sought and obtained to support participation by students and faculty from the other participating disciplines, complementing the support already available for students from the IECE program.

Structure of the Interdisciplinary Specialization

The team structure of the program serves as a driving force for curriculum content and for the structure within which that content is delivered. The interdisciplinary nature of the program is evident in each of the following components: 1) IECE students participate in coursework and seminars with students from other disciplines, taught by faculty from other disciplines; 2) IECE students complete an interdisciplinary internship as a team member with students and faculty from a variety of disciplines; 3) faculty from the various disciplines involved meet on a regular basis to address program issues; and 4) an advisory group with representatives from various community agencies and parents gives input on program content and process. Using a model similar to that of the University of Illinois, students are prepared in the traditional body of knowledge for their respective disciplines, specialized knowledge in the discipline regarding young children with disabilities and their families, and a common core of knowledge with students from other disciplines. In addition to students from the IECE program, a minimum of 15 students per year from social work, school psychology, and speech/communication disorders (5 students per discipline) complete an area of emphasis related to working with young children with disabilities (Jones, Stayton, Kersting, Lockett, & Forbes, n.d.). It is these students with whom the IECE students receive interdisciplinary training.

Students in the IECE master's program complete 36 semester hours of coursework over a 2-year sequence. This coursework addresses knowledge and skills related to young children and also provides a common body of knowledge and skills across disciplines. Table 2 outlines the program courses and the disciplines participating in each. During the second year of coursework, IECE students also participate in a minimum of three seminar sessions, one each in the fall, spring, and first summer semesters. These seminars include students from school psychology, social work, and speech/communication disorders with whom the IECE students will be completing the summer internship. The seminars focus on topics to be emphasized in the internship, including team structure and functioning, the individualized family service plan (IFSP) process, arena assessment, and curriculum issues. Emphasis is on both discipline-specific and cross-discipline roles in service delivery. Lecture, video presentations, role plays, simulations, and case studies are employed to develop knowledge and beginning-level skills in these content areas.

The 5-week summer internship is the culminating experience of the program. Offered at the child care/Head Start center during the second summer term, it involves 20–25 students from the four disciplines identified above. The center, located on the Western Kentucky University campus, serves children birth through 5 years of age in an integrated, full-day setting. Because it is a combination Head Start/child care program, services of educational, disabilities, parent involvement, and health and/or nutrition coordinators are available. The setting is already a familiar one to many of the students because throughout the year students from each of the four disciplines complete other practicum experi-

Table 2. Structural framework of Western Kentucky University's interdisciplinary specialization

Program content	Participating disciplines
Within-discipline knowledge and skills	
Organizing programs for interdisciplinary early childhood education	Interdisciplinary early childhood education
Assessment	Interdisciplinary early childhood education
Early childhood methods and materials	Interdisciplinary early childhood education
Early childhood special education curriculum and methods	Interdisciplinary early childhood education
Cross-discipline knowledge and skills	
Child development	Interdisciplinary early childhood education, child development
Language development	Interdisciplinary early childhood education, speech and communication disorders
Providing family-centered services	Interdisciplinary early childhood education, speech and communication disorders
Community services for children and families	Interdisciplinary early childhood education, social work
Interdisciplinary teaming and consultation	Interdisciplinary early childhood education, school psychology
Language intervention	Interdisciplinary early childhood education, speech and communication disorders
Interdisciplinary internship	Interdisciplinary early childhood education, child development, speech and communication disorders, social work, school psychology
Interdisciplinary seminars	Interdisciplinary early childhood education, child development, speech and communication disorders, social work, school psychology

ences in this setting. This program was chosen as the internship site for several reasons: 1) it is NAEYC accredited; 2) a variety of support services including program coordinators are available; 3) program staff and administrators are flexible in adapting program operations to include the interdisciplinary student and/or faculty teams; and 4) the site is one of the few available in the summer and is conveniently located on the university campus.

The program philosophy statement guides the internship experience just as it does the coursework. Students use learned skills to provide family-centered services in an inclusive setting as members of the team. Students are assigned to teams that include a minimum of one student from each of the four disciplines and a faculty member from one of the four disciplines. Teams are then assigned to an infant, toddler, or preschool room based on past experiences and professional interests. Each team is on-site for 5 hours per day, 5 days per week for 5 weeks. Each team member has a planning time during that 5-hour period with one or two other student team member(s) and a staff member. Initial orientation meetings with students and center staff emphasize that staff are to be considered members of the team and included in team activities. One faculty member is assigned to each team with the primary role being to facilitate effective team functioning. Each faculty member also provides individual supervision for students in his or her respective discipline. Regular meetings among faculty are used to coordinate supervision and grading.

As a team member, each student is required to serve as service coordinator for at least one child and family, plan and implement activities with children, plan and implement activities with families, participate in an arena assessment, participate in weekly team meetings, attend weekly seminars, and complete other activities identified by the student. Activities are individualized based on the background and professional development needs of each student. A self-rating of competencies specific to the internship is completed before and after the 5 weeks. Each student completes an individual plan based on the self-rating of competencies. For example, although all students must participate in the arena assessment, one student may want to be observed being the facilitator and request that role. Seminars during the internship period provide a vehicle for students to reflect on their team skills and functioning. Day-to-day issues regarding individual team member roles and team interactions are addressed in weekly team meetings. Students and center staff resolve these issues, with the faculty team member serving as a facilitator if necessary. Certain barriers have arisen from using an existing practicum site. Time to orient the staff to the philosophy and activities of the interdisciplinary practicum has been required, and students who already have worked together in courses or seminars may have difficulty integrating the staff into the team. Given the short time frame of the practicum, there is no assurance that staff will become an integral part of the team process.

In summary, the IECE master's program at Western Kentucky University has been designed to prepare students to work as team members in inclusive, family-centered settings. Critical features of the program include 1) a sequence of competency-based coursework and seminars that prepare students in discipline-specific knowledge and skills and cross-discipline knowledge and skills, 2) an interdisciplinary internship in which knowledge and skills are applied in a team setting with students from three other disciplines, and 3) a faculty member from each discipline who takes the lead in coordinating discipline-specific student activities and who works with other faculty members to implement and evaluate the program. Administrative support has undergirded the process since its inception, as is evident in the establishment of the original committee to develop the master's program. Of critical importance to the program has been the availability of an already existing internship site in which staff and administrators are flexible enough to accommodate interdisciplinary student teams in implementing a team-based, family-centered internship.

Contrast and Synthesis

Any program developing an interdisciplinary specialization will have its own ecology, determined by state, university, and departmental histories. Each initiative, therefore, must go through a process of identifying and adapting to its own unique contexts. The two approaches to training described in this chapter were used to illustrate two outcomes of this process of adaptation. Although many similar goals and ways of achieving an interdisciplinary focus are represented, these programs also demonstrate clear differences reflective of the unique supports and constraints that may influence program development and implementation for an individual site. In both programs, the preparation of students for team roles goes beyond an awareness and knowledge level, which might be achieved by having students merely participate together in courses taught in different departments. Rather, both programs emphasize the development of team skills and values, which are accomplished only through intensive participation together in an interdisciplinary team process. To accomplish this, faculty themselves have engaged in a similar process of team building as the programs were developed and continue to evolve.

In each of the programs described here, the interdisciplinary specializations began with federal grants to support student and faculty participation from multiple disciplines and to provide resources for team training activities. Klein and Campbell (1990) noted the extent to which early intervention training has been dependent on outside funding. Clearly, in these two cases, such funding was especially critical to accomplishing the more intensive interdisciplinary components of the training. The two programs also are similar in that the structure for interdisciplinary training was added within the context of existing professional training offered along traditional departmental lines; rather than creating new university structures, individual faculty from different departments joined forces to provide this training option to their students. The two programs also are based on similar models for organizing within- and cross-discipline content, as shown in Tables 1 and 2. The programs of study presented earlier are both designed for educators preparing to work with young children with disabilities and other unique needs, and both programs are based on areas of competence that have been identified for this profession by professional associations in ECSE and in early childhood education (DEC, ATE, & NAEYC, 1995; McCollum et al., 1989). The courses required by the two programs therefore appear quite similar. In addition, exposure to people and ideas from other disciplines is provided in both programs in part by having students from different disciplines participate in the same coursework. Despite these similarities, core elements were achieved in different ways, reflecting the unique contexts of each program. In Kentucky, the structure for discipline-specific and cross-discipline coursework is achieved by having IECE students take a relatively large proportion of the required coursework outside of education. This structure has been necessary in order to accommodate the discipline-specific accreditation standards for participating disciplines. In contrast, faculty in the Illinois program achieved the three-level model by developing interdisciplinary courses to address content needed across multiple disciplines. ECSE students take few Level 1 or Level 2 courses from faculty in other departments, in part because many of these courses historically have been offered by the Department of Special Education. Each of these approaches appears to have advantages and disadvantages. For instance, in the Kentucky program, it sometimes has proven difficult to maintain control of the program competencies, particularly if new faculty who are uninvolved with program management are assigned to teach courses. The students, too, sometimes have difficulty adjusting to the terminology and expectations in courses external to their own departments. Program faculty devote considerable time and energy to achieving coherence in the coursework that the students take. In the Illinois program, in contrast, the primary disadvantage has been the faculty resources required to develop and teach new interdisciplinary courses, whereas maintaining cohesive content has not been an issue.

Although in both programs an interdisciplinary team practicum comprises an important part of the training program, the way in which this has been accomplished also reflects the ecological context of each university. In each case, the practicum was developed to provide specific experiences not available to students within the communities in which the universities are housed, and team building is emphasized as students work together on interdisciplinary teams. Nevertheless, the team practicum in Kentucky is provided as a culminating experience during the summer after students have taken considerable coursework, whereas in Illinois it is taken concurrently with coursework during an academic semester. In addition, in Kentucky, 20–25 students participate in the practicum at the same time, with 4–5 students per team. In Illinois, not only is the total number of students smaller because fewer disciplines are housed on the campus, but the practicum is available in both fall and spring semesters. Hence, student teams usually consist of three students, with two teams operating groups during the same semester. In both universities, the timing and student population enrolled in this experience stem largely from practical considerations. In Kentucky, many of the students are enrolled part time and are employed during the school year; summer is the only time in which the interdisciplinary practicum is feasible. In Illinois, most of the students are enrolled full time during the academic year, and few summer courses are offered; the practicum therefore can last for an entire 14-week semester.

Differences in timing, site, and the number of students involved have had significant impact on the way that training is organized in each of the two sites. In Kentucky, although periodic interdisciplinary seminars prepare students for the practicum experience and acquaint them with one another, the students nevertheless may have had relatively little prior contact with individual team members and also have relatively little time (5 weeks) in which to engage in team building. Moreover, in Kentucky, the practicum utilizes an existing on-campus summer program for children, and classroom staff are present during the practicum and expected to be incorporated as team members. In Illinois, the team practicum was developed separately from any existing community program, and the model is one in which infants and toddlers participate in play groups with their parents. Students not only work together over an entire semester, but are well acquainted with one another prior to entering the practicum. In addition, because there are no cooperating professionals, all team members have equal status and are seeking to achieve the same learning goals. Although close interaction with families is emphasized in both sites, another major difference between the two sites is the presence of parents—the Kentucky practicum is integrated within an existing program for children, whereas the primary focus of the Illinois practicum is to support parent–child interaction and parents are always present.

Supervision in the two practicum sites also differs. Although both programs provide extensive on-site supervision, in Kentucky faculty from each department serve as practicum supervisors, providing team as well as within-discipline supervision of their own students across teams. In Illinois, doctoral students from different departments serve this role for the teams to which they are assigned; although they remain in the background, they are always present at the play groups because there are no collaborating staff. Faculty often are present as well, but as observers, as another goal of the practicum is to provide doctoral students with supervisory experiences. In each case, supervisory roles have been carefully delineated to support the interdisciplinary goals of the practicum. Clearly, the contexts of these two programs have had significant influence on the structure of these two different practica, as well as on the goals that can be addressed in each.

One final area of crucial importance in each of these two graduate programs is the new roles that faculty play. The success of each program is heavily dependent on there being, within each participating department, at least one faculty member committed to the interdisciplinary specialization. This individual serves as the link to faculty and students outside the department, as well as to those within the department. This faculty liaison role has been critical in achieving recruitment and advisement structures that are congruent with the specialization. However, interdisciplinary collaboration raises new issues, such as who should be involved in evaluating faculty for promotion and tenure. The amount of time committed to the specialization is significant and may not always be recognized by other faculty or administrators within the participating departments. In many ways, faculty who participate in these efforts are forging new ground; for these programs to succeed in the long run, new structures and systems undoubtedly will be necessary.

CONCLUDING REMARKS: FUTURE DIRECTIONS

Interdisciplinary training should respond to the following questions: with whom (e.g., which disciplines), for what content (e.g., awareness of what other disciplines do or collaborative skills and knowledge), using what kind of framework (e.g., within and across departments), with what intensity (e.g., a one-time exposure, a fully integrated program), in what contexts (e.g., coursework, practicum), and by whom (e.g., which faculty, from which departments)? An examination of the programs described in this volume indicates that key elements undergirding interdisciplinary training, as well as similar supports and challenges, may apply across disciplines.

Bailey (1989) listed several approaches that might be used to structure team training: additive models in which each student obtains dual training in two collaborating programs (e.g., Bailey, Farel, O'Donnell, Simeonsson, & Miller, 1986), integrated models in which students complete an area of specialization within a more traditional disciplinary program of study (e.g., Thorp & McCollum, 1994), and specialized programs in which students complete a sequence of coursework and practica designed specifically for the infant–toddler specialist (e.g., Geik, Gilkerson, & Sponseller, 1982). Interdisciplinary preparation also can occur at less intensive levels by focusing on joint seminars, individual courses, or practicum experiences rather than on programs of study. In some cases, faculty may choose to begin with less complex or less intensive models of collaboration training while working toward ones that are more comprehensive. An important lesson learned by the two programs described in this chapter was that the more comprehensive the model in terms of the levels (e.g., student, faculty, program) at which interaction occurs, the more likely it is that interdisciplinary understanding will occur and the more likely that skills supporting interdisciplinary interaction will be learned. However, the more comprehensive the model is, the more contextual barriers arise. It is clear from the range of models outlined in this book that creative solutions for overcoming barriers to interdisciplinary interaction can and have been developed. In part, these solutions have necessitated that faculty invent ways of adapting to existing structure, or of meeting disciplinary requirements in different ways. At times, faculty have had to develop their own expertise simultaneously with developing a specialization for their students. Thus, the model selected by each program will depend not only upon how much flexibility is available, but also on how willing faculty are to assume new roles.

ECSE may be somewhat unique among disciplines in ways that will influence how interdisciplinary training evolves. Early childhood special educators are in the position of being simultaneously the most frequent members of the early intervention team and those whose roles may be the least clearly defined and the most easy to change based on the circumstances of the particular state, geographic area, and setting in which they work. Yet, to be an effective member of an interdisciplinary team, early childhood special educators must be clear about their own contributions to the team. The attainment of a professional identity by the early childhood special educator working with children from birth to age 3 appears to have been particularly affected by the way in which the federal legislation distinguishes services at the infant–toddler level from services for preschoolers, and by the service and personnel certification structures that have been adopted by some states as this legislation is implemented. By federal definition, preschool services are under the state education agency. In contrast, federal legislation allows each state to define its own system of services for infants and toddlers (and thereby the roles of the individuals who work in the system), as well as to establish personnel standards separately from the certification system for public schools (McCollum & Bailey, 1991). Early childhood special educators may find it difficult to articulate the roles, teaching content, and teaching methodologies that they hold in common across infant–toddler and preschool levels. Although distinctions in roles and in training may be desirable for meeting the needs of different people, of all of the early intervention disciplines, ECSE is the one in which the sense of profession may be most influenced by federal and state legislation and related policy. Personnel preparation programs may be confronted with a special challenge in regard to assisting students to develop a professional identity.

The extent of variation that occurs in the generalist roles of the early childhood special educator may contribute significantly to difficulties encountered in clarifying the role of the early childhood special educator as this individual works among other disciplines. Nevertheless, these same generalist roles may provide an important link to other educators because early childhood special educators working at the preschool level, and educators who work with older children with special needs perform many similar roles in relation to professionals from other disciplines and to the services that they represent. Another link to education as a profession may come about as policies developed to support services to infants and toddlers and their families begin to work their way upward into preschool services, and potentially beyond the preschool level as well. Of particular note among the policies and practices being reexamined from this perspective are ones related to family-centered practice. Advocates for seamless services have recommended that states and programs use an IFSP in preference to the individualized education program throughout the early childhood period in order to maintain a focus on the role of the family. Such changes may influence interactions not only with families, but also among disciplines as they provide services to families. In addition, these changes may bring early childhood special educators closer together in the kinds of personnel preparation that they receive across universities.

A final link to the profession of education might be expected to occur as early childhood education and ECSE reexamine their relationship and as these disciplines learn from one another and become more blended in their practices, certification structures, and professional training. This blending may assist particularly in articulating and valuing the specialist aspects of the early childhood special educator's role by tying them to new emphases on the importance and processes of early development.

REFERENCES

Bailey, D.B. (1989). Issues and directions in preparing professionals to work with young handicapped children and their families. In J.J. Gallagher, P.L. Trohanis, & R.M. Clifford (Eds.), *Policy implementation and PL 99-457: Planning for young children with special needs* (pp. 97–132). Baltimore: Paul H. Brookes Publishing Co.

Bailey, D.B., Farel, A., O'Donnell, K., Simeonsson, R., & Miller, C. (1986). Preparing infant interventionists: Interdepartmental training in special education and maternal child health. *Journal of the Division for Early Childhood, 11*(1), 67–77.

Bailey, D.B., Palsha, S.A., & Huntington, G.S. (1990). Preservice preparation of special educators to work with infants with handicaps and their families: Current status and training needs. *Journal of Early Intervention, 14*(1), 43–54.

Bailey, D.B., Simeonsson, R.J., Yoder, D.E., & Huntington, G.S. (1990a). Infant personnel preparation across eight disciplines: An integrative analysis. *Exceptional Children, 56*(1), 26–35.

Bailey, D.B., Simeonsson, R.J., Yoder, D.E., & Huntington, G.S. (1990b). Preparing professionals to serve infants and toddlers with handicaps and their families: Current status and training needs. *Journal of Early Intervention, 14*(1), 43–54.

Bevins, S.B. (1992). *Survey of institutions of higher education in Illinois.* Unpublished doctoral dissertation, Department of Special Education, University of Illinois, Champaign.

Bricker, D. (1976). Educational synthesizer. In M.A. Thomas (Ed.), *Hey, don't forget about me* (pp. 84–92). Reston, VA: Council for Exceptional Children.

Bricker, D. (1989). *Early education of at-risk and handicapped infants, toddlers, and preschool children.* Palo Alto, CA: VORT Corp.

Bricker, D., & Slentz, K. (1988). Personnel preparation: Handicapped infants. In J.M.C. Wang, M.C. Reynolds, & H.J. Walberg (Eds.), *Handbook of special education: Research and practice* (Vol. 3, pp. 319–345). Elmsford, NY: Pergamon Press.

Bruder, M.B., & McLean, M. (1988). Personnel preparation for infant interventionists: A review of federally funded projects. *Journal of the Division for Early Childhood, 12*(4), 299–305.

Coleman, P.P., Buysse, V., Scalise-Smith, D.L., & Schulte, A.C. (1991). Consultation: Applications to early intervention. *Infants and Young Children, 4*(2), 41–46.

Division for Early Childhood of the Council for Exceptional Children (DEC), Association of Teacher Educators (ATE), & National Association for the Education of Young Children (NAEYC). (1995). *Personnel standards for early education and early intervention: Guidelines for licensure in early childhood special education.* Unpublished manuscript.

Fenichel, E.S., & Eggbeer, L. (1991). Preparing practitioners to work with infants, toddlers, and their families: Four essential elements of training. *Infants and Young Children, 4*(2), 56–62.

Geik, I., Gilkerson, D., & Sponseller, D.B. (1982). An early intervention training model. *Journal of the Division for Early Childhood, 5*, 42–52.

Hanson, M.J. (1990). *Final report: California early intervention personnel model, personnel standards, and personnel preparation plan.* San Francisco: California Early Intervention Personnel Study Project, Department of Special Education, San Francisco State University.

Individuals with Disabilities Education Act (IDEA) of 1990, PL 101-476. (October 30, 1990). Title 20, U.S.C. 1400 et seq: *U.S. Statutes at Large, 104*, 1103–1151.

Jones, E.L., Stayton, V.D., Kersting, F., Lockett, P., & Forbes, M. (n.d.). *Project TEAM: Interdisciplinary preparation of social work, school psychology, and speech/communication disorders students for early intervention.* Manuscript submitted for publication.

Klein, N.K., & Campbell, P. (1990). Preparing personnel to serve at-risk and disabled infants, toddlers, and preschoolers. In S.J. Meisels & J.P. Shonkoff (Eds.), *Handbook of early childhood intervention* (pp. 679–699). Cambridge, MA: Cambridge University Press.

Knowles, M. (1984). *The adult learner: A neglected species* (3rd ed.). Houston, TX: Gulf Publishing Co.

McCollum, J.A., & Bailey, D.B. (1991). Developing comprehensive personnel systems: Issues and alternatives. *Journal of Early Intervention, 15*(1), 51–56.

McCollum, J.A., Cook, R.J., & Ladmer, L.A. (1993). The staffing of early intervention programs in Illinois: A descriptive study of current personnel. *Illinois Council for Exceptional Children Quarterly, 43*(1), 15–28.

McCollum, J.A., & Hughes, M. (1988). Staffing patterns and team models in infancy programs. In J.B. Jordan, J.J. Gallagher, & P.L. Hutinger (Eds.), *Early childhood special education: Birth-three* (pp. 129–146). Reston, VA: Council for Exceptional Children.

McCollum, J.A., & Maude, S.P. (1994). Early childhood special educators as early interventionists: Issues and emerging practice in personnel preparation. *Yearbook in Early Childhood Education,* (Vol. 5, pp. 352–371). New York: Teachers College Press.

McCollum, J.A., McLean, M., McCartan, K., & Kaiser, C. (1989). Recommendations for certification of early childhood special educators. *Journal of Early Intervention, 13*(3), 195–212.

McCollum, J.A., Rowan, L.E., & Thorp, E.K. (1994). Philosophy as framework in early intervention personnel training. *Journal of Early Intervention, 18*(2), 216–226.

McCollum, J.A., & Thorp, E.K. (1988). Training of infant specialists: A look to the future. *Infants and Young Children, 1*(2), 55–65.

McCollum, J.A., & Yates, R.J. (1994). Technical assistance for meeting early intervention personnel standards: Statewide processes based on peer review. *Topics in Early Childhood Special Education, 14*(3), 295–310.

Miller, P.S. (1992). Segregated programs of teacher education in early childhood: Immoral and inefficient practice. *Topics in Early Childhood Special Education, 11*(4), 39–52.

Nash, J.K. (1990). Public Law 99-457: Facilitating family participation on the multidisciplinary team. *Journal of Early Intervention, 14*, 318–326.

Odom, S.L., & McEvoy, M.A. (1990). Mainstreaming at the preschool level: Potential barriers and tasks for the field. *Topics in Early Childhood Special Education, 10*(2), 48–61.

Rowan, L.E., McCollum, J.A., & Thorp, E.K. (1993). Collaborative graduate education of future early interventionists. *Topics in Language Disorders, 14*(1), 72–80.

Rowan, L.E., Thorp, E.K., & McCollum, J.A. (1990). An interdisciplinary practicum for infant-family related competencies in speech-language pathology and audiology. *Infants and Young Children, 3*(2), 58–66.

Sexton, D., & Snyder, P. (1991). *Louisiana personnel preparation consortium project for Part H.* New Orleans, LA: University of New Orleans.

Smith, B.J., & Powers, C. (1987). Issues related to developing state certification policies. *Topics in Early Childhood Special Education, 7*(3), 12–23.

Stayton, V.D., & Miller, P.S. (1993). Combining early childhood and early childhood special education standards in personnel preparation programs: Experiences in two states. *Topics in Early Childhood Special Education, 13*(3), 372–387.

Thorp, E.K., & McCollum, J.A. (1994). Defining the infancy specialization in early childhood special education. In L.J. Johnson, R.J. Gallagher, M.J. LaMontagne, J.B. Jordan, J.J. Gallagher, P.L. Hutinger, & M.B. Karnes (Eds.), *Meeting early intervention challenges: Issues from birth to three* (pp. 167–183). Baltimore: Paul H. Brookes Publishing Co.

Winton, P.J., & Bailey, D.B. (1990). Early intervention training related to family interviewing. *Topics in Early Childhood Special Education, 10*(1), 50–62.

5

PREPARING COMMUNICATION SPECIALISTS

Angela Losardo

Connie works as the communication specialist on a newly formed transdisciplinary team in a rural mountainous area of North Carolina. She has lived and worked in this area for most of her 20-year career and has long-standing relationships with all members of the local developmental evaluation team. Connie can remember a time when she interacted more often with other team members at the supermarket than through her professional work with children and families. The developmental evaluation team adopted a transdisciplinary model of service delivery 3 years ago and began to meet on a regular monthly basis.

At one of the monthly meetings, the county public health nurse mentions that a new family with three preschool-age children has moved into a house on the outskirts of town. She is quite certain that Michael, the youngest of the three children, has a language problem. The public health nurse routinely refers children to different members of the team based on the results of a screening and tracking program that the team adopted 3 years ago. Based on the team's recommendation, Connie makes the initial home visit to determine language and other assessment needs for Michael.

During the initial visit, Connie learns that Michael's mother, Mary, is a single mother who is struggling to find enough time in the day to manage all of her children's needs. She expresses concern that Michael is not talking like her other two children were when they were his age and that she does not know what to do to help him. Connie observes that although Michael does not use words, he is beginning to use communicative signals such as pointing to desired objects. She asks Mary to participate in the administration of an arena-style curriculum-based assessment in her home. Connie explains that two or three members of the team will observe Mary playing with her son and that Connie will act as the facilitator. Mary agrees to participate and the visit is arranged. Prior to the visit, Connie provides Mary with a copy of a measure developed specifically for families to familiarize her with the content of the assessment. The results of the assessment reveal that although Michael's chronological age is 30 months, his functioning is between 12 and 18 months in the social-communication domain and between 24 and 30 months in all other domains. Connie, Mary, and the other team members determine that Michael's primary need is in the area of language and communication.

On a separate visit to the home, Connie and Mary select and prioritize goals and objectives for Michael to focus on during the year, and they develop an individualized family service plan. They talk about simple ways they can work together to provide Michael with opportunities to practice his goals and objectives in the context of typical home routines and how they can monitor his progress toward selected targets. Mary appears pleased to be involved in all aspects of Michael's program without having to "take time away from the other children."

SINCE THE MID-1980S, the number of programs for infants and young children who are at risk and/or have disabilities and their families has grown steadily without accompanied increases in the number of trained personnel to work in these programs (Bricker & Slentz, 1988; McCollum & Thorp, 1988). A U.S. survey on the availability of adequately trained early intervention and early childhood special education personnel (Burke, McLaughlin, & Valdivieso, 1988) found that 32 of the country's 57 states and territories reported critical shortages. Similarly, personnel shortages exist among allied health personnel (e.g., communication specialists, occupational therapists, physical therapists) who are prepared to work with young children and their families. According to a survey conducted by Meisels, Harbin, Modigliani, and Olson (1988), most states and territories in the United States reported significant shortages of special education and allied health personnel for children birth through 5 and their families. Another survey (Yoder, Coleman, & Gallagher, 1990) reported similar shortages among allied health professionals. According to estimates of supply and demand for early intervention services, Yoder et al. reported a shortage in 1990 of 108,886 communication specialists in the United States.

The federal government reinforced its role in supporting services to young children and their families with the passage of PL 101-476, the Individuals with Disabilities Education Act (IDEA) of 1990 (a reauthorization of PL 94-142, the Education for All Handicapped Children Act of 1975). Referred to as the most significant federal policy for early childhood intervention (Meisels et al., 1988), Part H of IDEA reflects the government's emphasis on personnel development. Each state must have in place a comprehensive system of personnel development and ensure that adequately trained personnel are available to deliver early intervention services.

In light of the information on personnel shortages and the government mandate for establishing high-quality early intervention services, the need for properly trained communication specialists is significant. The need, however, goes well beyond simple supply and demand. Even if the numbers of speech-language pathology personnel were substantially increased, serious problems would remain. Communication specialists serving infants and young children with communicative impairments and their families are not adequately prepared (Crais & Leonard, 1990). According to a 1990 position statement drafted by the American Speech-Language-Hearing Association[1] (ASHA) Subcommittee on Speech-Language Pathology Service Delivery with Infants and Toddlers, communication specialists need training that will allow them to assume their roles within comprehensive, community-based programs that are family centered and coordinated with other early intervention services.

A telephone survey of 50 randomly selected speech-language pathology programs was conducted as part of the Carolina Institute for Research on Infant Personnel Preparation (Crais & Leonard, 1990). All programs were accredited by the Educational Standards Board of ASHA. Survey questions focused on specific

---

[1]As of January 1, 1997, the American Speech-Language-Hearing Association will be officially called the American Association of Speech-Language Pathology and Audiology.

areas of academic and clinical training needs for communication specialists at the bachelor's and master's degree levels. Results for both undergraduate and graduate groups indicated that the areas of study receiving the least attention included family assessment and intervention, values, and interdisciplinary team process. Although most of the programs reported the availability of practicum opportunities, *only* 40% of the 47 master's degree programs and 30% of the 23 bachelor's degree programs reported that they require practicum experiences with infants and families. If it is assumed that the quality and effectiveness of services are enhanced when speech-language pathology personnel are trained to work on teams that provide comprehensive and family-centered services in community-based programs, then the results of this survey are disturbing. Less than half of students are receiving the practical experience necessary to become effective professionals.

This chapter focuses on the transdisciplinary training needs of communication specialists who work with infants and young children and their families. It begins with a discussion of major changes in the field of speech-language pathology, which have broad implications for the training of communication specialists working with infants and young children and their families. The chapter then briefly reviews available preservice and in-service training programs in the area of speech-language pathology. The next section contains a discussion of certification and licensure requirements. Following that, general issues are explored that relate to teacher education across disciplines, as well as those issues more specifically related to the transdisciplinary training of communication specialists. In addition, a review of recommendations for the content and process of training of a model transdisciplinary personnel preparation program in the area of speech-language pathology is included.

MAJOR TRANSITIONS

Since the mid-1980s, major changes have occurred in the field of speech-language pathology that have broad implications for the preparation of communication specialists working with infants and young children and their families. These include changes in 1) the number and population of children becoming eligible for early intervention services, 2) the content and orientation of language development and intervention, 3) procedures for assessment and evaluation of language and communication, 4) approaches to intervention, and 5) the role of the communication specialist.

Numbers of Children Needing Early Intervention Services

The first area of change involves the increased numbers of children identified as needing early intervention services. Although accurate numbers of young children being identified as communicatively at risk, having delays, or having disabilities are difficult to determine, the National Institute of Neurological Disorders and Stroke (1988) estimated 15% of preschool-age children have speech disorders and 2%–3% have language disorders. According to figures of the National Joint Committee on Learning Disabilities (1987), over 60% of preschool-age children with learning disabilities have been identified as having speech or language disorders as their primary disability.

Moreover, in addition to children identified with speech or language problems as a primary disability, other children with disabilities requiring intermittent to extensive supports (e.g., those with mental retardation) have communication problems secondary to the primary problem. Abbeduto and Rosenberg (1992) reported that people with mental retardation experience performance delays in most fundamental areas of linguistic communication. Nearly 50% of children with mental retardation requiring intermittent supports and 90% of children with mental retardation requiring extensive supports exhibit some type of language disorder (National Institute of Neurological Disorders and Stroke, 1988).

In addition to the numbers of children with identified primary or secondary communication problems, there is an expanding population of infants who are considered biologically at risk (Goldson, 1993). As a result of advanced medical knowledge and technology, the mortality rate for infants with complex health care needs (e.g., low birth weight, prematurity) has dropped dramatically since the mid-1980s. Although data have shown that major disabilities are being prevented in infants who survive the newborn period (Bennett, 1987), one of the most frequently identified areas of concern for children with biological risk factors later in childhood is communication (Young, 1993).

Data indicate that infants and young children at risk for environmental reasons also are at risk for speech and language impairments (Beckwith, 1990). In 1987, 472,623 babies were born to teenage parents, increasing to 488,941 births in 1988, and to 517,989 births in 1989 (Center for Population Options, 1992). Brooks-Gunn and Furstenberg (1986) reported that adolescent mothers are generally less responsive to their children than adult mothers and that their styles of interaction with their children differ from the interactions of adult mothers, particularly in the area of vocalization. Infant–caregiver interactions are believed to have long-term effects on development of linguistic skills in children (Sparks, Clark, Oas, & Erickson, 1988). Communication specialists should be prepared to address the unique intervention and sometimes medical needs of these infants and their caregivers.

Content and Orientation of Language Development and Intervention

The second change in the field of speech-language pathology involves the content and orientation of language development and intervention. Dramatic growth has occurred in the understanding of early prelinguistic behaviors and its relationship to other critical domains of development (Bricker, 1992). Focus has shifted from language to communication for young children, with the acknowledgment that functional language systems evolve from earlier communicative, social, and cognitive behaviors (Bricker, 1992; Bricker & Carlson, 1981). The relationship between communication and other domains of development has important implications for intervention. Communication specialists must be skilled in developing comprehensive language and communication intervention programs that combine language and communication objectives with other targets in motor, social, and cognitive areas (Bricker, 1992; Fujiki & Brinton, 1994; Johnston & Heller, 1987).

Procedures Used in Assessment and Evaluation

The third area of change in speech-language pathology involves procedures used in the assessment and evaluation of language and communication disorders. Traditionally, professionals in the field of speech-language pathology have employed static assessment measures—a type of evaluation that determines what a child independently knows at any given point in time in a particular domain of behavior (Brown, Bransford, Ferrara, & Campione, 1983). Both norm-referenced and criterion-referenced assessments may be used as static measures of language performance.

Increasingly, professionals in the field of speech-language pathology are advocating the use of alternate forms of assessment, such as *curriculum-based* language assessment (Nelson, 1994) and *dynamic* assessment (Olswang, Bain, & Johnson, 1992; Palincsar, Brown, & Campione, 1994; Silliman & Wilkinson, 1994). Nelson (1994) distinguished curriculum-based language assessment from more general types of curriculum-based measurement by differences in their scope of purpose. Generally, a curriculum-based assessment is used to determine a child's instructional needs and to document progress over time. In contrast, a curriculum-based language assessment is used to determine whether a child has the necessary language skills and strategies for processing the language of the curriculum (Nelson, 1994). Special techniques (e.g., ethnographic recording) may be used to examine the linguistic and communicative abilities of a child in relation to the linguistic demands of different curricular contexts (Nelson, 1994).

Dynamic assessment is another alternative to the use of traditional psychometric procedures. In contrast to static assessment, dynamic assessment is a type of formative evaluation that determines a child's potential for learning, the level of environmental support the child needs in order to learn, and the strategies the child uses to learn (Minick, 1987). According to Lidz (1987), dynamic assessment is "an interaction between an examiner-as-intervener and a learner-as-active-participant, which seeks to estimate the degree of modifiability of the learner and the means by which positive changes in cognitive functioning can be deduced and maintained" (p. 4). Although models of dynamic assessment were originally developed for use with adolescents and school-age children, since the mid-1980s, several investigators have developed dynamic assessment measures and procedures appropriate for use with preschool-age children (Campione & Brown, 1987; Lidz & Thomas, 1987; Mearig, 1987; Tzuriel & Klein, 1985).

Approaches Used in Language and Communication Intervention

The fourth change in the field of speech-language pathology involves approaches used in language and communication intervention. Initially, curricular approaches and instructional methodologies used in early intervention programs evolved from the application of behavior analytic techniques used with older children and adults in institutions (Bricker & Carlson, 1981). Various adult-directed language intervention programs and procedures were developed in the 1970s that reflected the behavior analyst's position (Bricker & Bricker, 1974; Gray & Ryan, 1973; Guess, Sailor, & Baer, 1978; Kent, 1974). These programs focused primarily on the development of vocabulary and the structural aspects of language, namely syntactic structure. The prescribed methodology was effective in assisting young children in acquiring basic language forms, but targeted skills often failed to generalize to social contexts outside the controlled environment (Spradlin & Siegel, 1982; Warren & Kaiser, 1986).

Since the 1970s, approaches to intervention have shifted from using highly structured, adult-directed models to using more naturalistic, *learner-oriented models*. Learner-oriented models are those in which the interventionist follows the lead of children, and children's goals and objectives are embedded in ongoing interactions and activities (Bricker, 1992). Incorporating training into activities that are of interest to children capitalizes on children's motivation to participate in them and removes the need for artificial contingencies (Bricker, 1993). Various learner-oriented strategies have been developed that may be used to facilitate language and communication of young children within the context of typical communicative exchanges (Bricker & Cripe, 1992; Halle, Marshall, & Spradlin, 1979; Hart & Risley, 1975; Warren, McQuarter, & Rogers-Warren, 1984).

Role of the Communication Specialist

The fifth area of change in the field of speech-language pathology is the role of the communication specialist in service delivery. A 1990 ASHA position statement on the roles of communication specialists in service delivery to infants, toddlers, and their families emphasized the need for communication specialists to function as one member of a team consisting of family members and professionals from a variety of disciplines. Traditionally, communication specialists have adopted one of two approaches to service delivery: multidisciplinary or interdisciplinary. Using a multidisciplinary model, the communication specialist conducts assessment and intervention activities in isolation from other professionals. Consultations and meetings with family members are conducted on an individual basis. By design, communication specialists on multidisciplinary teams function as independent specialists.

A traditional interdisciplinary model is similar to the multidisciplinary model in many ways. Using the interdisciplinary model, the communication specialist conducts assessment and intervention activities separate from other team members but periodically meets with the family and other team members to share information. The isolated therapy or "pull-out" model is most consistent with the multidisciplinary and interdisciplinary models of service delivery.

A more recent approach to service delivery, the transdisciplinary model, attempts to build on the inadequacies of the multidisciplinary and interdisciplinary models. Using a team collaboration model, the communication specialist works with family members and other professionals to assess children and to develop an individualized family service plan (IFSP). All decision making is consensual. Depending on the child's concerns, a primary service provider is responsible for coordinating the plan with the family. For a child with significant language and communication problems, a teacher or a communication specialist may be assigned to implement the plan with consultation and direct assistance from other professionals when needed. An integrated therapy model in which children's goals and objectives are embedded in the natural context is more consistent with the transdisciplinary model.

Because of the increasing number of young children who are at risk, have communication delays, or have language or communication disorders, there is a growing demand for communication specialists who 1) understand the nature of early language development and its relationship to other critical domains of development, 2) are familiar with alternate assessment and evaluation procedures, 3) are prepared to work with young children in the sense of implementing appropriate and effective intervention programs, and 4) are prepared to work as members of a team to develop and implement such programs within the context of the child's usual environment.

PRESERVICE AND IN-SERVICE TRAINING PROGRAMS

The U.S. Department of Education, Office of Special Education Programs (OSEP), through the Division of Personnel Preparation, is the major source of federal support for interdisciplinary preservice and in-service training activities focused on people with disabilities. In 1990, OSEP funded a total of 34 interdisciplinary personnel preparation programs (28 master's degree programs, 2 preprofessional training programs leading to a master's degree, and 4 leadership programs) whose targets of training were graduate-level students in speech-language pathology (Guadagno, 1993).

At the preservice level, several different approaches have been employed to ensure that speech-language pathology personnel are adequately prepared to deliver quality services to infants and young children who are at risk and/or have disabilities and their families. Johnston and Heller (1987) reported on the development and evaluation of a curriculum module for graduate-level students in speech-language pathology who wish to specialize in language intervention with young children. The module includes coursework and practica activities related to preschool speech and language intervention. The coursework and practica were added to existing graduate program requirements. Of the 21 students who participated in an evaluation study, 7 completed the preschool curriculum module, 7 completed only part of the module, and 7 received no special training to work with preschool-age children. Students were tested using a video-based short essay examination to determine the program's success in training the targeted competencies. Results indicated that the performance of students who completed the curriculum module on the specially designed examination was higher than the performance of the other two groups. The authors concluded that completion of the curriculum module enhanced the professional ability of speech-language pathology majors to work with young children and their families.

McCollum and Thorp (1988) described an early intervention graduate program that offered cross-disciplinary coursework and practicum experiences for infancy specialization to students from several disciplines. The cross-disciplinary content for infancy specialization can serve as a major for graduate students in early childhood special education and as a minor for students from other disciplines (e.g., majors in speech-language pathology). Interdisciplinary practicum experiences are available to graduate students in the departments of speech-language pathology and early childhood special education. The practicum is part of a three-level model based on collaborative arrangements between the two departments (see Chapter 4).

Bricker, Losardo, and Straka (1995) described a preservice training program that offers a concurrent master's degree in communication disorders and sciences and early intervention. Students complete academic content and practicum requirements for both programs. A large part of this program focuses on interdisciplinary practicum experiences. Speech-language pathology students, working collaboratively with students from other disciplines (e.g., early intervention, school psychology), complete required practicum experiences in a variety of settings including classrooms, home environments, and clinics. Upon successful completion of all academic and practicum requirements, students are eligible to apply for a master's degree, the ASHA certificate of clinical competence, and a state teaching endorsement.

Extensive evaluation data were collected from the 22 speech-language pathology students enrolled in this program from 1989 to 1993. Major findings of this evaluation study indicated that the students' levels of knowledge and skill development in early intervention progressively improved across program competency areas and across terms in the program (Bricker et al., 1995).

Crais (1991) developed a model for embedding new training content in existing preservice speech-language pathology course requirements. Four modules were designed to introduce students to issues, beliefs, and practices related to working with young children with disabilities and their families. The four modules include the following:

1. Introducing terms and issues related to working with individuals with special concerns and their families
2. Working with families in the assessment process
3. Sharing assessment information and collaboratively setting goals with families
4. Evaluating and influencing the extent to which services are family centered

Each module begins with a list of student objectives and contains a content outline, suggested class and out-of-class activities, materials for producing handouts and transparencies, and suggested additional reading. Users are encouraged to modify or expand the content of each module to fit the needs of different groups of students.

Creative interdisciplinary models and programs such as these at the preservice level will presumably lead to more coordinated service delivery efforts by teams of professionals in community-based programs. However, preservice and in-service training activities must be coordinated to ensure that the personnel who currently provide services to young children with disabilities and their families are adequately prepared. ASHA has designed two in-service programs to enhance the preparation of experienced speech-language pathology professionals currently working in the field.

The first program, *The Infant Project: An Interdisciplinary Approach* (Catlett, 1991b), was designed to provide experienced speech-language pathology professionals with information on family-focused approaches to early intervention and strategies to train others. Funded by OSEP, each state had the opportunity to select a team of experienced professionals from various disciplines to participate in one of the project's three, 12-day training institutes. The training was provided by national leaders on family-centered early intervention services and consisted of both didactic and practical activities. Specific focus areas included early intervention services, interdisciplinary approaches, and service coordination. Team members were provided with information and strategies to conduct training events in their states for family members and other professionals.

Another program, *Building Blocks: An Early Childhood In-Service Education Program for Speech-Language Pathologists and Audiologists* (Catlett, 1991a), was a cooperative effort between ASHA and state speech-language-hearing associations. This popular program utilizes six instructional modules focused on key aspects of early intervention service delivery. Each 4-hour training module consists of presentations and practical activities supplemented with handouts and suggestions for additional reading materials. Efforts by ASHA and other professional organizations to conduct these types of in-service training activities will help ensure that professionals in the field keep abreast of important changes in the area of speech-language pathology and deliver quality early intervention services to infants and young children with disabilities and their families.

CERTIFICATION AND LICENSING

McCollum and Thorp (1988) noted that personnel preparation training content and process are often dictated by certification and licensure requirements. Below is a summary of Cooper's (1993) historical review of professional standards in speech-language pathology from the 1950s to the 1990s.

Prior to the 1950s, standards for communication specialists were defined and issued by state departments of education (Cooper, 1993). Teaching credentials for communication specialists were considered supplementary to general education credentials; that is, practitioners were required to complete all general education coursework in addition to specialized coursework in speech-language pathology (Minifie, 1994). The bachelor's degree was the minimum requirement for membership in ASHA; thus, little difference existed in the standards set by the national organization and state departments of education (Cooper, 1993).

During the 1960s, when more than three quarters of practitioners were employed in public schools, ASHA adopted new certification requirements for communication specialists and audiologists (Cooper, 1993). The new certificate of clinical competence required that an individual 1) complete a master's degree in speech-language pathology or audiology, 2) complete prescribed coursework in the major and minor professional areas, 3) pass a written national examination, and 4) complete 9 months of full-time work under the supervision of a certified communication specialist or audiologist. The disparity between standards for communication specialists set by state departments of education and ASHA was now significant.

By the end of the 1960s, the first state licensure law in speech-language pathology and audiology was passed by the Florida legislature. This law incorporated standards set by the ASHA certificate of clinical competence (Cooper, 1993). During the next 10 years, state legislatures in most states followed suit and adopted licensure requirements similar to the requirements for the certificate of clinical competence (Minifie, 1994). During this same time, more than half of the state departments of education upgraded their entry-level standards for practitioners to require that they have a master's degree (Cooper, 1993).

As of 1994, 42 states had licensure laws in speech-language pathology and audiology (Matthews & Frattali, 1994). Nearly half of those states that passed licensure laws requiring master's degrees still allow individuals with a bachelor's degree or less to provide services (Cooper, 1993).

MAJOR ISSUES

There are a multiplicity of issues related to teacher education across disciplines, as well as those issues more specifically related to the transdisciplinary training of speech-language pathology personnel. The following section discusses these general issues: 1) the need for changes in university training structures, 2) the need for research on preservice and in-service education of teachers, 3) the need for research on adult learning strategies used in preservice and in-service education of professionals, 4) the need for linkages between preservice and in-service training, and 5) the need for modifications or accommodations in learning environments for returning professionals who need additional academic and clinical preparation.

University Structures

The nature of coursework and practicum experiences in an interdisciplinary model does not fit into current university training structures (McCollum & Thorp, 1988). Interdisciplinary collaboration often requires restructuring of traditional patterns of training necessitated by different requirements within different departments (Rowan, Thorp, & McCollum, 1990). Even when restructuring is possible, the time required for institutions of higher education to establish new programs and train students can be prohibitive (Hanson & Lovett, 1992). To complicate matters further, institutions of higher education must prepare students to meet certification and licensing standards of various professional organizations. For example, ASHA requires that supervisory and field-based experiences for students in speech-language pathology be provided by a certified communication specialist.

Research on Personnel Preparation

As McCollum and Thorp noted in 1988, the data on the effectiveness of personnel preparation are extremely meager. This remains true in 1996. The literature contains numerous descriptions of innovative programs designed to prepare personnel to deliver quality services to infants and young children who are at risk and/or have disabilities and their families, but most often these descriptions focus on discussions of program rationales and training models. New research on effective strategies for preservice and in-service education of professionals is still needed (Bricker et al., 1995; Crais & Leonard, 1990).

Research on Adult Learning

In addition to the need for research on personnel preparation, investigation into adult learning strategies used in preservice education of professionals also is needed. Most of the research in this area has been conducted with in-service audiences. A meta-analysis of significant variables in staff development found that combinations of observation, micro-teaching, and video-audio feedback are among the most effective instructional techniques (Wade, 1985). Research is needed to examine optimal use of these strategies at the preservice level.

Preservice and In-Service Linkages

Linkages between preservice and in-service training efforts should take place at the state level. State policy for personnel development should include career-ladder or professional-advancement plans for professionals who are providing services in the field. At a time when there are severe shortages of personnel across disciplines, certification and licensure standards must be devised to ensure that present personnel who need training receive it, while ensuring that those professionals who are competent are not excluded (Brown & Rule, 1993).

Learning Environments

Since the 1970s, the demographic profile of the traditional student in higher education has changed dramatically (Kasworm, 1990; Long, 1987). Adult learners now comprise a significant proportion of the overall student population in the United States (Kasworm, 1990). Most adults who return to school do so as a result of family or career transitions (Schlossberg, Lynch, & Chickering, 1989). In addition, a number of professionals in the field are returning to school to upgrade their skills to meet state and professionally recognized standards (Crais & Leonard, 1990). Personnel preparation programs must make accommodations for these adult learners, such as adjustments in class schedules (e.g., evening and weekend classes) and modifications in locations of practicum sites (e.g., off-campus placements, professional's own worksite).

In addition to the above general issues regarding teacher education across disciplines, there is another set of more specific issues related to interdisciplinary training of speech-language pathology personnel that needs to be addressed. These include 1) identification of within- and cross-discipline knowledge and skill competencies needed by communication specialists to work effectively with infants and young children, 2) differences in academic and clinical preparation of bachelor's and master's level speech-language pathology personnel and how this relates to the qualified provider proviso regulation in IDEA, 3) certification and licensure requirements, 4) the amount and type of supervisory and field-based experiences required by ASHA for certification in speech-language pathology, and 5) the role of the communication specialist on teams in field-based activities.

Within- and Cross-Discipline Content

ASHA (1990) outlined the roles of communication specialists in service delivery to infants, toddlers, and their families. These roles have been defined as, but not limited to, the following:

1. Screening and identification
2. Assessment and evaluation

3. Design, planning, direct delivery, and monitoring of treatment programs
4. Service coordination
5. Consultation with, and referral to, agencies and other professionals providing services to young children and their families

Research is needed to identify and evaluate the specific knowledge and skill competencies needed by communication specialists to fulfill these roles. In addition, identification and evaluation of cross-discipline content for communication specialists who provide early intervention services are needed. Once specific within- and cross-discipline competencies have been identified, efforts must be made to provide communication specialists at the preservice and in-service levels with opportunities to communicate and interact with professionals from other disciplines (McCollum & Thorp, 1988).

Qualified Provider Proviso

According to the Crais and Leonard (1990) survey, significant differences exist between the master's degree and bachelor's degree levels of personnel preparation in both academic and clinical areas. In most academic content areas included on the survey, students with their master's degree received more training than students with their bachelor's degree. In clinical areas, only half of the bachelor's degree programs reported offering clinical opportunities with infants and toddlers and less than half provided experiences with families. The qualified provider proviso of IDEA requires personnel who provide services to young children and their families to meet the highest requirements in the state, which, for communication specialists in most states, is the master's degree. As mentioned previously, even in those states requiring master's level communication specialists to have their master's degree, emergency waivers or temporary credentials are available to personnel with a bachelor's degree but without additional preparation (Cooper, 1993). Yet, the ultimate success of IDEA requires availability and retention of fully qualified personnel.

Certification and Licensure

Several potentially divisive issues concerning certification and licensure requirements confront ASHA. Cooper (1993) challenged professionals in speech-language pathology to examine these issues and endorse a plan of action that recommends 1) a continuum of practitioner standards, from support personnel to specialist; 2) exemption-free licensure laws; and 3) a change in ASHA's governance structure from one of exclusion to inclusion.

The first recommendation involves the use of support personnel in speech-language pathology. Although the recognition and use of support personnel in other allied health professions is not uncommon (e.g., certified occupational therapy assistant), ASHA has traditionally used a single master's level practitioner system. Cooper (1993) recommended a continuum of practitioner standards ranging from support personnel to specialist, with different competencies required for each group. In a draft position statement, the ASHA Task Force on Support Personnel (1994) proposed that support personnel be used to provide activities adjunct to the primary services provided by a certified communication specialist. Appropriate training and supervision must be provided by professionals who are well qualified, and activities should be assigned only at the discretion of certified communication specialists or audiologists. These activities should be consistent with the scope of responsibilities for support personnel. This report showed ASHA's intent to move forward on this issue.

The second recommendation focuses on exemption-free licensure laws embodying ASHA's minimum standards for practitioners in speech-language pathology. Most, if not all, state departments of education requiring master's degrees continue to employ practitioners with only bachelor's degrees through emergency certification. Cooper (1993) has called for licensure laws that ensure the public receives services from consistently qualified speech-language personnel. The endorsement by ASHA of support personnel (e.g., professionals with a bachelor's degree) should strengthen efforts by state departments of education to respond to severe personnel shortages, while maintaining the quality of services provided to young children with communication impairments and their families.

The third recommendation involves changes to ASHA's governance structure. According to a 1994 demographic profile, ASHA's membership consists of two distinct groups, 56.3% who work in school facilities and 38% who are employed by health care facilities (ASHA, 1994). Professionals from within ASHA's membership have questioned whether the skill levels required for the certificate of clinical competence should be different for these two distinct specialty groups (Cooper, 1993). For example, Gonazlez Rothi (1993) asked whether it was necessary for a communication specialist who works in a public school setting to be proficient in treating swallowing disorders in individuals with compromised airways or able to assist in determining candidacy for neurosurgical intervention in seizure cases.

ASHA has undertaken efforts to restructure itself internally to become more of an "umbrella organization" for the increasing variety of related, but independent, professional organizations. Special interest divisions have been created to respond to the diverse and unique needs of these different interest groups. Based on recommendations of the ASHA Ad Hoc Committee on Specialty Certification (Rao, 1993), a Clinical Specialty Board was established to receive petitions from any of its special interest divisions, a related professional organization, or any other group to establish a specialty in a particular interest area.

ASHA's Supervisory Requirements

The amount and type of supervisory and field-based experiences required by ASHA for certification in speech-language pathology have recently come under fire from a variety of sources. ASHA's graduate program accreditation requirements include an established ratio of six full-time (or equivalent) students for each full-time (or equivalent) faculty member for master's degree programs. Many believe that ASHA's graduate program requirements—in particular the 6:1 student/faculty ratio—exacerbate the shortage of qualified professionals in the schools (Goldberg, 1993). Representatives from several U.S. organizations (e.g., the Council for Exceptional Children, the National Association of State Directors of Special Education, the Council of Administrators of Special Education) express concern that the 6:1 ratio and other policies of ASHA contribute significantly to the personnel shortages at the national level (Creaghead, 1994).

Role Definitions

McCollum and Thorp (1988) conducted a survey on team patterns in early inter-vention programs. They found considerable variation in personnel who were available to provide services and in the roles these personnel filled. Next to edu-cators, communication specialists comprised the second most frequently repre-sented discipline across programs. Personnel often fulfilled roles that were not strictly discipline specific. ASHA's requirements for certification in speech-language pathology must begin to reflect these trends. Communication special-ists will need information and clarification of their own professional roles, as well as information and practice on role sharing with professionals from other disciplines.

The issues specific to the development and implementation of interdisci-plinary personnel preparation programs for communication specialists are com-plex and require that ASHA work collaboratively with state institutions of higher education and state agencies. This need is underscored by Cunningham's (1993) warning that ASHA traditionally has been "a system that takes too long to respond, that is skewed toward the academic, and that does not anticipate changes, either positive or negative, that will affect the diverse membership" (pp. 55–56). New ground is being broken, and this will call for continued collabo-rative efforts among institutions of higher education and professional and/or state licensing bodies to produce a cadre of well-trained communication special-ists who can fill a variety of roles.

DESCRIPTION OF PRINCIPLES AND/OR RECOMMENDED PRACTICE

McCollum and Thorp (1988) suggested that the issues central to preparation of personnel who work with infants and young children and their families center on two major areas: the content of training and the process of training. The section below presents recommendations for academic content and practicum require-ments for interdisciplinary training programs designed to prepare communication specialists to work with young children and their families. These recommenda-tions are based on the assumption that communication specialists must be trained to work as team members to provide quality early intervention services that are comprehensive, community based, and family centered.

Program tracks are proposed as a means to provide students with specialized knowledge and experience to work effectively with young children with commu-nication impairments and their families. Training programs for communication specialists should be designed to offer students the option of specializing in dif-ferent tracks (e.g., early intervention, public school, clinic populations). Students who choose the early intervention track should be provided with academic and practical experiences to prepare them to perform the functions outlined in ASHA's (1990) position statement on service delivery.

To complete academic and practicum requirements for a master's degree in communication disorders and sciences, certification in speech-language pathology, and specialization in early intervention, the program of study should take stu-dents approximately 2 years to complete. The time required to complete the pro-gram depends on students experiential background and the number of credit hours taken per semester. Students without a bachelor's degree in speech-language pathology would need to complete all undergraduate-level speech-language pathology prerequisite coursework prior to admittance to a graduate program and thus extend program time to over 2 years.

Academic Content

The course of studies for an interdisciplinary personnel preparation program should be devised to ensure a balance between ASHA-mandated coursework and recommendations outlined in the 1990 position statement on the role of the communication specialist in service delivery to infants, toddlers, and young children and their families. Students who wish to complete ASHA's requirements for the certificate of clinical competence must complete at least 75 semester hours of academic coursework, 27 of which must be in the basic sciences and 36 of which must be in professional coursework. The remaining 12 hours may be distributed between the two areas. For students who choose the early intervention track, these 12 hours would need to be used for specialized early intervention coursework.

Core courses in speech-language pathology should provide essential information on communication sciences and disorders, speech-language development, and intervention strategies. IDEA has described separate service delivery systems for infants and toddlers (Part H) and for preschoolers (Part B). The early intervention core courses should address issues and techniques relevant to both age groups and service delivery systems for young children with disabilities and their families.

Practicum Requirements

Practicum requirements should provide the students with a range of experiences with young children who exhibit communication impairments and their families or children at risk for such problems and their families. Four practicum modules are proposed as a means to provide students with adequate opportunities to practice early intervention skill competencies in protected environments with the support and supervision of a well-trained clinician. The four modules include 1) screening, assessment, and evaluation; 2) direct provision of interventions; 3) consultation; and 4) service coordination. In developing a planned sequence for the training modules, flexibility should be paramount. For example, if a student has extensive experience working with young children with disabilities of different ages, placement in the practicum module, Direct Provision of Intervention, may be unnecessary. Instead, the student might choose a different module or add an optional module.

Screening, Assessment, and Evaluation

Assessment and evaluation procedures should underlie all intervention efforts. Examples of specific competencies in this area include the ability to 1) administer standardized screening and diagnostic instruments for the purposes of identification and referral of children to appropriate placements; 2) conduct interviews with family members to obtain developmental histories; 3) observe and assess infant–caregiver interactions; 4) conduct comprehensive developmental assessments; 5) use program-relevant measures such as curriculum-based assessments; 6) use curriculum-based language assessment and dynamic assessment techniques and procedures; 7) develop IFSPs based on families' concerns, priorities, and resources; and 8) employ daily or weekly data collection procedures.

Direct Provision of Interventions

Even if the communication specialist functions primarily as a consultant, he or she must also have the skills and knowledge necessary to intervene directly with young children in order to demonstrate effective training content and instructional strategies for family members and other early intervention personnel. Specific competencies for direct intervention include, but are not limited to, the ability to 1) develop functional intervention programs in which training targets are established in a developmental hierarchy; 2) choose among various curricular approaches and instructional strategies ranging from adult-directed to child-directed procedures; 3) conduct intervention using an integrated therapy model in a variety of settings including classrooms, homes, and hospitals and/or clinics; 4) provide small and large group instruction and individual instruction when needed; 5) use principles of behavior management; and 6) evaluate the effectiveness of the program for individuals and groups of children.

Consultation

Communication specialists must possess the skills to work collaboratively with families and other professionals from a variety of disciplines for all assessment-evaluation and intervention activities. Specific competencies for the consultant role include the ability to 1) develop partnerships with families and other professionals, 2) establish mutual concerns with families and other professionals about communicative development and intervention, 3) plan and implement communicative intervention programs with families and other professionals, 4) plan and employ practical and useful data collection systems with families and other professionals, and 5) assist family members and other professionals in integrating communicative training targets into daily classroom and home activities.

Service Coordination

From the perspective of effective programming for young children with special needs and their families, the concept of the communication specialist as an isolated professional is no longer acceptable. Communication specialists must seek assistance from a variety of resources, and this input must be synthesized into a cohesive program for the children and families. Some specific competencies include the ability to 1) understand roles of other disciplines, 2) serve as a liaison between multiple agencies that provide services for the child, 3) solicit and integrate diverse and sometimes conflicting information into a consistent approach for the child and family, 4) function as an advocate for families and provide limited counseling support, and 5) coordinate and monitor the delivery of early intervention services.

TRANSLATION OF RECOMMENDED PRACTICE TO THE FIELD

Whereas the previous section of this chapter focused on recommendations for the content of training, this section focuses on a recommended process for training. The literature provides descriptions of two model preservice training programs that utilize a well-defined and comprehensive approach to interdisciplinary training of students (Bennett & Watson, 1993; Bricker et al., 1995). These programs share exemplary training features. Both programs utilize adult-learning theory to guide the delivery of programmatic content, employ adult-learning principles to facilitate self-reflection and critical-thinking skills in students, and promote competency building through self-directed learning. These two programs recruit students with diverse academic and experiential backgrounds (e.g., social workers, occupational therapists, nurses) and require extensive practicum and field-based experiences. Academic and clinical training is provided using a team structure. Finally, specific training strategies, such as collaborative consultation, coaching model of supervision, cooperative learning, and team teaching, are used to facilitate learning. These strategies are believed to enhance the transfer of knowledge from classroom to field-based experiences and to future employment situations (Bricker et al., 1995). Suggestions for practical ways to integrate these strategies into the curriculum are discussed below.

Collaborative Consultation

Idol, Paolucci-Whitcomb, and Nevin (1986) defined collaborative consultation as

> an interactive process that enables teams of people with diverse expertise to generate creative solutions to mutually defined problems. The outcome is enhanced, altered, and produces solutions that are different from those that the individual team members would have produced independently. (p. 1)

Three guidelines for collaborative consultation include 1) development of a partnership, 2) establishment of mutual concerns, and 3) planning together (Hoskins, 1990).

Practicum experiences should be designed to provide communication specialists with ample opportunities to engage in collaborative consultation with professionals from other disciplines. For example, students should be trained to provide evaluation and treatment services within classroom and home environments, rather than removing children to isolated therapy settings. Use of an integrated therapy model would require communication specialists to share responsibility with center-based interventionists and other professionals for planning, implementing, and evaluating the outcomes of language and communication programs.

Coaching Model of Supervision

The coaching model of supervision is based on ideas articulated by Joyce and Showers (1982, 1983). This model involves a collegial approach to the analysis of teaching and requires the systematic application of four elements.

Discussion

The first element involves the discussion of the theoretical rationale behind an instructional approach or strategy. Information on curricular approaches and intervention strategies can be presented to students in coursework or in seminars associated with practicum experiences. During the initial presentation of information, terms should be clarified and a common language developed to facilitate communication among students with diverse educational and experiential backgrounds.

Demonstration

The second element of a coaching model involves the demonstration of the approach or strategy by an expert. Students should be provided with opportunities to observe program faculty, clinical supervisors, cooperating professionals, or other students in their practicum sites using the strategies. Further explanation will often be needed during this period to clarify when and how to apply the strategies most effectively with children.

Practice

The third element involves the practice of a new approach or strategy in a protected environment. Students should participate in activities that involve structured role-playing situations. Constructive feedback may be provided to students by the instructor, as well as by their peers. In addition, students should be required to practice new strategies in applied settings and to solicit feedback from their supervisors and cooperating professionals.

Integration

The fourth element of coaching involves integration of the new strategy into a student's existing teaching repertoire. Coaching is intended to provide companionship for students during the practice phase of the process. This can be provided in one of two ways: expert coaching and reciprocal coaching. Coaching by experts involves observation, support, and feedback given by personnel trained in early intervention (e.g., cooperating professional, supervisor). Reciprocal coaching involves two or more students who work together as a team. Students can observe one another using newly learned intervention strategies and provide constructive feedback. Feedback can be provided in writing or verbally, or some students might prefer to use videotape recordings of intervention activities.

Cooperative Learning

Cooperative learning is a teaching strategy that promotes interdependence among groups of individuals, knowledge of the process of group dynamics, and individual accountability (Johnson & Johnson, 1975). Cooperative learning requires that students be grouped into teams and assigned a common goal or task. Different cooperative formats may be used to accomplish the task. For example, all students may be assigned the responsibility for only one part of a task that cannot be accomplished without participation of all group members.

Traditionally, cooperative learning strategies have been used with school-age children to teach a variety of academic skills. These strategies have begun to be employed with graduate students in preservice training programs (Reynolds & Salend, 1989). For example, information can be presented to a large group of students on procedural or technical aspects of various intervention strategies. Students then can be divided into smaller groups and assigned responsibility for determining when it would be most appropriate to use one of the strategies and why. Following small group discussion, students can share the outcomes of their discussion with the larger group. Later, students can work in pairs, providing feedback to one another on when and how to implement the strategies appropriately across children, behaviors, and conditions in applied settings.

Team Teaching

Another strategy that can be used to facilitate learning within a team structure is team teaching. Team teaching involves two or more students who are assigned responsibility for teaching or executing an activity. Students may be paired together in several ways (e.g., randomly, based on experiential backgrounds, according to discipline, based on interest in particular topics). Activities can include teaching academic content to other students, making formal presentations to parent and professional groups, or working together in practicum settings to deliver instructional programs for children.

CONCLUDING REMARKS: FUTURE DIRECTIONS

The basic rationale behind the training of communication specialists is to systematically prepare them to work with families and other professionals to provide quality early intervention to young children with communication impairments. The most effective mechanism for developing and offering such programs can be accomplished only through collaboration among state policy makers, institutions of higher education, and professional organizations. The need for well-educated and well-trained communication specialists is increasing steadily. The demand exists both pragmatically and jurally. Educational institutions, professional organizations, and state governments must rise to the challenge of innovation and collaboration. Training must reflect both the interdisciplinary needs of communication specialists working with infants and young children and their families and the requirements of state licensure. This chapter has shown how a curriculum can be designed to accommodate such needs, the issues that should be addressed, and the research that should be undertaken in order to realize both the letter and the spirit of IDEA. The imperatives for progress in this area are clear. It remains for communication specialists to exercise their skills and imaginations in cooperative efforts of bringing the appropriate assistance to infants and young children with communicative impairments and their families.

REFERENCES

Abbeduto, L., & Rosenberg, S. (1992). Linguistic communication in persons with mental retardation. In S.F. Warren & J. Reichle (Series Eds.), *Communication and language intervention series: Vol. 1. Causes and effects in communication and language intervention* (pp. 331–359). Baltimore: Paul H. Brookes Publishing Co.

American Speech-Language-Hearing Association (ASHA). (1990). The roles of speech-language pathologists in service delivery to infants, toddlers, and their families. *Asha*, 32(Suppl. 2), 4.

American Speech-Language-Hearing Association (ASHA). (1994, July). *Demographic profile of the ASHA membership and affiliation certified in speech-language pathology only for the period January 1, 1994 through June 30, 1994.* Unpublished raw data. Subcommittee on Speech-Language Pathology Service Delivery with Infants and Toddlers.

American Speech-Language-Hearing Association (ASHA) Task Force on Support Personnel. (1994). *Proposed position statement and guidelines for the education/training, use, and supervision of speech-language pathology assistants and audiology assistants.* (Available from ASHA, 10801 Rockville Pike, Rockville, Maryland 20852.)

Beckwith, L. (1990). Adaptive and maladaptive parenting—Implications for intervention. In S.J. Meisels & J.P. Shonkoff (Eds.), *Handbook of early childhood intervention* (pp. 53–77). New York: Cambridge University Press.

Bennett, F.C. (1987). Infants at biological risk. In M.J. Guralnick & F.C. Bennett (Eds.), *Effectiveness of early intervention for at-risk and handicapped children* (pp. 79–112). New York: Academic Press.

Bennett, T., & Watson, A. (1993). A new perspective on training: Competency building. *Journal of Early Intervention, 17*(c), 309–321.

Bricker, D. (1992). The changing nature of communication and language intervention. In S.F. Warren & J. Reichle (Series Eds.), *Communication and language intervention series: Vol. 1. Causes and effects in communication and language intervention* (pp. 361–375). Baltimore: Paul H. Brookes Publishing Co.

Bricker, D. (1993). Then, now, and the path between: A brief history of language intervention. In S.F. Warren & J. Reichle (Series Eds.), A.P. Kaiser & D.B. Gray (Vol. Eds.), *Communication and language intervention series: Vol. 2. Enhancing children's communication: Research foundations for intervention* (pp. 11–31). Baltimore: Paul H. Brookes Publishing Co.

Bricker, D., & Carlson, L. (1981). Issues in early language intervention. In R. Schiefelbusch & D. Bricker (Eds.), *Early language: Acquisition and development* (pp. 477–515). Baltimore: University Park Press.

Bricker, D., & Cripe, J. (1992). *An activity-based approach to early intervention.* Baltimore: Paul H. Brookes Publishing Co.

Bricker, D., Losardo, A., & Straka, E. (1995). *Evaluation of an early intervention/early childhood special education personnel preparation program.* Manuscript submitted for publication.

Bricker, D., & Slentz, K. (1988). Personnel preparation: Handicapped infants. In M. Wang, H. Walberg, & M. Reynolds (Eds.), *The handbook of special education: Research and practice*, (Vol. 3, pp. 319–345). Oxford, England: Pergamon Press.

Bricker, W., & Bricker, D. (1974). An early language strategy. In R. Schiefelbusch & L. Lloyd (Eds.), *Language perspectives: Acquisition, retardation, and intervention* (pp. 431–468). Baltimore: University Park Press.

Brooks-Gunn, J., & Furstenberg, F.F. (1986). The children of adolescent mothers: Physical, academic, and psychological outcomes. *Developmental Review, 6*, 224–251.

Brown, A., Bransford, J., Ferrara, R., & Campione, J. (1983). Learning, remembering and understanding. In P. Mussen (Ed.), *Handbook of child psychology: Cognitive development* (Vol. 3, pp. 77–166). New York: John Wiley & Sons.

Brown, W., & Rule, S. (1993). Personnel and disciplines in early intervention. In W. Brown, S. Thurman, & L. Pearl (Eds.), *Family-centered early intervention with infants and toddlers: Innovative cross-disciplinary approaches* (pp. 245–268). Baltimore: Paul H. Brookes Publishing Co.

Burke, P., McLaughlin, M., & Valdivieso, C. (1988). Preparing professionals to educate handicapped infants and young children: Some policy considerations. *Topics in Early Childhood Special Education, 8*(a), 73–80.

Campione, J.C., & Brown, A. (1987). Linking dynamic assessment with school achievement. In C.S. Lidz (Ed.), *Dynamic assessment: An interactional approach to evaluating learning potential* (pp. 82–115). New York: Guilford Press.

Catlett, C. (1991a). Building blocks: An early childhood in-service education program for speech-language pathologists and audiologists. *Asha, 33,* 50–51.

Catlett, C. (1991b). Infant project—An interdisciplinary approach. *Asha, 33,* 50–51.

Center for Population Options. (1992). *Teenage pregnancy and too-early childbearing: Public costs, personal consequences.* Washington, DC: Author.

Cooper, E. (1993). The fractionation of our discipline. *Asha, 35,* 51–54.

Crais, E. (1991). *A practical guide to embedding family-centered content into existing speech-language pathology coursework.* Chapel Hill: Frank Porter Graham Child Development Center, University of North Carolina.

Crais, E., & Leonard, C. (1990). P.L. 99-457: Are speech-language pathologists prepared for the challenge? *Asha, 32,* 57–61.

Creaghead, N. (Ed.). (1994, March). *Status report.* (Available from Council of Graduate Programs in Communication Disorders and Sciences, Post Office Box 26532, Minneapolis, Minnesota 55426.)

Cunningham, D. (1993). Responses to Cooper. *Asha, 35,* 55–56.

Education of the Handicapped Act Amendments of 1986, PL 99-457. (October 8, 1986). Title 20, U.S.C. 1400 et seq: *U.S. Statutes at Large, 100,* 1145–1177.

Fujiki, M., & Brinton, B. (1994). Social competence and language impairment in children. In S.F. Warren & J. Reichle (Series Eds.), R.V. Watkins & M.L. Rice (Vol. Eds.), *Communication and language intervention series: Vol. 4. Specific language impairments in children* (pp. 123–143). Baltimore: Paul H. Brookes Publishing Co.

Goldberg, B. (1993). Recipe for tragedy: Personnel shortages in the schools. *Asha, 35,* 36–40.

Goldson, E. (1993). The medically fragile infant. In M. Krajicek & R. Tompkins (Eds.), *The medically fragile infant* (pp. 1–11). Austin, TX: PRO-ED.

Gonazlez Rothi, L. (1993). Responses to Cooper. *Asha, 35,* 56–57.

Gray, B., & Ryan, B. (1973). *Programmed conditioning for language (Monterey Language Program).* Palo Alto, CA: Monterey Learning Systems.

Guadagno, N. (1993). *1992–1993 directory of selected early childhood programs.* Chapel Hill, NC: National Early Childhood Technical Assistance System.

Guess, D., Sailor, W., & Baer, D. (1978). *Functional speech and language training.* Lawrence, KS: H & H Enterprises.

Halle, J.W., Marshall, A.M., & Spradlin, J.E. (1979). Time delay: A technique to increase language use and facilitate generalization in retarded children. *Journal of Applied Behavior Analysis, 12,* 431–440.

Hanson, M.J., & Lovett, D. (1992). Personnel preparation for early interventionists: A cross-disciplinary survey. *Journal of Early Intervention, 16*(2), 123–135.

Hart, B., & Risley, T. (1975). Incidental teaching of language in the preschool. *Journal of Applied Behavior Analysis, 8,* 411–420.

Hoskins, B. (1990). Collaborative consultation: Designing the role of the speech-language pathologist in a new educational context. In W.A. Secord & E.H. Wiig (Eds.), *Collaborative programs in the schools: Concepts, models, and procedures* (pp. 29–36). San Antonio, TX: The Psychological Corporation, Harcourt Brace Jovanovich.

Idol, L., Paolucci-Whitcomb, P., & Nevin, A. (1986). *Collaborative consultation.* Rockville, MD: Aspen Publishers, Inc.

Individuals with Disabilities Education Act (IDEA) of 1990, PL 101-476. (October 30, 1990). Title 20, U.S.C. 1400 et seq: *U.S. Statutes at Large, 104* (Part 2), 1103–1151.

Johnson, D.W., & Johnson, R.T. (1975). *Learning together and alone.* Englewood Cliffs, NJ: Prentice Hall.

Johnston, J.R., & Heller, A.B. (1987). Effectiveness of a curriculum for preschool language intervention specialists. *Asha, 21*(g), 39–43.

Joyce, B., & Showers, B. (1982). The coaching of teaching. *Educational Leadership, 40*(1), 4–10.

Joyce, B., & Showers, B. (1983). *Power of staff development through research on training.* Alexandria, VA: Association for Supervision and Curriculum Development.

Kasworm, C.E. (1990). Adult undergraduates in higher education: A review of past research perspectives. *Review of Educational Research, 60*(3), 345–372.

Kent, L. (1974). *Language acquisition program for the retarded or multiply impaired.* Champaign, IL: Research Press.

Lidz, C.S. (1987). *Dynamic assessment: An interactional approach to evaluating learning potential.* New York: Guilford Press.

Lidz, C.S., & Thomas, C. (1987). The preschool learning assessment device: Extension of a static approach. In C.S. Lidz (Ed.), *Dynamic assessment: An interactional approach to evaluating learning potential* (pp. 288–326). New York: Guilford Press.

Long, H.B. (1987). *New perspectives on the education of adults in the United States.* New York: Nichols.

Matthews, J., & Frattali, C. (1994). The professions of speech pathology and audiology. In G.H. Shames, E.H. Wiig, & W.A. Secord (Eds.), *Human communication disorders* (pp. 2–33). New York: Macmillan.

McCollum, J., & Thorp, E. (1988). Training of infant specialists: A look to the future. *Infants and Young Children, 1*(b), 55–65.

Mearig, J.S. (1987). Assessing the learning potential of kindergarten and primary-age children. In C.S. Lidz (Ed.), *Dynamic assessment: An interactional approach to evaluating learning potential* (pp. 237–267). New York: Guilford Press.

Meisels, S., Harbin, G., Modigliani, K., & Olson, K. (1988). Formulating optimal state early childhood intervention policies. *Exceptional Children, 55*(b), 159–165.

Minick, N. (1987). Implications of Vygotsky's theories form dynamic assessment. In C. Lidz (Ed.), *Dynamic assessment: An interactional approach to evaluating learning potential* (pp. 116–140). New York: Guilford Press.

Minifie, F.D. (1994). *Introduction to communication sciences and disorders.* San Diego, CA: Singular Publishing Group.

National Institute of Neurological Disorders and Stroke. (1988). *Developmental speech and language disorders: Hope through research* (NIH Publications No. 88-2757). Bethesda, MD: Author.

National Joint Committee on Learning Disabilities. (1987). Learning disabilities and the preschool child. *Asha, 29*(5), 35–38.

Nelson, N.W. (1994). Curriculum-based language assessment and intervention across the grades. In G.P. Wallach & K.G. Butler (Eds.), *Language learning disabilities in school-age children and adolescents* (pp. 104–131). New York: Macmillan.

Olswang, L.B., Bain, B.A., & Johnson, G.A. (1992). Using dynamic assessment with children with language disorders. In S.F. Warren & J. Reichle (Series Eds.), *Communication and language intervention series: Vol. 1. Causes and effects in communication and language intervention* (pp. 187–215). Baltimore: Paul H. Brookes Publishing Co.

Palincsar, A., Brown, A., & Campione, J. (1994). Models and practices of dynamic assessment. In G. Wallach & K. Butler (Eds.), *Learning disabilities in school-age children and adolescents* (pp. 132–144). New York: Merrill College Publishing.

Rao, P. (Ed.). (1993, November). *Special Interest Divisions Newsletter, 32*(2), 8–9. (Available from ASHA, 10801 Rockville Pike, Rockville, MD 20852.)

Reynolds, C., & Salend, S.J. (1989). Cooperative learning in special education teacher preparation programs. *Teacher Education and Special Education, 12*(3), 91–95.

Rowan, L., Thorp, E., & McCollum, J. (1990). An interdisciplinary practicum to foster infant-family and teaming competencies in speech-language pathologists. *Infants and Young Children, 3*(b), 58–66.

Schlossberg, N.K., Lynch, A.Q., & Chickering, A.W. (1989). Understanding adults' life and learning transitions. In N.K. Schlossberg (Ed.), *Improving higher education environments for adults* (pp. 13–33). San Francisco: Jossey-Bass.

Silliman, E., & Wilkinson, L. (1994). Observation is more than looking. In G. Wallach & K. Butler (Eds.), *Learning disabilities in school-age children and adolescents* (pp. 145–173). New York: Merrill College Publishing.

Sparks, S., Clark, M., Oas, D., & Erickson, R. (1988). *Clinical services to infants at risk for communication disorders.* Paper presented at the Annual Convention of the American Speech-Language-Hearing Association (ASHA), Boston.

Spradlin, J.E., & Siegel, G.M. (1982). Language training in natural and clinical environments. *Journal of Speech and Hearing Research, 47,* 2–6.

Tzuriel, D., & Klein, P.S. (1985). The assessment of analogical thinking modifiability among regular, special education, disadvantaged, and mentally retarded children. *Journal of Abnormal Child Psychology, 13*(4), 539–552.

Wade, R.K. (1985). What makes the difference in inservice teacher education? A meta-analysis of research. *Educational Leadership, 42*, 48–54.

Warren, S.F., & Kaiser, A.P. (1986). Generalization of treatment effects by young language-delayed children: A longitudinal analysis. *Journal of Speech and Hearing Disorders, 51*, 239–251.

Warren, S.F., McQuarter, R.J., & Rogers-Warren, A.K. (1984). The effects of mands and models on the speech and language of unresponsive language-delayed preschool children. *Journal of Speech and Hearing Disorders, 49*, 43–52.

Yoder, D., Coleman, P., & Gallagher, J. (1990). *Personnel needs: Allied health personnel meeting the demands of Part H, P.L. 99-457*. Chapel Hill: University of North Carolina.

Young, E. (1993). The NICU and early transitional care. In M. Krajicek & R. Tompkins (Eds.), *The medically fragile infant* (pp. 13–23). Austin, TX: PRO-ED.

6

PREPARING OCCUPATIONAL THERAPISTS

Barbara Hanft, Janice Posatery Burke, and Kathleen Swenson-Miller

The team members know they are not "getting through" to the McGregors about the safest way to feed 2-year-old Jamie, who has a closed brain injury resulting in hemiplegia and significant developmental delays. The occupational therapist is concerned that Jamie's choking will continue as long as Mrs. McGregor tries to feed Jamie on his back across her lap during each of his six daily feeding sessions. The nurse is worried about daily caloric intake and the social worker wonders if she should offer the McGregors respite care through temporary foster placement because the family appears overwhelmed trying to care for Jamie currently. A progress conference is held with the McGregors to talk about how Jamie is doing. During this discussion, the occupational therapist asks Mrs. McGregor about her expectations for Jamie over the next several months and is surprised to hear that she believes that Jamie will recover from his hemiplegia if only he would eat enough to gain back his strength. Finally, the occupational therapist and the social worker understand the McGregors' belief system; that is, feeding Jamie on his back is the best way to ensure that he will eat enough food to recover from his accident. They also realize they must gently redirect the McGregors in understanding the nature of Jamie's chronic condition and potential recovery and support them in caring for him in ways different from those they have used in the past.

IN 1986, THE U.S. CONGRESS enacted PL 99-457, the Education of the Handicapped Act Amendments.[1] Since then, the real work of implementation has focused on changing traditional professional practices, including those associated with teamwork. This challenge has proven particularly difficult because team practices are complex in nature and are based on long-standing traditions and assumptions held by the myriad of professionals who are involved. As the definition of a team has changed over time, many practitioners have been left wondering about their roles and their places on the team. In one survey, 77% of the occupational therapists in early intervention indicated that they worked on a team; yet, many respondents also said they were "unsure" if they were on a team because other team members were not in the same building and did not see one another every day (American Occupational Therapy Association [AOTA], 1988).

---

[1]Subsequently, in 1991, PL 102-119, the Individuals with Disabilities Education Act Amendments, was passed to reauthorize and expand PL 99-457.

In describing how the notion of *team* has changed over time, Maple (1987) wrote that it is essential for occupational therapists and other early intervention specialists to include families and their children as team members, rather than as recipients of the team's services. Maple asked a simple yet challenging question: "To work in coordinated, co-operative and goal-directed fashion sounds simple enough. Why then is it so difficult?" (1987, p. 145).

This chapter focuses on the challenges of defining teams in the era of family-centered, community-based care. It also identifies promising practices and approaches for preparing occupational therapy students, as well as updating professionals in practice, to function as members of family-centered, interdisciplinary, and interagency teams. The three major sections in this chapter discuss the 1) core philosophy of occupational therapy as it relates to early childhood; 2) recommended practice in preparing occupational therapists to serve on interdisciplinary, family-centered, and interagency teams; and 3) levels of professional preparation for occupational therapists to work with very young children, their families, and other professionals.

CORE PHILOSOPHY OF OCCUPATIONAL THERAPY

Historically, the profession of occupational therapy has been steeped in a concern for the everyday life and functioning of the individual. This includes expertise in understanding how a disability or chronic illness may interfere with occupational performance. Occupational performance reflects the behaviors that are manifested when individuals acquire and make use of motor, cognitive, and psychosocial skills to support their engagement in activities or *occupations* that are interesting and hold meaning for them (Reed, 1993).

The founders of the profession of occupational therapy represented diverse backgrounds including social work, medicine, psychiatry, and architecture. Their objective was to create a profession that would address the skills and habits that individuals with disabilities needed in order to productively interact in everyday life (Hopkins & Smith, 1993; Kielhofner & Burke, 1977). Through their work in hospitals for people with mental illness, the first occupational therapists recognized how an individual's daily living skills and habits deteriorated when he or she was removed from the stream of everyday life without the usual markers of time, place, and activity as guideposts.

Occupational therapists continue to be deeply committed to understanding the relationship among key variables related to human engagement in meaningful activities. Research within the field is focusing on questions such as the following:

How do different people "occupy" their time?
How do people feel as they engage in their occupation?
What are the ultimate effects of meaningful occupation on health and well-being?

When occupational therapists provide services, they attend to all human and nonhuman factors that contribute to the "fit" of an occupation to an individual. This includes consideration of the person, the activity or the occupation with which he or she is engaged, and the environment or context for the interaction.

A range of studies has explored how engagement in meaningful activity can affect a person's sense of well-being (i.e., duration of task, sense of pleasure in "doing," perceptions of the value of the task at hand, sense of the passage of time) (Csikszentmihalyi & LeFevre, 1989; Henry, Nelson, & Duncombe, 1984; Nelson, Thompson, & Moore, 1982).

Occupational therapists work in diverse practice settings, such as general, rehabilitation, and pediatric hospitals; community mental health centers; home health agencies; work rehabilitation programs; skilled nursing homes; private practices; school systems; early intervention programs; and neonatal intensive care nurseries. The top three employment settings are the school system, general hospitals, and rehabilitation hospitals or centers (AOTA, 1990).

Occupational Therapy in Early Childhood

Historically, occupational therapists worked with very young children with special needs alongside medically oriented professionals, such as physicians, physical therapists, and nurses (Poncher & Richmond, 1947; Tyler & Chandler, 1978). During the 1970s and 1980s, significant numbers of occupational therapists also joined educational teams in school settings (AOTA, 1990; Hanft, 1991a; Ottenbacher, 1991). In 1996, the majority of occupational therapists serving preschool-age children with disabilities (3–5 years old) work in the schools primarily with special educators, speech-language pathologists, and physical therapists. Lawler (1989) found that occupational therapists in early intervention settings (birth to 3 years old) worked most frequently with speech-language pathologists (91%), physical therapists (81%), teachers (74%), psychiatrists or psychologists (51%), and social workers (45%). Of these occupational therapists in early intervention settings, 68% of them worked on teams; nearly half of the therapists identified their team as interdisciplinary, 28% as multidisciplinary, and 16% as transdisciplinary.

Throughout the intervention process, the occupational therapist typically focuses on young children's *occupations* as manifested in play, social interaction, sensorimotor development, motor control, and adaptive skills, including feeding and toileting (Burke, 1993; Glass & Wolf, 1993; Gorga, 1989; Holloway, Glass, & Wolf, 1993; Stallings-Sahler, 1993; Swinth & Case-Smith, 1993). Working with family members to help them achieve desired outcomes for their children is also a primary goal (Case-Smith, 1991; Hanft, 1989b; Stewart, 1989). In a comprehensive interview of 118 occupational therapists specializing in early intervention, the following areas were most frequently identified as a focus for intervention: feeding and oral-motor skills, adaptive equipment, activities of daily living, sensory integration, parent training, splinting, fine motor development, and positioning (Lawler, 1989).

With the goal of facilitating maximum functional performance, the occupational therapist chooses meaningful *occupations* to develop skills and habits that will support the physical, cognitive, and psychosocial dimensions of the child's play, self-care, and behavior as a family member, preschooler, and playmate. Among an infant's meaningful occupations are skills and habits such as learning to use one's hands and eyes together in order to reach for and grasp a rattle, watching a turning mobile, settling down and going to sleep, drinking from a bottle, and rolling over to sit up and interact with toys and people. A preschooler's meaningful occupations may include using newly developed motor skills (e.g., squeezing, pinching, cutting, drawing); developing peer friendships; participating in setting the table for snack; exploring and developing gross motor capabilities by running, climbing, squatting, and jumping; and communicating ideas, feelings, and actions.

Occupational therapists also provide assistance to family members who are interested in acquiring skills to support their own occupational roles of parents and caregivers (Case-Smith, 1991; Parush & Clark, 1988; Zeitlin & Williamson, 1994). Skills that may enhance the parent and/or caregiver role include calming techniques to help quiet a fussy infant, handling skills to reduce high muscle tone interfering with movement and daily routines (e.g., diapering), and observing skills for reading the sensory cues of a child with a difficult temperament. Similarly, occupational therapists may work with siblings to facilitate their engagement in games and playful interactions with a brother or sister who has a developmental delay. As stated in professional documents of the AOTA,

> In collaboration with the parents, occupational therapy interventions may include activities such as seating and positioning for play, neuromuscular facilitation techniques to enable eating, facilitating parent skills in caring for and playing with their infant, and modifying the play space for accessibility. (1994, p. 4)

RECOMMENDED PRACTICE IN
PREPARING OCCUPATIONAL THERAPISTS

This section has two major purposes. The first is to identify and describe, through examples and scenarios, five major principles that must be built into professional preparation programs and in-service workshops in order to ensure that occupational therapy students and practitioners can work effectively on teams. These five principles are as follows:

- Principle 1: The family is the core of the interdisciplinary team.
- Principle 2: Families function as unique systems within social and cultural systems.
- Principle 3: Team members should provide options and choices.
- Principle 4: Team members share functions and information.
- Principle 5: Team members should understand each family story and expectations for service.

The second purpose is to highlight selected training activities that integrate each of the five principles. Recommended readings to support the training activities were selected to represent family, occupational therapy, and interdisciplinary perspectives. All training activities have been used successfully by the authors in preservice and in-service settings (Hanft, Burke, Cahill, Swenson-Miller, & Humphry, 1992). Many were first developed for a nationally recognized in-service project, *Family-Centered Care,* disseminated in 1990–1991 by AOTA with federal support (Hanft, 1991b). Regional workshops, led by teams of occupational therapists and parents of children with disabilities, were effective in promoting positive attitudes about working on interdisciplinary teams providing family-centered care as measured by pre- and post-attitude scales, follow-up telephone interviews, and mail surveys (Geissinger, Humphry, Hanft, & Keyes, 1993; Hanft, Geissinger, & Hunt, 1994; Humphry & Geissinger, 1993).

The occupational therapist's role on early childhood teams in medical and early education settings is evolving as teams themselves move from traditional to family-centered care (Case-Smith & Wavrek, 1993; Hanft, 1988). On traditional teams, membership has been limited to professionals who work together on a daily basis in one facility to identify and remediate a child's problems. Families are typically viewed as the recipients of the team's service. Family-centered teams, in contrast, include families as part of a team. In addition, members often come from different agencies and facilities within the community. All members collaborate to address family-generated outcomes and interventions.

The kind of training that occupational therapy students receive to work on family-centered, interdisciplinary teams has been the subject of study by several authors (Hanson & Lovett, 1992; Humphry & Link, 1990). One study found that 97% of the 36 bachelor's programs and 7 entry-level master's programs surveyed provided some instruction on team process, although the range varied greatly from 1 to 30 hours (Humphry & Link, 1990). Some clinical fieldwork experience with infants, such as site visits to an early intervention program or hands-on experience as part of a pediatric course, was required by 59% of the programs surveyed. The authors of this survey and their advisory board of pediatric experts recommended that students learn to work as part of an interdisciplinary team and participate in joint activities with other disciplines during their training.

Principle 1: The Family Is the Core of the Interdisciplinary Team

Whether the team provides service in a medical facility, school, home, or child care setting, recommended practice in occupational therapy identifies the child's family as the essential core of the early intervention team (AOTA, 1989; Case-Smith & Wavrek, 1993; Decker, 1992; Hanft, 1989b; Moersch, 1989; Schaaf & Mulrooney, 1989). This perspective of emphasizing the role of families as core members of the team has evolved since the 1970s as occupational therapists have become more involved in community services and have increasingly listened to parents share their dreams and desired outcomes for their children. Gradually, therapists have shifted from thinking of parents as extenders of therapy in their home to collaborating with families as core members of the child's team with full involvement in developing assessment, intervention, and transition strategies. In addition, occupational therapists must 1) develop and refine their communication skills, 2) examine personal and professional attitudes, 3) make programmatic changes in how intervention is provided to incorporate changes in public policy and recommended practice, and 4) expand knowledge about successful collaboration through clinical research (Stewart, 1989).

Therapists have realized that professionally driven recommendations and home programs that focused on remediating the child's "problems" were frequently abandoned when they were not considered meaningful by the family (Bazyk, 1989). Similarly, when therapists instructed parents on conducting therapy sessions at home, concerns arose about how such activities might pose conflicting role dilemmas for parents. Parents often believed their children were receiving the message, "You need to be fixed," and that this message directly interfered with their desire to enjoy, guide, and develop relationships with their children (Allen & Hudd, 1987; Tyler, Kogan, & Turner, 1974). As one mother observed, "I want to be Zak's Mom, not his therapist. . . . I do have a responsibility to help Zachary develop his motor skills, but I also have a responsibility to help him learn about life" (Lyon, 1989, p. 4). Below are two training activities with recommendations for reading in support of Principle 1.

Training activities

1. Discuss personal attitudes and values about working with families after completing the attitude survey *Issues in Early Intervention* (Humphry & Geissinger, 1993). Students can also complete this survey at the beginning and end of a course or workshop on teaming with families and reflect on any changes they have made.

2. Share a family photograph depicting a special event or gathering. Identify family members and their relationships. Describe the significance of the event or people pictured. Ask students to contrast the similarities and differences between their own family of origin and the families encountered in their training or employment site.

Recommended reading

Family perspective:	Pizzo, P. (1990). Parent advocacy: A resource for early intervention. In S. Meisels & J. Shonkoff (Eds.), *Handbook of early childhood intervention* (pp. 668–678). New York: Cambridge University Press.
Occupational therapy perspective:	Bazyk, S. (1989). Changes in attitudes and beliefs regarding parent participation and home programs: An update. *American Journal of Occupational Therapy, 43,* 723–728.
Interdisciplinary perspective:	Miller, L., Lynch, E., & Campbell, J. (1990). Parents as partners: A new paradigm for collaboration. *Best Practices in School Speech-Language Pathology, 1,* 40–56.

Principle 2: Families Function as Unique Systems within Social and Cultural Systems

Occupational therapists should recognize the multiple and complex cultural, social class, ethnic, and racial factors that influence family involvement with professionals. These factors affect how professionals and families from diverse cultures interact throughout the intervention process as they establish trusting relationships, communicate, ask questions, and find solutions. A survey of pediatric occupational therapists indicated that therapists perceive themselves to be more skilled in communicating with other professionals than with family members (Case-Smith, 1994). The skills defined as professional communication included consultation, establishing relationships with other disciplines, and collaboration. Skills in working with families included providing family support, assisting families in identifying their priorities, and considering families' cultural values. The following scenario typifies the experiences an occupational therapist may have when working in a community-based early intervention program with families from diverse cultural backgrounds:

A teenage single mother and her infant daughter (who has a history of irritability and nonorganic failure to thrive) are participating in a play group organized by an occupational thera-

pist in a drop-in family support program. During group discussion, the mother shares with the therapist that she lives with her sister and two nieces. The mother hopes to go to a full-time job training program but will need child care for her daughter in order to enroll in the program. To date, she has not kept any appointments for her daughter's developmental assessment. The child's pediatrician is concerned about the infant's slow development and poor weight gain.

The occupational therapist realizes that, in order to successfully engage this family in early intervention, it will be critical to integrate the efforts of a variety of family members as well as professionals from social services, education, and health agencies (Poulsen, 1993). The occupational therapist also recognizes that this mother has not responded to the programs that have been available to her thus far but is unsure why. The therapist knows that if she is to provide any real assistance to this mother, she needs to understand how the mother sees and defines the issues at hand. Together, the therapist and mother develop a tentative plan to identify the following:

- Issues that are of concern to the mother and her family
- Important people who can assist in understanding these concerns, including trusted family members and professionals who are skilled in working with infants
- The mother's goals for herself and her child
- What will help the mother achieve her goals, including who might provide important information and resources for economic, social, and educational support

Below are two training activities with recommendations for reading in support of Principle 2.

Training activities

1. View two segments from the MGM film *Moonstruck*, the story of how an Italian American family living in Brooklyn copes with the impending marriage of their daughter. Look for the unwritten family rules when the widowed daughter tells her parents she plans to remarry and during the kitchen scene at the end of the film when her fiancé's brother also proposes. How familiar or different are this family's structure, rules, and traditions to trainees' current family or family of origin?

2. Observe the physical structures (e.g., homes, buildings, stores, businesses), traffic flow, people, and activities of a defined area of the community and describe how an early intervention program could best meet the needs of the people living in this area. What additional information would be needed to answer this question and how could it be obtained?

Recommended reading

Family perspective: Turnbull, A.P., & Turnbull, H.R., III. (1990). *Families, professionals, and exceptionality: A special partnership* (2nd ed., pp. 52–76). Columbus, OH: Charles E. Merrill.

(continued)

Recommended reading. *(continued)*

Occupational therapy perspective:	Briggs, A., & Howe, M. (1988). Ecological systems model for occupational therapy. *American Journal of Occupational Therapy, 36*(5), 322–327.
Interdisciplinary perspective:	Darling, R. (1989). Using the social system perspective in early intervention: The value of a sociological approach. *Journal of Early Intervention, 13*(1), 24–35.

Principle 3: Team Members Should Provide Options and Choices

When professionals enable families to make choices regarding early childhood services, many individual preferences emerge. Some families cannot begin early intervention services soon enough. Others want to adjust privately to having a child with special needs before incorporating strangers into their circle, sometimes choosing not to participate at all in early intervention services. Therapists should listen to families' choices and then negotiate the type, location, and frequency of services. Sometimes the frequency of occupational therapy may be intensive, such as individual therapy with a newborn who has a brachial plexus injury. At the other end of the continuum, services may include monitoring the child's progress by checking periodically with the parents to review concerns and needs. Services could be provided in intervention programs, the family's home, a child care center, an outpatient program in a medical facility, or other community programs such as "baby swim" classes, family support and drop-in programs, infant Head Start, or a shelter for homeless families. The following example of recommended practice for giving families choices takes place in an interdisciplinary neonatal follow-up clinic in a university setting:

On this particular day, a family shares with the clinic coordinator that their biggest concern is their difficulty feeding their 6-month-old infant who was born prematurely. Thus, the primary focus of the follow-up visit is on feeding, although the infant's physical status and overall development are also examined. Even though the team consists of professionals from several different disciplines, as well as the parents, the developmental pediatrician and the occupational therapist take the lead with the family on this day because of the family's concern. The family, occupational therapist, and physician talk together and explore intervention options. As the occupational therapist listens to family members talk about their perceptions and their concerns regarding the child, he asks to see how the child eats. After asking permission to hold the baby, the therapist assesses the baby's oral-motor development and explores with the family the use of different positions to facilitate lip closure on the bottle. The physician completes a developmental assessment, and follow-up plans are made with the family to track the infant's eating patterns and weight gain.

The crucial variable defining this interaction is that the family is included in every step of the process as evidenced by their choice in direction for the session and their involvement in the assessment and development of a plan for intervention. Important information related to caring for the child is shared among team members, eliminating the need for the family to recount their story repeatedly with each additional professional contact. Below are two training activities with recommendations for reading in support of Principle 3.

Training activities

1. Ask students to schedule 1 day in the life of a family raising a child with a disability by organizing a set of index cards describing parents' work schedules, home routines, and child care activities (e.g., getting children off to school). Merge a second set of cards listing special needs (e.g., early intervention appointments, therapists' suggested home activities) with the first set. Finally, add a crisis card (e.g., the car breaks down, an older sibling breaks an arm) and reorder both sets of cards to accommodate a new schedule for the day. Which activities or routines get thrown out and why?

2. Distribute assessment results for an infant with delays. Have half of the students develop a traditional medical occupational therapy treatment plan for the infant and the other half an individualized family service plan (IFSP). Discuss the similarities and differences between the traditional plan and the IFSP.

Recommended reading

Family perspective:	Rocco, S. (1994). New visions for the developmental assessment of infants and young children: A parent's perspective. *Zero to Three, 14*(16), 13–15.
Occupational therapy perspective:	Miller, L. (1994). Journey to a desirable future: A values-based model of infant and toddler assessment. *Zero to Three, 14*(16), 23–27.
Interdisciplinary perspective:	Zeitlin, S., & Williamson, G. (1994). *Coping in young children: Early intervention practices to enhance adaptive behavior and resilience.* Baltimore: Paul H. Brookes Publishing Co.

Principle 4: Team Members Share Functions and Information

Family-centered care is based on the premise that parents and early intervention staff will work together in a collaborative way to determine the direction of early intervention outcomes and services for a child. Because each child and family is unique, the constellation of the early intervention services will vary depending on the concerns of the family and child. Like other professionals, the occupational therapist may play a primary role on one family's team and a more indirect, consultative role on another family's team. For example, when parents first begin an early intervention program for a very fussy infant, the family's priority may be to understand and manage their child's irritability. If this fussiness is due to a sensory processing disorder, the occupational therapist may be the most appropriate professional to work with the family (Humphry, 1989). If the family's priority centers on communication skills for their child, the occupational therapist may serve as a consultant to the team, monitoring the child's progress and providing input regarding secondary issues, such as appropriate play with toys, dressing skills, or environmental adaptations. This flexibility in the team members' roles, depending on the family's stated priorities at a given time, is a cornerstone of family-centered teams.

Interdisciplinary and interagency collaboration can be immensely helpful to the family for achieving specific goals for the child. For example, an occupational therapist in private practice may work in the home with a family who wants their child to feed himself during mealtimes. The occupational therapist explores with the family the context of how, where, when, and with whom the child eats in order to suggest specific ways to position the baby and offer food. In addition, the family may consult with a speech-language pathologist, possibly a member of their team from a nonprofit program, who provides strategies to facilitate communication with their child. A collaborative approach will provide opportunities for the family, the occupational therapist, and the speech-language pathologist to share their expertise and develop an intervention program that addresses the issues of self-feeding and using gestural communication to indicate food preference.

The product of such a rich collaboration among the occupational therapist, the speech-language pathologist, and the family is a coordinated, interrelated intervention strategy, which is clearly preferable to a model that would include two professionals from separate agencies working independently with the family. Below are two training activities with recommendations for reading in support of Principle 4.

Training activities

Students interview practicing occupational therapists (or listen to a panel discussion) to learn about the following:

1. Perspectives on family and/or therapist partnerships (e.g., decision making; identifying family concerns, resources, and priorities; choosing services; personal skills needed; working with families in stressful situations; impact of cultural values)

2. Experience collaborating with professionals in other facilities and/or settings (e.g., which professionals, where they work, mission of other facilities, how these other services complement the occupational therapy program, how and when to refer)

Recommended reading

Family perspective: Hunt, M., Cornelius, P., Levanthal, P., Miller, P., Murray, T., & Stoner, G. (1991). *Into our lives.* (Available from the Family Child Learning Center, 90 W. Overdale Drive, Tallmadge, OH 44278)

Occupational therapy perspective: Case-Smith, J., & Wavrek, B.B. (1993). Models of service delivery and team interaction. In J. Case-Smith (Ed.), *Pediatric occupational therapy and early intervention* (pp. 27–159). Boston: Andover Medical Publishers.

Interdisciplinary perspective: Kjerland, L., & Kovach, J. (1990). Family–staff collaboration for tailored infant assessment. In E.D. Gibbs & D.M. Teti (Eds.), *Interdisciplinary assessment of infants: A guide for early intervention professionals* (pp. 287–297). Baltimore: Paul H. Brookes Publishing Co.

Principle 5: Team Members Should
Understand Each Family Story and Expectations for Service

Listening to a family story is one way to understand family members' values and traditions as well as their dreams for the child's future. It also defines a collaborative interaction between family members and professionals leading to the identification of meaningful intervention strategies based on family-generated outcomes. Stories are ethnographic surveys of what people do and how they think (Mattingly & Fleming, 1993). Family stories are personal narratives that reflect the feelings, goals, needs, and values of the person telling the story. Eliciting family stories in a narrative interview provides a natural way for professionals to interact with family members by providing cues to answer the question, "Where and how can I enter this family's story and provide meaningful intervention?"

A family walks into an early intervention center and begins to smile warily as they quickly scan the environment. The room is colorful and full of comfortable chairs and toys. The parents have a new daughter, Christine, who is 2 months old and has Down syndrome. Their stereotyped image of early intervention had included visions of strange equipment, professionals in white coats, an austere environment, and antiseptic smells. As the early childhood educator, developmental pediatrician, and occupational therapist sit down with the parents over a cup of coffee, the parents begin to share their dreams for Christine. Part of the family story includes an animated description of the sports activities of the family members. They ask tentatively, "This may seem silly to you, but skiing is an important family activity for us. When Christine is older, is there any hope that she could go skiing with our family?"

This family's story leads the team to develop several outcome statements that focus on active group activities for Christine and her three brothers and sisters to share. Such family stories serve as guides for assessment and intervention planning and ensure that the family receives information and services that are meaningful to them. Below are two training activities with recommendations for reading in support of Principle 5.

Training activities

1. Ask students to explore the health practices and beliefs regarding disability and wellness of different cultural groups residing in their community. Information can be gathered by speaking with members of each cultural group as well as to doctors, dentists, nurses, educators, psychologists, or religious and community leaders. Discuss how a family's cultural practices and beliefs affect expectations about early intervention services.

2. Spend a defined amount of time (e.g., Saturday afternoons, Wednesday evenings for several weeks) with a family willing to provide practical experience in daily care for a child with special needs. Elicit the family's story by asking about and observing routine activities and special roles family members play. Listen for cues about what family members hope for and expect to happen in the future as their child grows older. Keep a journal of observations and personal reactions.

(continued)

(continued)

Recommended reading	
Family perspective:	Watson, C. (1994). Behind every dedicated parent is a person who needs support. *Developmental Disabilities Special Interest Newsletter, 17*(4), 5.
Occupational therapy perspective:	Hanft, B. (1994). The "good" parent: A label by any other name would not smell as sweet. *Developmental Disabilities Special Interest Newsletter, 17*(4), 5.
Interdisciplinary perspective:	Mattingly, C., & Fleming, M. (1993). *Clinical reasoning: Forms of inquiry in a therapeutic practice.* Philadelphia: F.A. Davis.

PROFESSIONAL PREPARATION OF OCCUPATIONAL THERAPY PERSONNEL

There are two career paths in occupational therapy: one as a registered occupational therapist (OTR) and the other as a certified occupational therapy assistant (COTA). All occupational therapy personnel must meet AOTA standards for entry-level practice, including clinical fieldwork requirements.

Entry-Level Preparation

OTRs can enter the profession with either a bachelor's or master's degree; COTAs must complete a 2-year program and earn an associate degree. The minimum standards for accrediting programs that prepare individuals to enter occupational therapy as OTRs or COTAs are specified in the *Essentials and Guidelines for an Accredited Educational Program for the Occupational Therapist* (AOTA, 1991a, 1991b). These essentials require that COTAs and OTRs have coursework and clinical experience with individuals of all ages from a variety of disability groups because occupational therapy personnel are expected to practice in diverse settings with individuals of any age who have physical and/or mental impairments. Table 1 identifies the requirements for entry-level practice in occupational therapy acquired through academic coursework, clinical fieldwork, and successful completion of a national certification examination. In addition to AOTA's requirements ensuring that students in programs across the country will receive similar coursework, licensure or some other form of state regulation is required in all states except Colorado.

Fieldwork

In occupational therapy programs, two levels of fieldwork are required. *Level I* fieldwork is short-term clinical fieldwork. This type of fieldwork is designed to enrich didactic coursework through directed observation and participation in selected aspects of the occupational therapy process. *Level II* fieldwork involves full-time affiliations (6 months for OTRs and 2 months for COTAs) in practice settings in which occupational therapists typically work. Requirements for Level II fieldwork stipulate that students have experience working with individuals

Table 1. Requirements for entry-level practice in occupational therapy

Requirements	Registered occupational therapist	Certified occupational therapy assistant
Academic coursework	Graduation from a program accredited by the Accreditation Association Committee of the American Occupational Therapy Association; entry level as an OTR can be at either the bachelor's or master's level	Graduation from a 2-year community college accredited by the Accreditation Association Committee of the American Occupational Therapy Association
Clinical fieldwork	1. Short-term clinical fieldwork (Level I) as needed to enrich academic coursework	1. Short-term clinical fieldwork (Level I) as needed to enrich academic coursework
	2. 6 months (a minimum 940 hours) of full-time affiliation with direct supervision (Level II)	2. Minimum 2-month full-time affiliation with direct supervision (Level II)
National exam given by the American Occupational Therapy Certification Board	Successful completion of a national exam for registered occupational therapists	Successful completion of a national exam for certified occupational therapy assistants

across the life span who have various psychosocial and physical performance problems.

Fieldwork is provided in various medical, education, and social services settings, primarily in hospitals, rehabilitation units, schools, and psychiatric facilities. Although Levels I and II fieldwork are an essential part of the professional preparation process, there is no requirement that academic courses or fieldwork focus on working with young children and their families in early intervention or preschool settings. A random sample of 250 pediatric therapists reported that 64% of the therapists had Level II fieldwork experience with children during their professional preservice preparation (AOTA, Commission on Education, 1991).

Preparation in Pediatrics and Interdisciplinary Teamwork

In occupational therapy, work with children from birth to 18 years of age is called *pediatric* practice. Although specific early childhood courses and clinical fieldwork are not required for entry-level practice in occupational therapy, all students must study typical and atypical development across the life span. The AOTA has issued recommendations for pediatric practice entitled *Guidelines for Curriculum Content in Pediatrics* (AOTA, Commission on Education, 1991). These guidelines specify the knowledge and skills entry-level OTRs must possess to work effectively with children of all ages and their family members. Although these guidelines reflect the recommended practices discussed above, they focus on more than interdisciplinary, family-centered teamwork. The guidelines are divided into two sections addressing entry-level practice: 1) academic coursework and accompanying Level I fieldwork for clinical enrichment, and 2) Level II fieldwork or full-time clinical practicum. A summary of recommended entry-level guidelines for academic courses and fieldwork for pediatric OTRs is presented in Table 2.

Table 2.   Summary of guidelines for entry-level practice for pediatric occupational therapists

Topic	Academic and Level I fieldwork	Level II fieldwork
Typical and atypical development	Concepts and theories of child development Stages of development in sensory motor, perceptual, cognitive, and social and/or emotional development Critical developmental variables Appropriate life tasks and roles, evaluation and treatment	Interpret information related to developmental status and provide assistance to caregivers in adapting environment.
Family issues	Family systems theory, including life cycle Ecology of family life within society Emotional and social impact of disability on family life and of family member's dysfunctional behavior on the child	Establish rapport with caregivers. Engage in collaborative consultation.
Pediatric diagnoses	Etiology, characteristics, effect on performance, principles of medical and educational intervention Principles of occupational therapy assessment and intervention, strategies for gaining information Diagnoses most frequently encountered by pediatric occupational therapists: cerebral palsy, mental retardation/developmental disorders, learning disabilities/attention deficit disorder, pervasive developmental disorders, emotional and behavioral disturbance	Use appropriate resources to recognize and identify diagnoses in specific children. Interpret impact of diagnosis on life stages.
Intervention process, including assessment	Understand commonly used approaches: developmental, perceptual-motor, compensatory, biomechanical, occupational behavior and/or human occupation Introduction to advanced approaches: neurodevelopmental training, behavioral, psychodynamics, sensory integration	Select appropriate approach for a specific child.
Assessment	Assessment methods and procedures for performance areas and components outlined in *Uniform Terminology for Occupational Therapy* (AOTA, 1994) Psychometric qualities and developmental performance components of normal and criterion-referenced tests	Select assessment in collaboration with primary caregiver for specific child. Administer, score, and interpret tests for each performance component or area

(continued)

Table 2. *(continued)*

Topic	Academic and Level I fieldwork	Level II fieldwork
	Clinical observations of performance Effects of child behavior on test results Interpretation of functional performance Documentation	from *Uniform Terminology for Occupational Therapy* (AOTA, 1994). Report in jargon-free language.
Treatment planning and implementation	Knowledge of age-appropriate performance areas and components in the domain of pediatric occupational therapy Application, including treatment approaches, performance objectives, and intervention strategies to specific case study Interrelationship of age, disability, family issues, service delivery model, setting, and team goals, and their impact on treatment goals	Apply academic and Level I fieldwork requirements to specific child. Implement and adapt intervention activities based on a specific child (with supervision). Recognize when to refer
Management of pediatric occupational therapy services	Characteristics, mission, finances, and structure of typical service provision settings (medical, community, education, home) and impact on occupational therapy services Recognition of impact of legislation and payment sources on occupational therapy intervention Models of team interaction (multi-, inter-, and transdisciplinary) and service delivery (direct → consultation)	Identify family needs and desired outcomes with service setting and models of delivery. Identify impact of legislation on occupational therapy intervention for specific child.

Source: AOTA, Commission on Education. (1991).

Advanced Training in Pediatrics

A third section identified in AOTA's *Guidelines for Curriculum Content in Pediatrics* describes education and experience beyond entry-level preparation. Topics covered include understanding how a variety of diagnoses and developmental problems may interact and influence a child's occupational behavior over time; developing skills in advanced approaches, such as sensory integration; developing assessment procedures for an entire program, not just an individual child; working with infants and caregivers in neonatal intensive care units; and serving as a service coordinator and participating in state and regional early childhood committees and boards. Occupational therapists develop advanced skills in pediatrics through graduate training, continuing education outside of universities, on-the-job training, and relationships with mentors.

Following entry-level preparation at the master's or bachelor's level, occupational therapists can seek a master's degree in a specialty of occupational therapy (e.g., working with very young children with disabilities). Of all the occupational therapists in the United States, 13% have earned a graduate degree; however, among those occupational therapists who work in early intervention, 27% have graduate degrees (AOTA, 1990; Hanft, 1991b). This difference most likely reflects the general view within the profession that practice in early intervention is considered to be a specialty area and therefore warrants advanced education and training in order to ensure effective intervention (AOTA, 1989; Case-Smith, 1994; Hanft, 1989a). Graduate education for therapists practicing in early intervention is typically completed in related fields, such as special education or child development, as well as pediatric occupational therapy.

Among the most influential training programs designed to facilitate interdisciplinary team skills and expertise in developmental disabilities are those offered by universities with interdisciplinary centers serving individuals with neurodevelopmental and related disorders (i.e., university affiliated programs). These centers were initially established in 1962 with federal funds to provide preservice training, research, and service to individuals with developmental disabilities. Such interdisciplinary centers, as well as other early intervention projects, have trained therapists in team skills that ensure equality among members, effective strategies for communicating, and development of family-centered strategies (Bruder, Brinckerhoff, & Spence, 1991; Hiranaka, 1992).

In 1992, the AOTA initiated a process to designate specialization in pediatrics for practicing occupational therapists. Therapists who have worked for 5 or more years in pediatrics and who meet specific criteria related to teaching, mentoring, research, and continuing education are eligible to take a written examination. Questions cover pediatric occupational therapy theory, as well as assessment and treatment for infants, children, and adolescents in medical, education, and early intervention settings. As of 1995, 240 therapists had taken the pediatric specialty certification exam.

CONCLUDING REMARKS: FUTURE DIRECTIONS

This chapter has focused on three major topics: 1) defining occupational therapy and emphasizing intervention in early childhood settings, 2) discussing principles of recommended practice for interdisciplinary teamwork, and 3) professional preparation of occupational therapists and certified occupational therapy assistants to work with children. Five principles have been identified that reflect the recommended practice for preparing occupational therapists to work effectively on interdisciplinary, early childhood teams with family members and colleagues.

1. The family is the core of the interdisciplinary team.
2. Families function as unique systems within social and cultural systems.
3. Team members should provide options and choices.
4. Team members share functions and information.
5. Team members should understand each family story and expectations for service.

Selected readings and learning activities for students are provided for each of the five principles of recommended practice to illustrate supportive training practices.

Traditional teams focus almost exclusively on providing direct intervention to remediate children's delays, maintain their skills, and/or adapt the environment. In contrast, recommended practice in occupational therapy in early childhood views family members as equally important consumers of occupational therapy services. Although therapists provide developmental assessment and direct intervention for individual children, they also assist family members and other colleagues in achieving desired outcomes for the child. Collaboration with the family and other team members is an ongoing process and ultimately leads to the identification of *meaningful* outcomes toward which all team members should work. Collaborative teamwork requires that all team members share information and develop joint goals and intervention plans, rather than have each team member develop and work on his or her own goals and intervention activities. "When professionals work collaboratively with families, not only are families empowered, but professionals gain new insight that enables them to teach, treat and understand in different ways" (AOTA, 1989, p. 17).

REFERENCES

Allen, D., & Hudd, S. (1987). Are we professionalizing parents? Weighing the benefits and pitfalls. *Journal of Mental Retardation, 25,* 133–137.

American Occupational Therapy Association (AOTA). (1988). *Occupational therapy and early intervention.* Unpublished survey results. Rockville, MD: Author .

American Occupational Therapy Association (AOTA). (1989). *Guidelines for occupational therapy services in early intervention and preschool services.* Rockville, MD: Author.

American Occupational Therapy Association (AOTA). (1990). *Member data survey.* Rockville, MD: Author.

American Occupational Therapy Association (AOTA). (1991a). *Essentials and guidelines for an accredited educational program for the certified occupational therapy assistant.* Rockville, MD: Author.

American Occupational Therapy Association (AOTA). (1991b). *Essentials and guidelines for an accredited educational program for the occupational therapist.* Rockville, MD: Author.

American Occupational Therapy Association (AOTA). (1994). *Uniform terminology for occupational therapy* (3rd. ed.). Rockville, MD: Author.

American Occupational Therapy Association (AOTA), Commission on Education. (1991). *Guidelines for curriculum content in pediatrics.* Rockville, MD: Author.

Bazyk, S. (1989). Changes in attitudes and beliefs regarding parent participation and home programs: An update. *American Journal of Occupational Therapy, 43,* 723–728.

Briggs, A., & Howe, M. (1988). Ecological systems model for occupational therapy. *American Journal of Occupational Therapy, 36*(5), 322–327.

Bruder, M., Brinckerhoff, J., & Spence, K. (1991). Meeting the personnel needs of PL 99-457: A model interdisciplinary institute for infant specialists. *Teacher Education and Special Education, 14*(2), 77–87.

Burke, J. (1993). Play: The life of the infant and young child. In J. Case-Smith (Ed.), *Pediatric occupational therapy and early intervention* (pp. 198–221). Boston: Andover Medical Publishers.

Case-Smith, J. (1991). The family perspective. In W. Dunn (Ed.), *Pediatric occupational therapy: Facilitating effective service delivery.* Thorofare, NJ: Slack.

Case-Smith, J. (1994). Defining the specialization of pediatric occupational therapy. *American Journal of Occupational Therapy, 48*(9), 791–802.

Case-Smith, J., & Wavrek, B.B. (1993). Models of service delivery and team interaction. In J. Case-Smith (Ed.), *Pediatric occupational therapy and early intervention* (pp. 27–159). Boston: Andover Medical Publishers.

Csikszentmihalyi, M., & LeFevre, J. (1989). Optimal experience in work and leisure. *Journal of Personality and Social Psychology, 58*(5), 815–822.

Darling, R. (1989). Using the social system perspective in early intervention: The value of a sociological approach. *Journal of Early Intervention, 13*(1), 24–35.

Decker, B. (1992). A comparison of the individualized education plan and the individualized family service plan. *American Journal of Occupational Therapy, 46*(3), 247–252.

Education of the Handicapped Act Amendments of 1986, PL 99-457. (October 8, 1986). Title 20, U.S.C. 1400 et seq: *U.S. Statutes at Large, 100,* 1145–1177.

Geissinger, S., Humphry, R., Hanft, B., & Keyes, L. (1993). Assessing changes in professional attitudes: Effects of continuing education. *Journal of Continuing Education in the Health Professions, 13,* 99–116.

Glass, R., & Wolf, L. (1993). Feeding and oral-motor skills. In J. Case-Smith (Ed)., *Pediatric occupational therapy and early intervention* (pp. 225–288). Boston: Andover Medical Publishers.

Gorga, D. (1989). Occupational therapy treatment practices with infants in early intervention. *American Journal of Occupational Therapy, 43*(11), 731–736.

Hanft, B. (1988). The changing environment of early intervention services: Implications for practice. *American Journal of Occupational Therapy, 42,* 724–731.

Hanft, B. (1989a). Early intervention: Issues in specialization. *American Journal of Occupational Therapy, 43*(7), 431–434.

Hanft, B. (Ed.). (1989b). *Family-centered care: An early intervention resource manual.* Rockville, MD: American Occupational Therapy Association.

Hanft, B. (1991a). Impact of federal policy on pediatric health and education programs. In W. Dunn (Ed.), *Pediatric occupational therapy: Facilitating effective service provision* (pp. 273–284). Thorofare, NJ: Slack.

Hanft, B. (1991b). *Training occupational therapists in early intervention* (Final report). Rockville, MD: American Occupational Therapy Association.

Hanft, B. (1994). The "good" parent: A label by any other name would not smell as sweet. *Developmental Disabilities Special Interest Newsletter, 17*(4), 5.

Hanft, B., Burke, J., Cahill, M., Swenson-Miller, K., & Humphry, R. (1992). *Working with families: A curriculum guide for pediatric occupational therapists.* Chapel Hill, NC: Carolina Institute for Research on Infant Personnel Preparation.

Hanft, B., Geissinger, S., & Hunt, M. (1994). *Involving families in preparing professionals to provide family-centered care: Perspectives of parents and professionals.* Unpublished paper.

Hanson, M., & Lovett, D. (1992). Personnel preparation for early interventionists: A cross-disciplinary survey. *Journal of Early Intervention, 16*(2), 123–135.

Henry, A., Nelson, D., & Duncombe, L. (1984). Choice making in group and individual activity. *American Journal of Occupational Therapy, 38*(4), 245–251.

Hiranaka, C. (1992, Sept. 2). Preparing for leadership roles in developmental disabilities. *OT Week,* 6.

Holloway, E., Glass, R., & Wolf, L. (1993). Early emotional development and sensory processing. In J. Case-Smith (Ed.), *Pediatric occupational therapy and early intervention* (pp. 163–197). Boston: Andover Medical Publishers.

Hopkins, H., & Smith, H.D. (Eds.). (1993). *Willard and Spackman's occupational therapy* (8th ed.). Philadelphia: J.B. Lippincott.

Humphry, R. (1989). Early intervention and the influence of the occupational therapist on the parent-child relationship. *American Journal of Occupational Therapy, 43*(11), 738–742.

Humphry, R., & Geissinger, S. (1993). Issues in early intervention: Measuring attitudes about family-centered care. *The Occupational Therapy Journal of Research, 13*(5), 163–182.

Humphry, R., & Link, S. (1990). Entry-level preparation of occupational therapists to work in early intervention program. *American Journal of Occupational Therapy, 44*(9), 828–833.

Hunt, M., Cornelius, P., Levanthal, P., Miller, P., Murray, T., & Stoner, G. (1991). *Into our lives.* (Available from the Family Child Learning Center, 90 W. Overdale Drive, Tallmadge, OH 44278)

Individuals with Disabilities Education Act Amendments of 1991, PL 102-119. (October 7, 1991). Title 20, U.S.C. 1400 et seq: *U.S. Statutes at Large, 105,* 587–608.

Kielhofner, G., & Burke, J.P. (1977). Occupational therapy after 60 years: An account of changing identity and knowledge. *American Journal of Occupational Therapy, 31*(10), 675–689.

Kjerland, L., & Kovach, J. (1990). Family–staff collaboration for tailored infant assessment. In E.D. Gibbs & D.M. Teti (Eds.), *Interdisciplinary assessment of infants: A guide for early intervention professionals* (pp. 287–297). Baltimore: Paul H. Brookes Publishing Co.

Lawler, M. (1989). A descriptive study of the clinical practice patterns of occupational therapists working with young children. *American Journal of Occupational Therapy, 43*(11), 755–764.

Lyon, J. (1989). I want to be Zak's Mom, not his therapist. *Developmental Disabilities Special Interest Newsletter, 12*(1), 4.

Maple, G. (1987). Early intervention: Some issues in cooperative team work. *Australian Journal of Occupational Therapy, 34*(4), 145–151.

Mattingly, C., & Fleming, M. (1993). *Clinical reasoning: Forms of inquiry in a therapeutic practice.* Philadelphia: F.A. Davis.

Miller, L. (1994). Journey to a desirable future: A values-based model of infant and toddler assessment. *Zero to Three, 14*(16), 23–27.

Miller, L., Lynch, E., & Campbell, J. (1990). Parents as partners: A new paradigm for collaboration. *Best Practices in School Speech-Language Pathology, 1*, 40–56.

Moersch, M. (1989). Parent and family involvement. In P. Pratt & A. Allen (Eds.), *Occupational therapy with children* (pp. 132–146). St. Louis: C.V. Mosby.

Nelson, D., Thompson, J., & Moore, J. (1982). Identification of factors of affective meaning in four selected activities. *American Journal of Occupational Therapy, 36*(6), 381–387.

Ottenbacher, K. (1991). Conflicting views: Who knows best? In C. Royeen (Ed.), *School-based practice for related services* (Lesson 2). Rockville, MD: American Occupational Therapy Association.

Parush, S., & Clark, F. (1988). The reliability and validity of a sensory development questionnaire. *American Journal of Occupational Therapy, 42*, 11–16.

Pizzo, P. (1990). Parent advocacy: A resource for early intervention. In S. Meisels & J. Shonkoff (Eds.), *Handbook of early childhood intervention* (pp. 668–678). New York: Cambridge University Press.

Poncher, H., & Richmond, J. (1947). Occupational therapy in pediatrics. *American Journal of Occupational Therapy, 1*, 276–280.

Poulsen, M. (1993). Strategies for building resilience in infants and young children at risk. *Infants and Young Children, 6*(2), 29–40.

Reed, K. (1993). The beginnings of occupational therapy. In H.L. Hopkins & H.D. Smith (Eds.), *Willard and Spackman's occupational therapy* (8th ed., pp. 26–43). Philadelphia: J.B. Lippincott.

Rocco, S. (1994). New visions for the developmental assessment of infants and young children: A parent's perspective. *Zero to Three, 14*(16), 13–15.

Schaaf, R., & Mulrooney, L. (1989). Occupational therapy in early intervention: A family-centered approach. *American Journal of Occupational Therapy, 43*(11), 745–754.

Stallings-Sahler, S. (1993). Sensory integration: Assessment and intervention. In J. Case-Smith (Ed.), *Pediatric occupational therapy and early intervention* (pp. 309–341). Boston: Andover Medical Publishers.

Stewart, K. (1989). Collaborating with families: Reflections on empowerment. In B. Hanft (Ed.), *Family-centered care: An early intervention resource manual* (Section 2, pp. 71–77). Rockville, MD: American Occupational Therapy Association.

Swinth, Y., & Case-Smith, J. (1993). Assistive technology in early intervention: Theory and practice. In J. Case-Smith (Ed.), *Pediatric occupational therapy and early intervention* (pp. 342–368). Boston: Andover Medical Publishers.

Turnbull, A.P., & Turnbull, H.R., III. (1990). Family interaction. In A. Turnbull & R. Turnbull (Eds.), *Families, professionals and exceptionality: A special partnership* (2nd ed., pp. 52–76). Columbus, OH: Charles E. Merrill.

Tyler, N., & Chandler, L. (1978). The developmental therapists: The occupational therapist and physical therapist. In E. Allen, V. Holm, & R. Schiefelbusch (Eds.), *Early intervention—A team approach* (pp. 169–198). Baltimore: University Park Press.

Tyler, N., Kogan, K., & Turner, P. (1974). Interpersonal components of therapy with young cerebral palsied. *American Journal of Occupational Therapy, 28,* 395–400.

Watson, C. (1994). Behind every dedicated parent is a person who needs support. *Developmental Disabilities Special Interest Newsletter, 17*(4), 5.

Zeitlin, S., & Williamson, G. (1994). *Coping in young children: Early intervention practices to enhance adaptive behavior and resilience.* Baltimore: Paul H. Brookes Publishing Co.

7

PREPARING PHYSICAL THERAPISTS

Irene R. McEwen
and M'Lisa L. Shelden

The traditional picture of physical therapy with young children shows a smiling child sitting or lying on a large, colorful ball. Although the picture is still visually appealing, it represents a bygone mode of intervention. The ball belongs to an era when pediatric physical therapists focused on children's balance reactions, muscle tone, and other neuromusculoskeletal impairments, assuming that improved movement during therapy sessions would carry over to meaningful functional skills in real-life environments. Partially as a result of increased knowledge of motor learning principles, physical therapists are now more likely to be found working in natural environments with other team members on functional activities that are individually meaningful to children and their families. A physical therapist might, for example, go to a grocery store with a family to help solve the problem of seating a child who lacks postural control in a grocery cart or work with a child care provider to promote a child's motor development during typical daily activities.

WHEN INFANTS AND YOUNG CHILDREN have neuromuscular, musculoskeletal, or cardiopulmonary impairments, physical therapists are often members of their early intervention teams. Unlike some of the other team members, physical therapists are usually not extensively prepared to work with children, and they often receive little exposure to or experience with infants and families in their professional preparation programs; therefore, they must build on their academic foundations with additional educational experiences following graduation. This chapter describes a series of professional and postprofessional educational activities that help physical therapists to gain the attitudes, skills, and knowledge they need to work effectively with infants and young children, families, and other team members. The major roles that physical therapists must learn to assume when providing early intervention services are listed in Table 1 (Cochrane, Farley, & Wilhelm, 1990).

Preparation of this chapter was partially supported by a Preparation of Related Services Personnel grant (#H029F30020) from the U.S. Department of Education, Office of Special Education and Rehabilitative Services. The contents, however, do not necessarily represent the policy of the agency, and no official endorsement should be inferred.

Table 1.   Major roles of physical therapists working with infants and preschool-age children and their families

1. Screening for neuromusculoskeletal, cardiopulmonary, and general developmental dysfunction
2. Assessing children's neuromusculoskeletal status and motor skills for differential diagnosis
3. Assessing children's cardiopulmonary status
4. Designing, implementing, and monitoring therapeutic interventions
5. Evaluating intervention effectiveness and modifying programs as needed
6. Identifying with the family their strengths, priorities, and concerns
7. Developing family recommendations and monitoring their implementation
8. Participating in interdisciplinary planning
9. Consulting with the family members and caregivers
10. Consulting with and referring to other professionals and community agencies
11. Serving as service coordinators
12. Recommending or fabricating adaptive equipment and mobility devices
13. Recommending or implementing environmental modifications

Adapted by permission from Cochrane, Farley, & Wilhelm (1990).

Physical therapists working in early intervention need certain disciplinary and cross-disciplinary expertise that is unique to infants and young children, their families, and early intervention teams; general knowledge and skill in pediatric physical therapy are not sufficient. Little data or other information exist, however, about the preparation of physical therapists to work specifically in early intervention programs. For this reason, this chapter includes content related to general pediatric specialization in physical therapy (including birth to age 21), which is an essential basis for subspecialization in early intervention. When available, information specific to early intervention is reviewed. Although some chapters of this book define the term *early intervention* to include children older than 2 years, the term as used in this chapter refers to programs and services for children from birth to 2 years old and their families. This chapter focuses on this age range because, according to Part H of PL 101-476, the Individuals with Disabilities Education Act (IDEA) of 1990, physical therapy as an early intervention service for children between birth and 2 years old is philosophically and legally different from physical therapy as a related service for children 3 years and older (described in Part B of the law).

OVERVIEW OF PHYSICAL THERAPY EDUCATION

There are three general types of personnel preparation programs for physical therapists: professional education, postprofessional graduate education, and postprofessional continuing education. Physical therapy education also includes 2-year associate degree programs for physical therapist assistants who work under the supervision of physical therapists. Although physical therapist assistants can be valuable members of early intervention teams, particularly in center-based programs, this chapter focuses on preparation of physical therapists.

Professional Education

The term *professional education* is used to designate preparation of physical therapists for their first professional degree, which can be at the bachelor's, master's, or doctoral level. These programs were formerly called *entry-level* in physical therapy and are often referred to as *preservice* in teacher education programs.

In early 1995, there were 140 accredited physical therapist professional education programs in the United States and 32 developing programs in the process of accreditation (American Physical Therapy Association [APTA], personal communication, January 9, 1995). Of the accredited programs, 64 were bachelor's degree programs and 76 were master's degree programs. There has been a trend since the 1970s toward the master's degree as the professional-level degree, a trend that the APTA has encouraged. Newly developing programs are usually at the master's (or doctoral) degree level, and established baccalaureate-level programs are continuing to convert to master's degree programs as institutional support for the change is secured. Prior to the 1960s, certificate programs for students with degrees in other fields were common, but APTA now lists only four schools that offer a certificate option ("Education Programs," 1994).

The first professional-level doctoral program, at Creighton University in Nebraska, accepted its inaugural class of students for the doctor of physical therapy (D.P.T.) degree in 1993. D.P.T. programs emphasize clinical practice and are therefore different from Ph.D. programs, which have a research orientation. Some physical therapists now see the D.P.T. as the appropriate professional-level degree, but this opinion has generated a great deal of discussion and controversy within the profession (Soderberg, 1993). Those who support the professional-level D.P.T. believe that doctoral-level education is essential to prepare physical therapists with the expertise required for contemporary practice. Others believe that such problems as increased costs, lack of an adequate number of qualified faculty, and confusion resulting from multiple professional-level degrees outweigh any advantages (Hummer, Hunt, & Figuers, 1994). The trend toward doctoral-level education is just beginning, so it will be interesting to examine the bachelor's, master's, and doctoral program options available in the 21st century.

Postprofessional Graduate Education

Physical therapists who have a professional-level degree or certificate can pursue postprofessional master's or doctoral degrees. Postprofessional programs often focus on one or more specialized areas of practice, such as pediatrics, musculoskeletal disorders, or sports physical therapy. This is in contrast to professional-level programs, which must cover the broad scope of physical therapy practice. In December 1994, APTA published a list of postprofessional programs in the United States and Canada that included 48 master's degree programs and 13 doctoral degree programs ("Education Programs," 1994).

Postprofessional Continuing Education

Many physical therapists acquire the expertise they need to work effectively with infants and young children and their families through continuing education. As discussed later in this chapter, professional-level education prepares physical therapists to provide services across the broad scope of practice, and pediatric content is often extremely limited. It is only after they are licensed professionals that many physical therapists have an opportunity to gain expertise in pediatrics and develop a subspecialty in early intervention (Stuberg & McEwen, 1993).

Short courses, in-service courses at a place of employment, conference presentations, and self-study are common sources of continuing education (Reynolds, 1994a). Fellowships, clinical residencies, and courses that are several weeks or months in length are also highly valued by many therapists (Long & Sippel, 1995). Information about continuing education courses is disseminated widely in general physical therapy publications, publications of the APTA Section on Pediatrics, and publications of cross-disciplinary organizations to which some pediatric physical therapists belong, such as the Council for Exceptional Children, Division for Early Childhood, and the American Academy for Cerebral Palsy and Developmental Medicine.

A growing number of states now have professional development requirements for license renewal, thus ensuring that therapists participate in a minimum amount of continuing education to maintain a license to practice. The effect of this requirement on practice, however, is controversial (Hruska & Harden, 1994), with much of the debate centered on the lack of quality control of the continuing education experiences.

Accreditation

Professional-level programs must be accredited if their graduates are to be eligible for licensure. Program accreditation is conducted through APTA's appointed and independently functioning body, the Commission of Accreditation in Physical Therapy Education (CAPTE). CAPTE is recognized by the Council on Postsecondary Accreditation and the U.S. Department of Education as the sole authority in the United States to accredit physical therapist and physical therapist assistant education programs. As of 1996, only professional-level education programs are accredited through APTA. Neither postprofessional master's nor doctoral degree programs are included in the accreditation program, although these programs are usually affiliated with colleges or universities that are accredited by regional and national accrediting associations.

The APTA Department of Education is developing guidelines for accreditation, approval, or other types of recognition for continuing education courses and clinical residencies. This effort is in response to APTA members' requests for help in knowing which continuing education courses meet certain standards of quality. The provision of continuing education has become a major business within the profession and most physical therapists highly value it, but the quality of the offerings varies greatly.

LICENSURE AND CERTIFICATION

Licensure and certification are two credentialing processes in physical therapy. A license is required to practice, whereas certification in specialty areas of physical therapy is voluntary.

Licensure

Following graduation, physical therapists must become licensed before they can practice in any of the 50 states, the District of Columbia, Puerto Rico, or the U.S. Virgin Islands. Each state or other entity administers its own licensure regulations, so physical therapists must apply and qualify for a separate license in each locale in which they work. Regardless of where they practice, physical therapists must pass an examination that was developed by the Committee on Licensure Examinations of the Federation of State Boards of Physical Therapy, which is administered by the Professional Examination Service. Passing scores and additional requirements vary somewhat from state to state. The examination is given three times a year, in March, July, and November ("State Licensing Agencies," 1994).

After becoming licensed, physical therapists can use the letters P.T. after their names. Since 1978, APTA has recommended the use of P.T., rather than R.P.T. or L.P.T., unless required by state law (APTA, 1994). This recommendation is based on the fact that one must be licensed to be a physical therapist (making the L redundant), and the R indicates recognition by a registry that ceased to exist once licensure was required by all states.

Pediatric Clinical Specialist Certification

Physical therapists with advanced skills in pediatrics can pursue clinical specialist certification through the American Board of Physical Therapy Specialties (ABPTS). ABPTS is a component of APTA that oversees clinical specialist certification in the following seven areas of physical therapy practice: cardiopulmonary, clinical electrophysiologic, geriatric, neurologic, orthopedic, pediatric, and sports physical therapy.

Each area has a three-member specialty council that is responsible for development of examinations and other certification requirements, using guidelines established by ABPTS. The content of examinations is based on an analysis of advanced clinical practice, conducted at least every 10 years. The last analysis of pediatric practice was reported in *Description of Advanced Clinical Practice: Pediatric Physical Therapy* (ABPTS, Pediatric Specialty Council, 1994), which defined advanced clinical practice in the pediatric area and the specific knowledge and skills required of pediatric specialists.

Physical therapists who receive pediatric clinical specialist certification can use the professional designation P.C.S. following P.T. after their names. Certification is limited to 10 years, after which therapists must meet recertification requirements to maintain their clinical specialist certification.

Certification for Early Intervention and Public School Programs

Some states require that physical therapists working in public schools or early intervention programs have additional certification specific to those settings. Washington State, for example, requires Educational Staff Associate certification for all nonteaching professional staff. To become certified to work in schools or early intervention programs, physical therapists usually need additional courses and/or experiences that provide knowledge and skill needed in these specialized settings.

MAJOR ISSUES AND BARRIERS IN PERSONNEL PREPARATION

There are a number of issues to consider and barriers to overcome if an adequate number of physical therapists who are well-qualified to work with infants and young children and their families are to be prepared. Some of the most important issues and barriers include 1) the content of professional education programs, 2) the availability of postprofessional education in pediatric physical therapy, 3) the content of continuing education courses, 4) the shortage of physical therapists and physical therapy faculty, and 5) the location of many physical therapy programs. Each of these issues is discussed below.

General Professional Education Content

Physical therapy professional education programs prepare students to be competent generalists, capable of entering any of the many settings in which physical therapists practice. Sports medicine clinics, outpatient orthopedic practices, nursing homes, and hospitals are but a few of the practice sites in which students must be prepared to work. Unique aspects of pediatric practice, including disciplinary and cross-disciplinary content related to early intervention programs, must compete for space in the curricula of a profession in which less than 10% are pediatric practitioners (APTA, personal communication, July 26, 1994).

The *Accreditation Handbook* (APTA, 1990) includes little that is unique to pediatric practice and much that is only marginally related. Programs are required to document, for example, that graduates of the program can implement a comprehensive treatment plan that includes, but is not limited to, 25 types of treatment. Of these, usually only "developmental activities" are unique to children. The value of content in other areas that could be important, such as "patient/family education," depends on how faculty view the family in the intervention process. The criterion that a graduate's plan of care must include "collaboration with patients, families, those individuals responsible for the patient, and colleagues" (p. B-31) also opens the door for content related to family-guided, team-oriented collaboration, but it need not.

Professional Education Content Specific
to Working with Infants, Young Children, and Families

In 1989, the Carolina Institute for Research on Infant Personnel Preparation (1993) conducted a study to determine the unique issues associated with preparation of professionals from multiple disciplines to work with infants and toddlers with disabilities and their families. Based on data from professional preparation programs in physical therapy and other disciplines, the researchers concluded that at the time of the survey, most of the instruction related to assessment and intervention with infants and toddlers was inadequate for effective practice, and that little time was spent on family assessment, team processes, or case management. Across disciplines, the greatest educational needs were related to family issues and team collaboration (Bailey, Simeonsson, Yoder, & Huntington, 1990).

Data specific to physical therapy strongly reflect the overall findings of the study. Cochrane et al. (1990) reported that although most of the professional-level programs they surveyed provided some instruction in topics related to infants, the number of clock hours varied widely and many students received little or no instruction in family-related topics or clinical experience working with families.

The Education Committee of the APTA Section on Pediatrics reported similar findings from a survey of professional-level physical therapy education programs. The survey was conducted to identify curriculum structure and content in pediatric physical therapy during the 1990–1991 academic year (Cherry & Knutson, 1993). Nearly all of the programs who responded to the survey (76 of 123 programs, for a 62% return rate) reported that their programs require content related to child development (97%), pediatric disorders (99%), and management of pediatric conditions (93%). The amount of time spent teaching these three content areas varied widely, however, ranging from a few hours to more than 60 hours, with most programs spending between 11 and 20 hours in each of the areas. There was a trend toward a greater amount of time spent on child development topics than on pediatric disorders and management of pediatric conditions.

Experiences *with* children were more limited than content *about* children. Laboratory experiences in assessment of children were required by 82% of the programs, optional in 5% of the programs, and not available in 13% of the programs reporting. Only 51% of the programs offered laboratory experience in treatment of children, 20% provided optional experience, and 29% provided no laboratory experience. Most of the students who had laboratory experiences in assessment and treatment of children spent 2–4 hours in these areas, with somewhat more time usually spent on assessment than on treatment. Laboratory experiences in physical therapy education are part of students' didactic coursework and are often supervised by academic faculty. By contrast, clinical affiliations are required field-based experiences, from several days to several weeks in length, that are supervised by volunteer clinical instructors[1] who work in the clinical settings. Of the programs surveyed, 8% reported that they required clinical experiences in pediatric settings, 85% offered the students a choice of one pediatric clinical affiliation, and pediatric clinical affiliations were available by lottery in the remaining 7% of programs.

Although most of the data Cherry and Knutson (1993) reported concerned pediatric physical therapy in general, some of the data are more specific to early intervention. These data suggest that fewer professional-level students receive academic content related to important features of early intervention than receive general pediatric information and experiences.

Only 58% of programs reporting taught family-centered care, with a mean of 0.8 hours spent on this topic (range 0–10). The roles of other professionals were taught in 84% of programs (mean 1.5 hours, range 0–30 hours) and consultation by 52% of programs (mean 0.7 hours, range 0.2–5 hours). Individualized educa-

---

[1]Clinical instructors are physical therapists who agree to supervise and teach students in their practice settings. Neither they nor their employers are usually paid by the student or the school for this instruction.

tion program (IEP) content was taught by 70% of programs (mean 1.7 hours, range 0–6 hours) and individualized family service plan (IFSP) content by 52% of programs (mean 1 hour, range 0–3 hours). Because this was a survey of content taught during the 1990–1991 academic year, which was before many states had implemented IFSP requirements, it is likely that the number of programs teaching IFSP content has risen to the number of programs teaching IEP content (70%).

Clinical instructors can fill some of the important gaps in academic content for students who have clinical affiliations in an early intervention setting. The appropriateness of the experiences, however, will depend on the knowledge and skill of the instructor, which probably will not reflect up-to-date practices unless the therapist has had *recent* postprofessional education. Most therapists were, and many still are, prepared to provide discipline-specific treatment, focusing almost entirely on the individual's neuromusculoskeletal and cardiopulmonary problems. In pediatric physical therapy there has been gradual movement toward a more child- and family-centered team approach since the mid-1970s, following the enactment of PL 94-142, the Education for All Handicapped Children Act of 1975, and the passage of PL 99-457, the Education of the Handicapped Act Amendments of 1986. There has also been considerable change in many assessment and intervention strategies since the early 1990s, away from traditional developmental approaches toward more functional, systems-oriented approaches that incorporate motor learning principles (Lister, 1991).

Pediatric Postprofessional Graduate Education

Effgen (1993) surveyed 21 master's degree programs listed by APTA as having a specialty in pediatrics or developmental disabilities. She found that many of the programs had few, if any, courses in pediatrics or developmental disabilities and no pediatric curriculum. She concluded that there are no more than nine universities in the United States "where a potential graduate student can get [postprofessional] master's [level] . . . education in pediatric physical therapy" (p. 137). Effgen found only one physical therapy doctoral program with pediatric specialization.

Because there are few postprofessional programs in pediatric physical therapy, many physical therapists interested in working with children and obtaining a postprofessional degree do their graduate work in a related area, such as education, psychology, or basic biomedical sciences (Effgen, 1993). This is especially true at the doctoral level. The scarcity of postprofessional graduate education in pediatric physical therapy can be seen as a positive situation because it leads many therapists to pursue degrees in related areas with professionals of other disciplines, thus enhancing their opportunities to develop transdisciplinary communication, knowledge, and skills. The lack of postprofessional programs is also a problem because it limits opportunities for therapists to gain up-to-date specialized disciplinary knowledge and skill, to advance disciplinary knowledge through research, and to share this information through teaching (Effgen, 1993).

Continuing Education

Physical therapy continuing education courses typically involve discipline-specific content with "hands-on" experiences to improve technical skills. Attendees are usually physical therapists, although it is common for occupational therapists and physical therapists to attend the same courses, especially when the emphasis is pediatrics. Historically, most of the continuing education courses attended by physical therapists working with infants and young children with disabilities have emphasized skill attainment or refinement in such areas as neurodevelopmental treatment, sensory integration, myofascial release, and splinting. These and similar content areas often reflect child-focused services that, when combined with a paucity of cross-disciplinary training opportunities, limit implementation of family-centered practices when working with infants and young children with disabilities. Therapists need child-focused clinical information, but family-focused, team-oriented content must be a foundation for all continuing education if physical therapists are to become capable of providing appropriate, high-quality early intervention services (Bailey, McWilliam, & Winton, 1992).

Shortage of Physical Therapists

It is widely known that there is a shortage of physical therapists in most areas of practice and in nearly every part of the United States (Glickman, 1993). Although there are indications that health care reform efforts have reduced the shortage somewhat, there is still an unmet need for physical therapists that has implications for preparation of physical therapists to work in early intervention programs.

One important implication is that the shortage of physical therapists has resulted in a great influx of applicants to professional education programs, applicants who, pragmatically, wish to enter a profession that the U.S. Department of Labor lists as one of the professions that will be in greatest demand until at least the year 2010. Rozier and Hamilton (1991) found that good salary, job availability, and an opportunity for work variety are the primary reasons that students chose physical therapy as a career. Because of the demand, the typical physical therapy professional education program receives many more applications than it has spaces for students. Students often apply year after year, hoping they will eventually be accepted.

Highly competitive admission to physical therapy professional programs makes it unrealistic to focus recruitment efforts on preprofessional students with interest in working with children and hope that they will be admitted. Instead, physical therapy faculty with interest in pediatrics usually also attempt to recruit and support students from within the program, and potential employers may provide scholarships and other incentives for students to join them when they graduate.

A related issue is that early intervention programs must compete with employers that often pay much higher salaries for physical therapy graduates, such as hospitals and home health agencies. Early intervention programs must also compete with areas of practice that are more attractive to many students and that some graduates consider to be more prestigious than a pediatric option, such as sports physical therapy or outpatient orthopedics practice. Because there is a great deal of demand for graduates and students can anticipate at least several good job offers while they are still in school, the number of students who wish to take a pediatric elective course or clinical affiliation, if available, may be limited.

Shortage of Faculty

Frustrated applicants, parents, and potential employers often ask why the physical therapy profession does not simply increase the number of education programs so all qualified students can be admitted. Although the number of programs has increased considerably since the mid-1980s to 140 programs in 1995 (APTA, personal communication, January 9, 1995), a primary factor limiting further growth is a critical shortage of physical therapy faculty (APTA, 1988). Few physical therapists enter the profession intending to become academicians and until relatively recently, few had master's or doctoral degrees. One of the major efforts of the APTA since the mid-1980s has been to increase the number of physical therapy faculty and the number of faculty with doctoral degrees (APTA, 1988; 1994).

The faculty shortage has affected pediatric physical therapy as well as other areas of practice. Cherry and Knutson (1993) found that many physical therapy education programs use adjunct or part-time faculty to teach pediatric content. They also found that, on average, only about half of the programs have faculty members who teach in the pediatric area more than 50% of the time. In some programs, pediatric content is taught by faculty whose primary interest and expertise are not in working with children and families, often because pediatric faculty cannot be found (Stuberg & McEwen, 1993). Obviously, the quality of these students' academic preparation in pediatrics is likely to be limited and it will probably be dated if faculty attempt to use their own pediatric education as a foundation for their teaching.

Location of Physical Therapy Education Programs

Traditionally, physical therapy has its strongest links with the health care field and many physical therapy programs are located in or near medical schools. Although there is a trend toward locating programs in other settings (Young, 1989), the academic health center location of many physical therapy programs can isolate students and faculty from non–health-related disciplines. This isolation, whether caused by tradition, attitudes, or distance, can require considerable effort and planning to promote communication and learning with students and faculty of other disciplines that provide early intervention services.

PRINCIPLES OF RECOMMENDED PRACTICE

Following an analysis of personnel preparation in physical therapy and seven other disciplines providing early intervention services, Bailey et al. (1990) concluded that it is unrealistic to expect development of specialized early intervention tracks within most preservice programs, except perhaps in special education and speech-language pathology. Given the need to work within existing programs, Bailey and his colleagues made four high-priority recommendations pertaining to young children and their families:

1. Students should be introduced to legislative mandates and receive an overview of available programs and services to help make them aware of early intervention as a career option.

2. Students should be exposed to real programs and services, as a way to "hook" them into this area of practice.
3. Instructional and clinical experiences in working with families should be increased, not necessarily with an exclusive early intervention focus.
4. Instructional and clinical experiences in which students work with professionals of other disciplines should be increased—again, not necessarily with a focus on early intervention.

These priorities are consistent with recommendations that pediatric physical therapists have proposed to expand relevant content in professional education programs, to recruit students to work with children and families, and to provide physical therapists with the information, attitudes, and skills they need to work effectively with children and their families (Effgen, 1992; Gandy, 1993).

To provide for the continuing education needs of providers of services for infants and toddlers with disabilities and their families, the Carolina Institute for Research on Infant Personnel Preparation (1993) recommended a change in the way that training was traditionally planned and implemented. Rather than each agency or profession carrying out its own professional development activities, a more effective model would coordinate training resources, priorities, and funds across traditional disciplinary boundaries. The various Part H partners (e.g., education, health, mental health, human services) need to develop transdisciplinary preservice and in-service training in collaboration with the professional organizations serving the members of their disciplines.

Through their professional and postprofessional educational activities, physical therapists can acquire attitudes and skills that have been identified as necessary for working effectively in certain pediatric settings. Competencies have been defined for therapists working in neonatal intensive care units (NICUs) (Scull & Deitz, 1989), early intervention (APTA, Task Force on Early Intervention, 1991), and educational environments (K. Martin, 1989). In its *Description of Advanced Clinical Practice: Pediatric Physical Therapy*, the ABPTS Pediatric Specialty Council (1994) also delineates competencies for physical therapists working with children and their families. This document serves as a basis for the examination for pediatric clinical specialist certification and, although it is not specific to early intervention, the competencies identified in 1994 reflect the increased emphasis on early intervention, families, and team-oriented service delivery since the mid-1980s.

Most of the NICU, early intervention, and educational environment competencies, and those defined in *Description of Advanced Clinical Practice: Pediatric Physical Therapy*, are not expected of entry-level therapists, as therapists are not expected to acquire such competencies in their professional-level programs. The competencies are meant to serve as guidelines for personnel standards, and a combination of professional and postprofessional education is required to achieve competence in these specialized areas of practice.

TRANSLATION TO PRACTICE IN THE FIELD

Translating recommended practices in early intervention education to practice in the field requires change at all levels of physical therapy education: professional, postprofessional graduate, and continuing education. Regardless of the educational level, the elements that Fenichel and Eggbeer (1991) described as essential in preparation of personnel to work with infants and young children and families should be considered:

1. Peer support within and across disciplines
2. A common basic level of knowledge across disciplines relative to typical issues of infants and toddlers with disabilities and their families
3. The need for direct observation and interaction with children and their families in a supervised training environment
4. The need for individualized supervision, which supports the idea of developing mentoring programs at the local level affording therapists the opportunity to develop skills in particular areas within the context of family-centered recommended practice

Professional-Level Education Programs

As mentioned previously, the time given to pediatric content in professional-level curricula is limited and many programs lack faculty with expertise in pediatrics, especially in working with infants and families. Even with these constraints, one effective way to begin teaching content necessary for physical therapists to work with young children and their families is to infuse team-oriented, child-, patient-, and family-centered attitudes and skills throughout the curriculum (Bailey et al., 1990; Cochrane et al., 1990). A change within the physical therapy profession that makes this infusion highly feasible is that the profession as a whole is beginning to recognize that regardless of the age or diagnosis of the individual, it is important to 1) involve the individuals, families, and other caregivers in determining goals and implementing intervention; 2) identify functional outcomes of intervention that are meaningful to the individuals and their families; 3) consider environmental influences on outcomes; and 4) promote collaboration among disciplines (Payton, Nelson, & Ozer, 1990; Reynolds, 1994b). Physical therapists and other professionals working with children and families have understood the importance of these issues for a long time, largely because of special education legislation and recommended practices (McEwen, 1994). Managed care and other health care reform approaches appear to be playing a similar role in raising the awareness of professionals working in varied health care settings with individuals of all ages.

In addition to infusing early intervention principles throughout the curriculum, faculty who can teach pediatric content must be recruited and appropriate clinical education experiences must be made available if physical therapy students are to be prepared to provide a basic level of early intervention services. Suggestions to address each of these issues are discussed below.

Infusing Early Intervention–Related Content Throughout the Curriculum

A working conference of pediatric physical therapy educators, convened by Cochrane et al. (1990) to examine early intervention personnel preparation, developed content recommendations for all professional-level physical therapy education, whether infused throughout the curriculum or taught as separate courses. Their recommendations are listed in Table 2.

Table 2. Recommended pediatric content for physical therapy professional-level curricula

1. Family-focused topics including family dynamics, family systems theory, and cultural and economic variations in family patterns
2. Service coordination including the role of the service coordinator, community resources, and child and family advocacy
3. Life-span issues including transitions, crisis intervention, and typical and atypical development with integration across developmental domains
4. Communication style with team and families, including team processes and interprofessional competencies
5. Federal laws including Part H of PL 101-476, the Individuals with Disabilities Education Act, and the development of the IFSP
6. Treatment of the child through the family
7. Issues related to prevention of dysfunction
8. Selection criteria for standardized assessment

Adapted by permission from Cochrane et al. (1990).

The recommended topics in Table 2 are *not* exclusive to working with young children and most should be of concern to physical therapists working with people of all ages. One content topic that was not included by Cochrane et al. (1990), perhaps because it is the topic on which the most time is typically spent in professional education programs, is child development (Bailey et al., 1990; Cherry & Knutson, 1993). Although knowledge of child development is important, it clearly is not sufficient for physical therapists to work effectively with infants and young children, families, and other team members.

Sparling and Sekerak (1992) provided one example of how a family-centered approach to physical therapy across the life span was embedded in the curriculum at the University of North Carolina at Chapel Hill. Content was incorporated primarily into four courses: 1) Human Growth and Development, a 3-credit course that focuses on the family unit over the life span; 2) Clinical Education, a 2-credit course that includes family assessment and practice with one family; 3) Neuromuscular Assessment and Treatment II–Pediatrics, which provides 21 contact hours in assessment and goal setting for children and parents; and 4) Psychiatry and Mental Health, a 2-credit course that covers the broad continuum of mental health issues and the cyclical nature of an individual developing within a family unit. A curriculum guide, including content for each course along with overheads, handouts, and other materials, is available from the Carolina Institute for Research on Infant Personnel Preparation (Sparling, 1992).

The University of Oklahoma Health Sciences Center (OUHSC), Division of Rehabilitation Sciences, has developed a curriculum that may also serve as an example for other institutions attempting to infuse content related to early intervention across the curriculum. Some of the ways in which this has been accomplished reflect the recommendations of Bailey et al. (1990) that all students should be introduced to legislative mandates and programs for children, have practical experiences with children and families, learn family-oriented service delivery across the life span, and have academic and clinical experiences with professionals of other disciplines.

Physical therapy students enter the OUHSC bachelor's degree program in their junior year, following completion of prerequisites at the main University of Oklahoma campus or another college or university. Table 3 lists the courses of the 2-year professional preparation program and the content in each that is related to working with children, families, and teams. The occupational therapy and physical therapy curricula have become increasingly integrated, which has had an obvious impact on the students' knowledge of and respect for the contribution of each other's discipline. As of 1996, occupational and physical therapy faculty and students are together for Dynamics of Human Motion, Pediatric Seminar, Neurobiology, Research in Allied Health, Therapeutic Exercise III, and portions of Theory and Methods I. These courses have been so successful that faculty are making plans to combine other courses or parts of courses in the future.

Faculty Models for Providing Pediatric Content

Because of the faculty shortage and the relatively small proportion of pediatric content in most professional education programs, many programs do not have full-time tenured or tenure-track faculty with pediatric expertise teaching pediatric content. Large programs and programs with postprofessional pediatric graduate studies are often better able to recruit and support traditional full-time faculty than are small programs without a graduate track in pediatrics, but recruitment is difficult for most programs (Stuberg & McEwen, 1993).

Several alternatives to traditional faculty models have been proposed to ensure that pediatric content is included in professional curricula and that it is taught by therapists with pediatric expertise (Stuberg & McEwen, 1993). In addition, these alternatives may also be useful for acquiring faculty with particular expertise in early intervention. One alternative is to recruit physical therapists working in facilities associated with a university to teach part time. At an academic health center, for example, there may be a pediatric hospital or a pediatric rehabilitation center or the campus may have therapists working in other facilities that serve children and their families.

Part-time adjunct faculty can also be recruited from the pediatric clinicians in the local community or from the clinicians and academicians living virtually any place in the world. These part-time faculty could offer a few lectures and/or laboratory sessions of a class or could be responsible for an entire course. When faculty are from outside the local area, creative scheduling can concentrate a course into a week or even a weekend. One program, for example, had an out-of-state therapist teach the didactic portion of a 3-hour pediatric elective course during two week-long visits, spaced 6 weeks apart. The students had 15 contact hours during each visit, with laboratory experiences in pediatric sites with local clinicians before and between the two visits. A full-time faculty member without pediatric expertise coordinated the course and facilitated development of course objectives by the visiting faculty and local clinicians who provided laboratory experience (Stuberg & McEwen, 1993).

Regardless of how pediatric content is provided, students must have high-quality experiences if they are to learn to provide safe and effective services, become collaborative team members, and be "hooked" into working with children and their families. An important part of a quality experience is having faculty available to advise students, to serve as positive role models, and to support students as they decide upon and take their first jobs. This aspect of faculty

Table 3. Infusion of content with direct application to early intervention in a professional-level (bachelor's degree) physical therapy curriculum at the University of Oklahoma Health Sciences Center

Semester and course title	Number of credits	Requisite status	Early intervention–related content	Lab hours required	Clinical hours required
Fall semester					
Theory and Methods I	3	R[a]	Age-related considerations of basic physical therapy assessments and procedures (e.g., range of motion, strength testing, transfers)	3	8
Human Development	2	R	Infant and child development in a systems-based approach to development across the life span; developmental aspects of motor learning; students administer the Denver II (Frankenburg et al., 1992) and write a report	0	0
Theory and Application I	1	R	Introduction to child-, patient-, and family-centered functional goals of intervention	0	0
Dynamics of Human Motion	3	R	Developmental aspects of cervical and trunk biomechanics and respiration, introduction to cross-disciplinary collaboration	4	0
Human Anatomy	5	R	Congenital cardiovascular defects	0	0
Modalities	1	R	Indications and contraindications for using modalities with children	0	0
Spring semester					
Orthopedics	4	R/E[b]	Neonatal musculoskeletal development, common pediatric orthopedic conditions, differential diagnosis; development of balance across the life span; designing goals and treatment specific to "life roles", requires a paper, which may be on a pediatric orthopedic topic	2	0
Neurobiology	4	R	Embryology of the nervous system, neural tube defects, and other congenital neurological disorders	0	0

(continued)

Table 3. (continued)

Semester and course title	Number of credits	Requisite status	Early intervention–related content	Lab hours required	Clinical hours required
Clinical Education I	1	R/E	Optional 3-day affiliation in a pediatric setting; academic portion includes psychosocial aspects of disability in the family, teamwork, systems change, and family- and patient-centered goals and services	0	24
Therapeutic Exercise I	3	R	Exercise prescription for children and teaching of exercise to children; introduction to motor learning principles, which support family-centered services and cross-disciplinary service delivery models	3	0
Theory and Methods II	3	R	Family and patient education, home program considerations for caregivers	0	0
Pathology	3	R	Organ-specific developmental diseases and common pediatric disorders	0	0
Pediatric Seminar	1	E[c]	Introduction to pediatric practice settings and major issues involved in pediatric practice	0	8
Summer term					
Therapeutic Exercise II	1	R	Development of mature gait	0	0
Electrotherapy	2	R	None		
Research in Allied Health	1	R/E	Required project, which may be on a pediatric topic	0	0
Clinical Education II	2	R/E	Optional 6-week, full-time clinical affiliation in a pediatric setting	0	200
Fall semester					
Therapeutic Exercise III	5	R	Systems-based approach to team-oriented, child-, patient-, and family-centered functional goals, assessment, and intervention for children and adults with neurological impairments; rules and regulations of the Individuals with Disabilities Education Act, Medicaid, and other legislation; team processes, transition, standardized assessment, consultation, and assistive technology	24	9

Course	Credits		Type[a][b][c]	Description	
Clinical Education III	1	0	R	Six full days working with children with neurological impairments	48
Seminar in Physical Therapy	3	0	R/E	Emphasis on all clinically related topics on functional goals, family considerations, and teamwork; required major course project, which may be on a pediatric topic	0
Pharmacology	2	0	R	Human conception; drugs frequently prescribed for children (e.g., for seizures, hyperactivity, spasticity)	0
Administration	2	0	R	Program planning; contracts, consulting, and quality assurance	0
Physical Therapy for Children with Developmental Disabilities	3	0	E	Knowledge, skills, and attitudes needed to work in early intervention and school programs; includes legislation and regulations, family systems, team processes, family-centered team approaches to assessment and intervention, IEP and IFSP, consultation, community resources, and transition	20
Spring Semester					
Clinical Education IV	8	0	R/E	Of the 24 weeks of full-time clinical affiliations, students who take the pediatric elective class spend 6 weeks in a pediatric setting (may be in an early intervention setting); others may choose a 6-week pediatric affiliation	240

[a] R = Required course.

[b] R/E = Required course with elective pediatric experiences, as specified.

[c] E = Elective course.

151

responsibility often requires more thought and planning if the faculty teaching pediatric content are part time.

Clinical Education Experiences

In addition to academic experiences that prepare students to work with infants and young children and their families, students need opportunities to participate in appropriate clinical experiences. Clinical education is an essential component of physical therapy education, with most students spending more than 80 weeks in clinical settings during their professional education (Gandy, 1993). Clinical education provides students with opportunities not only to practice what they have learned in the classrooms and laboratories, but also to develop attitudes and skills that are difficult to teach in an academic setting, such as working effectively with professionals of other disciplines and learning to appreciate people whose cultures and values are different from their own.

Although few physical therapy programs require students to have a clinical affiliation in pediatric settings (Cherry & Knutson, 1993; Gandy, 1993), opportunities for such clinical affiliations are critical for both educating physical therapists and recruiting them to work with children when they graduate (Stuberg & McEwen, 1993). Because clinical educators are volunteers, it is often difficult for academic coordinators of clinical education to find adequate numbers of clinical sites for students (Gandy, 1993). In pediatrics it can be especially difficult because some potential clinical educators view pediatrics as beyond entry level and, if they agree to accept students, will take only those who have acquired specialized pediatric skills (Gandy, 1993; T. Martin, 1989). Martin maintained that "placement criteria involving prior experience and/or special coursework, while well meaning, may actually decrease the numbers of students who are exposed to and eventually work in pediatrics" (p. 15). To increase the number of pediatric clinical sites and improve students' experiences in those sites, she suggested the following:

1. Every pediatric therapist must be willing to take students without making unrealistic prerequisite demands;
2. Clinical sites must be willing to establish clear goals and objectives that fill the gaps in academic preparation; and
3. Clinical affiliations should be an integral part of the continuum of academic preparation rather than a separate entity. (p. 15)

All students must be prepared to provide safe and effective services for infants, young children, and their families. Particularly in rural areas, one physical therapy generalist often must serve the needs of people across the life span with a variety of conditions. Services for children and families in early intervention and special education are the only physical therapy services that are mandated by law, and all graduating physical therapists must be prepared to meet basic needs with only their professional-level education (Cherry & Knutson, 1993; Gandy, 1993).

Postprofessional Graduate Education

Postprofessional graduate education offers physical therapists opportunities for transdisciplinary studies and a specialized focus that are not possible in professional education programs. The decision to pursue postprofessional graduate education is often influenced by a desire for advanced knowledge and skill in assessment and intervention care, for increased self-confidence, or to move into another area of professional activity, such as teaching, program administration, or research (Effgen, 1993). Because all postprofessional graduate programs do not offer the same opportunities to accomplish the varied professional goals that students have, it is important for students to investigate as many programs as are realistically possible for them to attend. Because there are so few pediatric physical therapy graduate programs, the selected program is likely to be in a related discipline.

Like many other professionals, physical therapists who return to graduate school have become accustomed to a standard of living that is usually not possible to maintain as a traditional full-time graduate student. For this reason, graduate programs are increasingly scheduling classes and other activities in concentrated blocks and/or after working hours. At least one pediatric graduate program in the United States schedules classes on weekends, which are attended by people from all over the country who have found the content to be good and the expense of flying to the courses less than the cost of attending classes in their own communities. Another program, which has students commuting from all parts of a relatively large state, attempts to schedule all classes on the same day of the week and coordinates the day with classes students take in outside areas, such as special education. Distance learning through televised instruction and other means is also increasing.

Many postprofessional graduate programs in physical therapy and related areas can provide grant support for students wishing to pursue graduate study in working with infants, young children, and their families. A major source of grant funding to programs is the U.S. Department of Education, Office of Special Education Programs (OSEP), through its Training of Personnel for the Education of Individuals with Disabilities Program. Grants are competitive and are awarded for a number of training activities.

Other major sources of grant funding for personnel preparation programs that could be of value to physical therapists are the Administration on Developmental Disabilities, through its University Affiliated Programs, and the Maternal and Child Health Bureau (Campbell, 1994). Grants from these agencies and OSEP usually provide tuition and stipends for students and may provide other supports, such as some professional travel and thesis or dissertation expenses.

Continuing Education

There are a number of ways in which physical therapists can pursue professional development apart from formal degree programs. A 1994 APTA study found that in addition to continuing education courses, common professional development activities were reading journals, conducting personal research, writing for peer-reviewed journals, and working on professional committees (Reynolds, 1994a). The most popular format for professional development was a small-group session during working hours or weekends, offered in the participants' home community.

Because it is difficult to increase the amount of early intervention content in professional preparation programs, Bailey et al. (1990) believe that "an important priority is significant investment in . . . continuing education programs" (p. 34).

Continuing education is important not only for preparing recent graduates of professional programs (Hanson & Lovett, 1992), but also for updating the thousands of physical therapists and other professionals who may have worked with children in the past but have not had an opportunity to gain the specialized knowledge and skills needed to work with infants, young children, and their families. New information affecting physical therapy, early intervention, and special education practices requires current and readily available opportunities for ongoing professional development.

Winton (1990) maintained that a comprehensive, long-term, systematic approach to continuing education must be employed for change to occur in intervention practices of personnel working with infants, young children, and their families. One comprehensive, long-term continuing education program that has been built on cross-disciplinary and family-centered practices is the Oklahoma Statewide Training and Regional Support (STARS) program. This program began as a part of the SoonerStart Early Intervention Program and is designed to meet the present and projected personnel preparation needs under Part H of PL 101-476, the Individuals with Disabilities Education Act.

The current goals of the STARS program are to 1) develop a cadre of highly skilled individuals prepared to work with infants, young children, and their families; 2) provide a coordinated training package that allows both individuals and local and/or community teams to establish goals for training, and then through training opportunities, obtain the information or level of expertise desired; 3) decrease the need for statewide training as local facilitators are prepared to conduct community-based training while state-level trainers maintain a supportive role; 4) enable families by providing them technical and procedural information through training opportunities that will permit them to function as equal team members; and 5) ensure knowledge of the federal regulations and state policies and procedures as mandated in Parts B and H of IDEA.

Overview of STARS

This program provides a mechanism for participants to develop competencies in two major areas—team functioning and technical skills. Embedded within these two areas is a "train-the-trainer" model, known as facilitators' training, which supports the goal of moving training from the state to the community level.

The following are the 10 key elements the STARS training philosophy embraces:

1. Training involves all major stakeholders (team members), who include administrators and families.
2. Within the team training component, team members participate together.
3. Information is presented through all learning modalities.
4. The cultural, racial, ethnic, and socioeconomic diversity of all participants is respected.
5. Training is experiential.
6. Training builds on the experiences, knowledge, and expertise of the participants.
7. Training is based on the participants' expectations, questions, concerns, and issues about selected topics.

8. Training is not a "one-shot" meeting; rather it is a process that occurs through a series of workshops with time between each workshop for the team to apply the information (Bailey et al., 1992).
9. Trainers and trainings are flexible.
10. Strategies are provided for team development, decision making, and problem solving (Gallagher, Shield, & Staples, 1990).

The majority of training occurs at the local level, while topics presented by national speakers are at the state level.

Team Training Component

The team training component of the STARS program consists of workshops organized within six modules: *family-centered services, appreciating individual differences, gathering information, individualized family service plans (IFSPs), service delivery/service coordination,* and *team building* (American Speech-Language-Hearing Association, 1990; Bailey et al., 1992; Crais, Geissinger, & Lorch, 1992). The training content within each module is presented by state agency/program staff, local team facilitators, consultants, and national trainers. Teams develop an individualized team training plan, outlining their team goals and training plans, and then prioritize by team consensus the topics on which they would like to receive training.

Technical Training Component

The technical training component consists of five modules: *multidisciplinary motor mastery program, specific evaluation tool training, medical issues, issues in infant/toddler development,* and *assistive technology.* The technical trainings are presented by state agency and/or program staff, trained regional staff, consultants, and national trainers. Individuals develop an individualized excellence plan outlining professional development goals and training plans, then prioritize the courses with which they will be fulfilled.

Facilitators' Training

As suggested by Bailey et al. (1992), each team of facilitators consists of a parent, an early intervention service provider, a resource coordinator or administrator, and faculty members from regional colleges and universities who train students to work with infants and toddlers with disabilities (e.g., special education, occupational and physical therapy, nursing, speech-language pathology). The trained facilitators then transfer the training to their local program and university. Training the facilitators on the team-training modules consists of an annual statewide workshop and an annual follow-up conducted by state agency trainers. The facilitators' training for the technical training module consists of local workshops conducted by state trainers or consultants. These workshops are specific to the technical information needs identified by the local program staff and families.

Overall, the STARS training program has been found to be cost effective, to improve skills in both functioning as a team and providing family-centered services, and to provide training for virtually every early intervention employee, contract provider, and family wishing to participate. It is funded by the three primary SoonerStart state agencies (Department of Education, Department of Health, and Department of Human Services) to meet Part H requirements for a comprehensive system of personnel development. Each agency assumes costs for its own employees and supports families. Travel, lodging, and food are provided, if necessary. In addition, each agency supports the program through in-kind contributions of clerical support, audiovisual and meeting room expenses, purchase and duplication of training materials, and provision of qualified instructors. Rush, Shelden, and Stanfill (1995) have described the implementation of this statewide system of training.

CONCLUDING REMARKS: FUTURE DIRECTIONS

In 1994, the APTA Section on Pediatrics celebrated its 20th anniversary. To commemorate the event, a special issue of *Pediatric Physical Therapy* was published, which reviewed past and current practices in pediatric physical therapy and projected the future. In her review of the articles in the issue, Heriza (1994) identified three major interrelated shifts in practice over the past 20 years. These shifts, which continue in 1996, are 1) from neuromaturational theories of development to systems-based models, 2) from center-based and child-centered services to family-centered services in natural environments, and 3) from neurodevelopmental frameworks for assessment and intervention to a disablement model that focuses on goal-related functional activities in task-specific environments. *Disablement* is a term that "reflects all of the diverse consequences that disease, injury, or congenital abnormalities may have on human functioning at many different levels" (Jette, 1994, p. 380). The World Health Organization (1980) defined four levels of disablement: pathology, impairment, disability, and handicap. This and similar models provide a useful framework for structuring assessment and intervention at a level that is likely to be the most effective. The concept of task-specific environments is from systems-based models of motor development and motor control, which maintain that movement is organized to accomplish tasks under specific conditions. Movement organized to sit on a chair, for example, is different from movement organized to sit on a therapy ball.

In contrast to the changes in practice, Spake (1994) concluded that there has been little change in pediatric professional-level education since the mid-1970s. To promote essential change, she urged the profession to define and recognize pediatric physical therapy as a clinical science, to develop curricular models for incorporating pediatric content into educational programs, to mandate defined minimal pediatric content for all programs, and to expand clinical education opportunities in pediatric settings.

Change also is overdue in postprofessional physical therapy education, particularly in continuing education courses. Nearly all of the continuing education offerings listed in physical therapy publications deal with assessment of neuromusculoskeletal impairments and therapeutic techniques. There are few courses that assist physical therapists in making the shift toward systems-based, family-centered, and team-oriented assessment and intervention that are directed toward individually meaningful, functional outcomes.

Physical therapy education at all levels (professional, postprofessional, and continuing education) needs to ensure that physical therapists are effectively accomplishing the shifts in practice identified by Heriza (1994) and that they can provide services that are consistent with early intervention legal mandates and contemporary practices. Both now and in the future, physical therapists need the ability to more effectively 1) work with families of diverse cultural backgrounds; 2) use alternative practice models, such as consultative and teaching models, rather than focusing on hands-on models; 3) share their roles with others and provide services beyond traditional professional boundaries; 4) participate in transition services; and 5) provide assistive technology services (Heriza, 1994; McEwen, 1994).

REFERENCES

American Board of Physical Therapy Specialties (ABPTS), Pediatric Specialty Council. (1994). *Description of advanced clinical practice: Pediatric physical therapy*. Alexandria, VA: Section on Pediatrics, American Physical Therapy Association.

American Physical Therapy Association (APTA). (1988). *Action plan to address the faculty shortage*. Alexandria, VA: Author.

American Physical Therapy Association (APTA). (1990). *Accreditation handbook*. Alexandria, VA: Author.

American Physical Therapy Association (APTA). (1994). *House of delegates policies*. Alexandria, VA: Author.

American Physical Therapy Association (APTA), Task Force on Early Intervention, Section on Pediatrics. (1991). Competencies for physical therapists in early intervention. *Pediatric Physical Therapy, 3*, 77–80.

American Speech-Language-Hearing Association. (1990). *ASHA Infant Project*. Rockville, MD: Author.

Bailey, D.B., McWilliam, P.J., & Winton, P.J. (1992). Building family-centered practices in early intervention: A team-based model for change. *Infants and Young Children, 5*(1), 73–82.

Bailey, D.B., Simeonsson, R.J., Yoder, D.E., & Huntington, G.S. (1990). Preparing professionals to serve infants and toddlers with handicaps and their families: An integrative analysis across eight disciplines. *Exceptional Children, 57*, 26–35.

Campbell, S.K. (1994). The Maternal and Child Health connection. *Pediatric Physical Therapy, 6*, 154–156.

Carolina Institute for Research on Infant Personnel Preparation. (1993). *Executive summary*. Chapel Hill: Frank Porter Graham Child Development Center, University of North Carolina.

Cherry, D.B., & Knutson, L.M. (1993). Curriculum structure and content in pediatric physical therapy: Results of a survey of entry-level physical therapy programs. *Pediatric Physical Therapy, 5*, 109–116.

Cochrane, C.G., Farley, B.G., & Wilhelm, I.J. (1990). Preparation of physical therapists to work with handicapped infants and their families: Current status and training needs. *Physical Therapy, 70*, 372–380.

Crais, E.R., Geissinger, S.B., & Lorch, N.H. (1992). Inservice needs and preferences of speech-language pathologists working with infants and toddlers with special needs and their families. *Infant–Toddler Intervention, 2*, 263–276.

Education for All Handicapped Children Act of 1975, PL 94-142. (August 23, 1977). Title 20, U.S.C. 1400 et seq: *U.S. Statutes at Large, 89*, 773–796.

Education of the Handicapped Act Amendments of 1986, PL 99-457. (October 8, 1986). Title 20, U.S.C. 1400 et seq: *U.S. Statutes at Large, 100*, 1145–1177.

Education programs. (1994). *Physical Therapy, 74*, 1140–1159.

Effgen, S.K. (1992). Editorial: Family-centered physical therapy. *Pediatric Physical Therapy, 4*, 53–54.

Effgen, S.K. (1993). Postentry level preparation for pediatric physical therapy. *Pediatric Physical Therapy, 5*, 135–138.

Fenichel, E.S., & Eggbeer, L. (1991). Preparing practitioners to work with infants, toddlers, and their families: Four essential elements of training. *Infants and Young Children*, 4(2), 56–62.

Frankenburg, W.K., Dodds, J., Archer, P., Bresnick, B., Maschka, P., Edelman, N., & Shapiro, H. (1992). *Denver II* (2nd ed.). Denver, CO: Denver Developmental Materials.

Gallagher, J., Shield, M., & Staples, A. (1990). *Personnel preparation options: Ideas from a policy options conference*. Chapel Hill: Carolina Policy Studies Program, University of North Carolina.

Gandy, J.S. (1993). Survey of academic programs: Exploring issues related to pediatric clinical education. *Pediatric Physical Therapy, 5*, 128–133.

Glickman, L.B. (1993, April). Brave new world. *PT—Magazine of Physical Therapy, 1*, 62–67.

Hanson, M.J., & Lovett, D. (1992). Personnel preparation for early interventionists: A cross-disciplinary survey. *Journal of Early Intervention, 16*, 123–135.

Heriza, C.B. (1994). Pediatric physical therapy: Reflections of the past and visions for the future. *Pediatric Physical Therapy, 6*, 105–106.

Hruska, R., & Harden, B. (1994, May). Should continuing education be a requirement for relicensure? *PT—Magazine of Physical Therapy, 2*, 72–73.

Hummer, L.A., Hunt, K.S., & Figuers, C.C. (1994). Predominant thoughts regarding entry-level doctor of physical therapy programs. *Journal of Physical Therapy Education, 8*, 60–66.

Individuals with Disabilities Education Act (IDEA) of 1990, PL 101-476. (October 30, 1990). Title 20, U.S.C. 1400 et seq: *U.S. Statutes at Large, 104*(Part 2), 1103–1151.

Jette, A.M. (1994). Physical disablement concepts for physical therapy research and practice. *Physical Therapy, 74*, 380–386.

Lister, M.J. (Ed.). (1991). *Contemporary management of motor control problems: Proceedings of the II STEP Conference*. Alexandria, VA: Foundation for Physical Therapy, Inc.

Long, T.M., & Sippel, K. (1995, January). A pediatric clinical residency. *PT—Magazine of Physical Therapy, 3*, 56–63.

Martin, K. (1989). Physical therapy in educational environments: Update on national guidelines. *Pediatric Physical Therapy, 1*, 214–216.

Martin, T. (1989). Message from the chair: New beginnings. *Pediatric Physical Therapy, 1*, 15–16.

McEwen, I.R. (1994). Special education legislation and pediatric physical therapy: Past and future influences. *Pediatric Physical Therapy, 6*, 152–153.

Payton, O.D., Nelson, C.E., & Ozer, M.N. (1990). *Patient participation in program planning: A manual for therapists*. Philadelphia: F.A. Davis.

Reynolds, J.P. (1994a, May). Professional development: A new role for APTA. *PT—Magazine of Physical Therapy, 2*, 48–50.

Reynolds, J.P. (1994b, April). Patient-focused care. *PT—Magazine of Physical Therapy, 2*, 52.

Rozier, C.K., & Hamilton, B. (1991). Why students choose physical therapy as a career. *Journal of Physical Therapy Education, 5*, 51–55.

Rush, D.R., Shelden, M.S., & Stanfill, L. (1995). Facing the challenges: Implementing a statewide system of inservice training in early intervention. *Infants and Young Children, 7*, 55–61.

Scull, S., & Deitz, J. (1989). Competencies for the physical therapist in the neonatal intensive care unit (NICU). *Pediatric Physical Therapy, 1*, 11–14.

Soderberg, G.L. (1993). The twenty-seventh Mary McMillan lecture: On passing from ignorance to knowledge. *Physical Therapy, 73*, 797–808.

Spake, E.F. (1994). Reflections and visions: The state of pediatric curricula. *Pediatric Physical Therapy, 6*, 128–132.

Sparling, J.W. (1992). *A guide for embedding family information in an entry-level physical therapy curriculum*. Chapel Hill: Frank Porter Graham Child Development Center, University of North Carolina.

Sparling, J.W., & Sekerak, D.K. (1992). Embedding the family perspective in a physical therapy curriculum. *Pediatric Physical Therapy, 4*, 116–121.

State licensing agencies. (1994). *Physical Therapy, 74*, 1160–1162.

Stuberg, W., & McEwen, I. (1993). Faculty and clinical education models of entry level preparation in pediatric physical therapy. *Pediatric Physical Therapy, 5,* 123–127.

Winton, P.J. (1990). A systematic approach for planning inservice training related to Public Law 99-457. *Infants and Young Children, 3*(1), 51–60.

World Health Organization. (1980). *International classification of impairments, disabilities, and handicaps.* Geneva, Switzerland: Author.

Young, R.H. (1989). The scenario-planning technique: Proposed application to physical therapy education. *Journal of Physical Therapy Education, 3,* 34–39.

8

PREPARING NURSES

Ann W. Cox

While working as an obstetrical nurse in a hospital in the 1970s, I became rather fond of a couple having their first child. At delivery, the couple's new son was diagnosed with myelomeningocele and rushed to a tertiary care center about 60 miles away to undergo surgery. The mother remained in our hospital for several days, unsure of the immediate outcome for her new son, Andy, and questioning the staff about his future. At the time, I was developing a home-based child development program in our county and thought that our new program would be beneficial for this family.

Andy did well following surgery and returned home in 3 weeks. I called Andy's mother one evening to inquire whether she would be interested in participating in our new home-based child development program. She asked, quite astutely, how our program would differ from the services provided by her community health nurse. As I began to explain our services, it became clear that much of what we had to offer was being addressed by the community health nurse. In addition, the community health nurse had already connected the family with resources to address their identified needs. The only support that Andy's mother believed would be gained from our program was the opportunity to connect with other families.

Andy and his family eventually did become involved in the child development program, through collaboration with the community health nurse. The nurse remained the primary interventionist with the family, as a meaningful and supportive relationship had already been established. Our program provided technical assistance for the nurse as she continued to support the family's adjustment to Andy's health care and developmental needs. This collaborative relationship became the model that our program followed as we continued to build working relationships throughout the community.

I lost contact with this family about 2 years after they moved out of the state. Andy was growing and developing well at the time, and the family was expecting another child. Upon reflection, several important lessons were learned from this experience. First, Child Find begins early for some families, often while in the hospital following delivery. Hospital personnel need to know about resources in their communities with which to link families. Second, timing is everything, and the sensitive, competent professional must be able to match services and supports with the family's expressed needs. Third, those who specialize in early child development are not always the most appropriate or initially trusted professionals chosen by families for assistance and support. It is vital that each family's choices are respected and supported. Finally, building community connections is preferred to competition for service identity because the benefits that these relationships bring will expand options that can be made available to families. Community health nurses, as demonstrated by this case scenario, make excellent community collaborators and links with families.

THE EDUCATION OF THE HANDICAPPED Act Amendments of 1986, PL 99-457, established a program to provide early intervention services for infants and toddlers
from birth to 3 years old who have developmental disabilities and their families;
PL 102-119, the Individuals with Disabilities Education Act Amendments of
1991, later reauthorized PL 99-457. The law also included the option to provide
services for children from birth to 3 years old who are at risk for developmental
delays. Furthermore, PL 99-457 established programs for preschoolers with disabilities. With this legislation, Congress provided opportunities for all eligible
young children and their families to receive the benefits of early intervention
services through statewide comprehensive systems of services that are family
centered, multidisciplinary, and collaborative. This radical departure in service
delivery from discipline- and system-specific, professionally driven services challenges the staff of all professional education programs to rethink the ways in
which they prepare professionals for future roles.

Nursing was identified in the legislation as 1 of 14 qualified disciplines to
provide early intervention services. In addition, the Department of Health serves
or co-serves as the lead agency for Part H in 19 states (Association of Maternal
and Child Health Programs, 1992). Thus, nurses working in state maternal and
child health programs are active participants in the early intervention system.
To provide guidance, nursing services were further delineated and defined by the
law to include the following:

> (a) . . . The assessment of health status for the purpose of providing nursing care including
> identification of patterns of human response in actual or potential health problems; (b) provi-
> sion of nursing care to prevent health problems, restore or improve functioning and promote
> optimal health and development; and (c) administration of medications, treatments, and regi-
> mens prescribed by a licensed physician. (*Federal Register*, 1989, p. 119)

The purpose of this chapter is to investigate the historical context of nursing
in the provision of services to young children and their families; the status of
nursing practice in 1996; nursing education, licensure, and certification; challenges to providing early intervention services to children from birth to 6 years
old; opportunities for nursing preparation in early intervention; and recommended educational practice in early intervention for nurses.

HISTORICAL CONTEXT OF NURSING AND SERVICES

Nursing has always been guided by a distinctive philosophy of health care characterized by a holistic approach toward health care problems, a balance between
health promotion and illness care, delivery of care in multiple settings, and an
ethical responsibility to advocate for the individual. A review of the history of
nursing indicates that nursing has participated in the health care of children
since the late 1800s (Lerner & Ross, 1991). In the 19th century, the issue of abandoned children raised the awareness of the impact that social problems had on
the health problems of the day. Standards of nursing care during that period focused on feeding, cleanliness, and enhancement of growth and development.

By the 20th century, state governments were beginning to focus on the
needs of the poor. Child health received special attention with the first White
House Conference on Child Welfare in 1910. The Children's Bureau was estab-

lished in 1912 with the focus of improving services for the health and hygiene of mothers and children. Hundreds of nurses were employed to provide these families with health education, health screening, and health monitoring through home visitation. Children began to receive health and developmental screening, immunizations, medications, and an assortment of psychosocial interventions and referrals through the development of organized public health nursing. The mission of public health nursing was, and is, congruent with the need to prevent, reduce, or minimize disability among children (Bender, 1990).

Today, nursing is the largest health care profession (Redman, 1994). Nurses in child-related settings frequently serve on teams to address the needs of young children and their families and to deliver services through an assortment of programs such as the Early and Periodic Screening, Diagnosis, and Treatment Program; Head Start; primary health care; school health; Children with Special Health Care Needs (CSHCN); child development centers; outpatient and health department clinics; and home health services. Nurses are active participants on comprehensive, multidisciplinary teams addressing early identification and treatment services for a range of children and families. Similar to the delivery of services in acute care pediatric settings, nurses approach community services for young children within a holistic framework that is inclusive of the wishes, desires, and abilities of the family. The broad concern of nursing has consistently been optimal functioning in their environment.

Most nurses, however, still begin their careers in hospitals. The Division of Nursing of the American Nurses' Association (American Nurses' Association, 1990) reported that 68% of the nation's 1.67 million working nurses are employed in hospitals, whereas 20% of nurses work in ambulatory care, community-based agencies, and long-term care. Other nurses work in nursing education programs, administration, and governmental agencies. As health services move away from the acute care tertiary center, new roles with concomitant responsibilities are emerging for all health care professionals. Additional knowledge, skills, and abilities are required to prepare the health professional for these emerging roles. Nursing education must respond to the need for changes in personnel preparation. It is essential, however, to have a basic understanding of the educational system for nursing in the United States in order to understand the response of nursing education to provide health services to eligible infants, toddlers, and preschool children and to identify strategies for changing systems.

THE STATUS OF NURSING PRACTICE

Since the late 1960s, nursing has been defining the profession's independent contribution to health care practice. Widely accepted now is the fact that nursing practice centers around potential or actual functional abilities of individuals (Carpenito, 1987). Disease prevention, health promotion, and health restoration are terms commonly used to define the focus of nursing practice. Like most professions, however, nursing engages in various levels of independent, dependent, and interdependent practice as it works with infants and young children and their families.

The Nursing Process

The nursing process is the underlying scheme that provides order and direction to nursing care and is the essence of professional nursing practice. The nursing process entails 1) data collection (screening and assessment), 2) diagnosis, 3) planning, 4) treatment or intervention, and 5) evaluation. A constant feedback loop exists between evaluation and all other steps of the process.

The nursing process is supported by standards that provide guidelines for practice. These standards require the systematic, continuous collection of health data from which a nursing diagnosis is derived. Nursing diagnoses provide the basis for the construction of a plan of nursing care expressed in terms of potential or actual problems encountered by the individual. The treatment phase involves nursing actions that are selected and performed with the individual's participation. The selected interventions are directed toward the promotion, maintenance, or restoration of health and serve to maximize the health of the individual. The degree of progress toward goals is mutually determined by the individual requiring care and the nurse and may result in reassessment, reordering of priorities, establishment of new goals, and revision of the plan of care.

The nursing process is supportive of the child-focused, family-centered philosophy of early intervention in that active participation of child, family, and professional is sought at all levels of decision making. Furthermore, nursing's orientation has moved from categorical disease diagnoses to the functional abilities of individuals in relation to potential or actual health states.

Interdependence in Nursing Practice

Because nurses work with professionals from a variety of other disciplines and frequently on teams, there is a significant part of the practice that is interdependent and collaborative. In order to serve young children and their families effectively, practitioners must become comfortable with the notion of interdependence; they need to acknowledge the limits of their own knowledge and skills, to learn from families and colleagues, and to trust the collaborative process (Fenichel & Eggbeer, 1991). Infants and young children with disabilities often exhibit complex challenges that require the expertise of many disciplines working together with families. Thus, although one discipline may assume a leadership role, it is critical that other disciplines play a supportive role. Much of the multidisciplinary and interagency nature of working with early intervention teams requires interdependent functioning among all team members, not just nurses.

Nursing Education, Licensure, and Certification

The term *professional nurse* refers to the registered nurse. Other designations, such as licensed practical nurse, vocational nurse, or nursing assistant or aide, are not specifically addressed in this chapter.

In most states, the highest standard for nurses in early intervention is the registered nurse. A few states require the standard of a registered nurse to include a bachelor of science degree in nursing (Shishmanian, 1990). The registered nurse licensure indicates that the nurse was educated as a generalist and may lack the specific knowledge and abilities to practice within early intervention systems without additional continuing education and experiences leading to credentialing required by the state's Comprehensive System of Personnel Development. Advanced practice or specialist nursing occurs at the master's or doctoral level. These nurses declare a specialty and pursue an organized and systematic curriculum of scientific concepts, specialty knowledge, and supervised clinical practice.

Professional Education Program

Generalist Education

Entry-level or generalist nursing education prepares nurses to work in a variety of settings. There are three predominant entry-level programs to prepare the nurse graduate to become a registered nurse:

1. Diploma degree (3-year non-college or non-university program)
2. Associate degree (2-year college program)
3. Bachelor's degree (4- to 5-year college or university-based program)

Generic nursing education includes coursework in the biological, behavioral, and social sciences. Basic courses include biology, anatomy and physiology, pharmacology, pathophysiology, nutrition, growth and development, systems theory, and interpersonal relationships. Furthermore, generalist nursing curricula include content and application coursework in health promotion and health restoration with children and families. Nurses prepared at the bachelor's degree level receive education in community health, including principles of interdisciplinary and interagency service coordination or case management and nursing research (American Nurses' Association Early Intervention Consensus Committee, 1993).

In 1992, two thirds of the annual graduates in nursing completed their basic nursing education in an associate degree program (Moses, 1992). Community health nursing practice is generally not an emphasis in 2-year associate degree programs; thus, graduates generally do not receive content and practice in teamwork or interagency collaboration. The emphasis of these programs is generally on health restoration and disease management. Diploma education programs have been decreasing in number as associate degree programs have been increasing.

Enrollment has increased in almost all generalist education programs, although it has leveled off in the mid-1990s. There is a trend for nurses educated in diploma and associate degree programs to return for a bachelor's degree. Programs for registered nurses to receive their bachelor of science degree in nursing had 20%–25% increases in enrollment for the 1994–1995 school year (Berlin & Bednash, 1995). In a 1994 survey of the 650 university and 4-year colleges that granted bachelor's and master's degrees in nursing, Berlin and Bednash (1995) reported that 133,464 students were enrolled in baccalaureate nursing programs. This represented an average increase of 4,565 students per year from 1990, although the fall 1994 growth was the smallest annual gain in 5 years (2.6%) (Berlin & Bednash, 1995).

A shortage of nurses following the year 2000 has been predicted. Several factors seem to influence this prediction. First, the average age of registered nurses in 1992 was 43, which was 2 years older than it had been in 1988 (U.S. Department of Health and Human Services, 1992). Thus, losses in the nursing field are expected as a result of more nurses retiring. Second, the demand for nurses is expected to increase in all employment sectors with the largest increase in the nursing home sector (Silvestri, 1993). Third, there is a predicted decline in enrollment throughout the country, and therefore there is an expected decline in the graduation classes of the future (U.S. Department of Health and Human Services, 1992). The implications of this predicted nursing shortage for early intervention, when coupled with market expansion in other areas of nursing practice, are troubling.

Advanced Practice Education

According to Jones (1994), the term *advanced practice* has been used in nursing to suggest a movement beyond the basic preparation in nursing. Typically this occurs through further academic preparation at the master's or doctoral degree level. Advanced practice nurses are prepared to engage in research, develop and test theory, and synthesize and utilize a broad range of knowledge, theories, and skills in clinical practice (American Nurses' Association, 1990). There are approximately 361 master's programs and 61 doctoral programs in nursing in the United States. As many as 16 additional doctoral programs are in the planning stage (Berlin & Bednash, 1995). The clinical nurse specialist and the nurse practitioner are the most popular clinical advanced practice roles in nursing.

Clinical Nurse Specialist

The clinical nurse specialist role developed from a need to decrease fragmentation of health care services and improve patient care (Jones, 1994). In 1986, the American Nurses' Association Council of Clinical Nurse Specialists published *The Role of the Clinical Nurse Specialist*. Within this document, the role of the clinical nurse specialist included the 1) assessment of health status; 2) diagnoses of human responses to actual or potential health problems; 3) planning, along with the individual specific therapeutic interventions, to meet mutually agreed-upon goals; and 4) evaluation of patient care outcomes. In addition, the clinical nurse specialist is seen as an educator, a consultant, a researcher, and an administrator (American Nurses' Association Council of Clinical Nurse Specialists, 1986).

Nurse Practitioner

The major impetus for the development of the role of the nurse practitioner grew out of a shortage of physicians during the 1950s (Jones, 1994).

> The intent of the first practitioner demonstration project was to determine the safety, efficacy, and quality of a new model of nursing practice designed to improve health care to children and families and to develop a new nursing role—that of the nurse practitioner. (Ford, 1979, p. 517)

Initially, nurse practitioners were educated in programs offered through continuing education departments. As an advanced practitioner, recognized by the newly formed Council of Nurses in Advanced Practice (American Nurses' Association, 1991), educational requirements for nurse practitioners now include completion of a graduate degree in a specialty area of nursing practice. The major activities of nurse practitioners have included screening, completing health histories, performing physical and psychological examinations, managing care during wellness and illness, teaching, consulting and collaborating, conducting patient follow-up and referrals, promoting positive health, managing personnel, and administration (Jones, 1994). In short, nurse practitioners provide primary health care for various populations, including infants and young children as well as families.

In the mid-1990s, programs leading to advanced practice as nurse practitioners (36.8%) and clinical nurse specialists (28%) enroll two thirds of all nursing master's degree candidates (Berlin & Bednash, 1995). Within both advanced practice roles, nurses can specialize in a variety of areas supportive of infants and young children and their families in early intervention. The length of these advanced practice education programs varies from a minimum of 12 months to several years.

Licensure and Certification

Licensure

To become registered nurses, applicants must pass an examination following completion of their accredited generalist nursing education program. States develop their own acceptable criteria for licensing, and therefore each applicant is licensed only in the state in which he or she passes the examination. Nurses cannot legally practice in a state without being registered in that state. A system of reciprocity has been developed among many states in order to facilitate the registration process when nurses relocate.

Each state regulates the profession through the development and implementation of a *Nurse Practice Act*. This act describes the scope of nursing practice and the standards for licensure in a particular state. In addition to the basic registered nurse licensure, many states have developed continuing education requirements for nurses to maintain their licensure. These requirements vary greatly among states and are part of the periodic review of nurses for renewal of licensure (Cox, 1995).

Certification

Beyond basic licensure, nurses can obtain certification in specialty areas. The American Nurses' Association, Divisions of Practice, introduced the concept of certification in the late 1960s, ultimately resulting in the establishment of the American Nurses' Association Certification Program in 1973 (Jones, 1994). The American Nurses' Association Credentialing Center was established in 1990 and offers certification in 21 clinical areas. More than 90,000 nurses are certified by the Advanced Practice Credentialing Center through certification examinations (Wharton, 1992). Generalist certification historically has been available to all nurses; however, by 1998, a minimum of a bachelor's degree will be required to take the certification examination. It is anticipated that the master's degree in nursing will be required for all specialist certification by the year 2000 (Jones, 1994). In addition to the American Nurses' Association Credentialing Center, other specialty nursing organizations offer certification for nurses in specific specialty areas, such as developmental disabilities and neonatal nursing.

Initial steps have been completed to develop a certification for nurses in early intervention services. IDEA has reinforced the need for a description of nursing's scope of practice and the development and adoption of standards of practice for nurses providing early intervention services. In order to respond to this need, an Early Intervention Consensus Committee was formed by the American Nurses' Association Council on Maternal–Child Health Nursing in 1990. The intent of this committee was to describe nursing's scope of practice and develop standards supportive of nursing's diverse and significant contributions to the care of infants and young children and their families.

The 1993 *National Standards of Nursing Practice for Early Intervention Services* (American Nurses' Association Early Intervention Consensus Committee, 1993) clearly delineates the scope of practice based on the level of educational preparation the nurse must have and outlines recommended practices and each element of the nursing process as it relates to infants and young children and their families. Table 1 presents a comparison of the scope of recommended practices in early intervention of the nurse generalist (registered nurse) and the advanced practice nurse.

The publication of the *National Standards of Nursing Practice for Early Intervention Services* is the first step toward professionally recognized certification for nurses in early intervention. The adoption by the American Nurses' Association of the standards of care listed in Table 2 will establish clear outcomes for nurses in early intervention and will greatly influence nursing education. However, the American Nurses' Association has not acted on these proposed standards.

CHALLENGES TO EARLY INTERVENTION NURSING EDUCATION

The ability of nursing educators to respond to the mandates to prepare well-qualified nursing personnel for an evolving early intervention system is constrained by the economic, political, and sociodemographic realities within health and human services and higher education systems in the United States. The realities within the services arena find that many nurses are not prepared to work within an interdisciplinary, interagency context (Bailey, Simeonsson, Yoder, & Huntington, 1990), and that nursing licensure, as defined within the Nurse Practice Act of a state, may be jeopardized by certain inter- and transdisciplinary early intervention models (Sobsey & Cox, in press). Within higher education, problems include compressed and streamlined nursing curricula, shortages of qualified faculty, limited interdisciplinary clinical experiences, and reduced incentives to embrace nontraditional, interdisciplinary educational practices within the typical college or university structure (Brandt & Magyary, 1989).

Health and Human Services Systems

What might the nurse generalist or advanced practice nurse experience upon graduation when considering employment in early intervention? Salaries are considerably lower in community-based early intervention jobs when compared with hospital-based nursing (Shishmanian, 1990). Furthermore, the increased longevity of Americans means that today's nursing students will spend 75% of

Table 1. Recommendations of the Early Intervention Consensus Committee on scope of practice in early intervention of the nurse generalist and the advanced practice nurse

Nurse generalist	Advanced practice nurse
Registered nurses who provide early intervention services must be licensed under the Nurse Practice Act in the state in which the services are provided.	All of the recommendations for the registered nurse apply to the advanced practice nurse (APN).
Registered nurses who provide early intervention services should participate in credentialing processes required by the state.	In addition:
Registered nurses who provide early intervention services should participate in appropriate continuing education as outlined in the state plan for a comprehensive system of personnel development.	APN who specializes in early intervention is qualified to provide a comprehensive nursing assessment, nursing interventions, and consultation.
	APN contributes to the interdisciplinary process in the team's evaluation of the infant/child.
Registered nurses will participate in Child-Find activities and provide direct nursing care to prevent health problems, restore or improve functioning, and promote optimal health and development.	APN provides service coordination for children and families with complex health needs.
Registered nurses participate as members of interdisciplinary teams providing early intervention services.	APN participates in the social and political processes advocating for quality, family-centered, culturally appropriate services for infants and children at risk for or with special health or developmental needs and their families.
Registered nurses who provide early intervention and service coordination should at a minimum hold a bachelor's degree *and* have received additional education and supervised clinical experience to learn principles and demonstrate competence in early intervention and service coordination.	APN actively participates in the development and implementation of public awareness programs addressing the need for and availability of early intervention services.
	APN seeks positions of leadership on voluntary governmental and advisory boards affecting services rendered to infants and children at risk for or with special health or developmental needs and their families.
	APN contributes to the development of theory and research-based practice.

Adapted from American Nurses' Association Early Intervention Consensus Committee. (1993). *National standards of nursing practice for early intervention services.* Lexington: University of Kentucky College of Nursing; adapted by permission.

their working lives treating people older than 65 years of age (U.S. Department of Health and Human Services, Public Health Service, 1991). Thus, a tremendous number of graduates will find the job market pulling them into gerontology, not early intervention. The rise of multiculturalism also is affecting the field of nursing. African Americans and Hispanics now comprise 25% of school-age children in the United States; by the year 2000, it is projected that ethnic groups will represent 47% of the school-age population (Task Force on Women, Minorities, and the Handicapped in Science and Technology, 1988). Yet, the proportion of students from racial or ethnic groups who are enrolled in college and university nursing programs remained stable in 1994–1995 with 16.9% of the students earning bachelor's degrees and 11.4% of the students earning master's degrees (Berlin & Bednash, 1995). Clearly, efforts to address multiculturalism within

Table 2.   Standards of care and professional performance for nurses in early intervention

The nurse

- Systematically collects, records, and analyzes comprehensive and accurate data.
- Analyzes assessment data, utilizes scientific principles and professional judgment, and collaborates with the family in determining appropriate nursing diagnoses.
- In collaboration with the family, identifies expected outcomes that support the health and development of infants and children and the values and priorities of their families.
- In collaboration with the family and the interdisciplinary team, participates in the development of the individualized family service plan.
- In partnership with the family, implements actions identified on the individualized family service plan that promote, maintain, or restore health and development.
- In collaboration with the family and interdisciplinary team, evaluates the progress of the infants and children and their families toward attainment of outcomes.
- Is accountable for promoting quality of care in early intervention services and systems.
- Participates in self-evaluation.
- Maintains appropriate knowledge and skills in order to effectively implement the standards of practice and specialty guidelines for early intervention services.
- Contributes to the professional development of peers, colleagues, and others.
- Collaborates with the family and other members of the interdisciplinary and interagency team in providing care to infants and children and their families.
- Applies appropriate, scientifically sound empirical research and theory as a basis for nursing practice decisions.
- In collaboration with the family and the interdisciplinary team, pursues strategies to enhance access to and utilization of adequate health care and educational services.

Adapted from American Nurses' Association Early Intervention Consensus Committee. (1993). *National standards of nursing practice for early intervention services.* Lexington: University of Kentucky College of Nursing; adapted by permission.

nursing education programs and through recruitment strategies should be a priority.

Health care reform initiatives in the 1990s have meant that hospitals are no longer the center of the health care system. Significant changes in priorities include shifts from acute patient care to a continuum of care, from treating illness to maintaining wellness, and from caring for the individual patient to accountability for the health status of defined populations (Ferguson, 1994). The nationwide move toward managed health care options, however, may signify that fewer team-based, interdisciplinary options will be supported unless actual cost-effectiveness is demonstrated. The fear is that more discipline-specific, fragmented approaches will prevail. And with cost containment driving the system, service coordination may serve a gatekeeping function rather than enhance a family-centered perspective.

Higher Education System

As these changes in service delivery occur, the educational systems, particularly higher education, are undergoing radical changes. Within nursing, faculty are learning how to do more with less. As faculty shorten and streamline curricula, they are finding it difficult to 1) cover content previously believed to be essential for basic nursing education, 2) require electives, and 3) expand content into areas of emerging need. This means that recommended practice concepts in early intervention (e.g., service coordination, teamwork) are either addressed minimally or completely omitted in basic generalist education programs (Holditch-Davis, 1989).

One of the driving forces for this curriculum compression is related to the high cost of education and the desire to remain competitive in recruiting students. Clearly, fewer federal and state dollars will be available to assist students with tuition in coming years.

A shortage of faculty who are familiar with and experienced in early intervention and interdisciplinary practice exists. One solution is to cultivate faculty from within agencies to deliver content and supervise students. A tremendous shift in nursing programs to the use, even at the preservice level, of clinical faculty who are often unpaid is under way.

At the college or university level, programs are organized within a departmental model. The philosophical commitment to interdisciplinary learning within higher education is unlikely to be successful unless supported by a formalized structure that extends across the school and throughout departments (Brandt & Magyary, 1989). Although there is often a willingness among faculty to collaborate, resource allocation and formal organizational linkages doom many efforts to failure.

Conceptually, interdisciplinary programs are consistent with the desire to reduce redundancy within colleges and universities, streamline and increase student enrollment in classes, and prepare future professionals for the realities of the working environment. Consideration must be given to joint or adjunct faculty positions held across different schools; to promotional and merit incentives for cross-discipline collaboration in teaching, clinical, and research activities; and to a cross-school budgetary process for the joint sponsorship of courses, faculty positions, and interdisciplinary teaching methods (Brandt & Magyary, 1989).

OPPORTUNITIES FOR NURSING PREPARATION IN EARLY INTERVENTION

Given the move toward community-based interagency systems of services that are responsive to individual and family needs, education in nursing at all levels must begin to emphasize teamwork, service coordination, and family- and/or person-centered services. The expansion of these services to infants and young children and their families inherent within IDEA legislation challenges all disciplinary education programs to identify relevant content and application opportunities for their students.

For nursing, as well as many other discipline-specific programs, the challenge to prepare personnel is compounded by existing shortages of trained professionals (Hebbeler, 1994), creating a pressing need to systematically identify and develop educational programs and opportunities for professionals within both disciplinary and team contexts. In order to identify opportunities to expand early intervention content, it is essential to understand the level of nursing content in this area.

Early Intervention Content within Generalist Curriculum

All generalist nursing education programs contain content on child health care needs and on families. This pediatric content is largely organized by age group (birth to 18 years old) and addresses health promotion (well-child content) and health maintenance and restoration (illness content). An important emphasis is on the role of the family as the primary care provider of children. Of significance, the Carolina Institute for Research on Infant Personnel Preparation (1993) identifies nursing as one of only two disciplines surveyed that provides content and clinical opportunities for working with families within their generalist education program.

The application or clinical portion of the child health curriculum varies considerably among degree programs (diploma, associate, and bachelor's) and among programs that lead to the same degree. For example, some associate degree programs require clinical experience only within acute care settings whereas others add a community pediatric experience (e.g., in health departments, child care centers). However, not all students receive direct clinical experience with every age group within the pediatric populations. The bachelor's degree student will also receive content and clinical experience in community health nursing. Again, the broad nature of this content emphasizes the community health care needs of all individuals and clinical experiences with some but not all age groups. However, concepts and experiences in community service coordination and interagency collaboration are emphasized.

A review by the author indicates that most child health nursing texts introduce students to IDEA, including the Part H regulations, the role of nursing in early intervention and in schools, and service coordination. Few programs, however, are able to provide clinical experiences that emphasize the integration of family-centered service coordination and interdisciplinary and interagency teamwork principles that are essential for implementing early intervention services. In a survey of 74 nursing schools, Holditch-Davis (1989) found that most schools provide content to beginning nurses in the areas of typical infant and young childhood development, family assessment, selected disability conditions in childhood, and values and ethics. Information on service coordination, teamwork, and family-centered service was minimal.

Clearly, all generalist education programs are constrained by the need to cover essential didactic content and provide clinical experiences with all populations within a limited amount of time. Child health content typically is allocated for either a single quarter or a semester within the curriculum, as is community health within the bachelor's degree programs.

In summary, the typical graduate in nursing will have received basic content on early childhood growth and development, health promotion of young children, health and developmental assessment, conditions placing the young child at risk, management of chronic conditions and disabilities that affect the young child, and working with families of young children. These graduates may or may not have had actual supervised clinical experiences with young children and their families. Nor will they typically receive planned opportunities to learn about other disciplines with whom they will be expected to interact if they enter the field of early intervention.

Although it is highly unlikely that generalist nursing education programs will develop specialized early intervention tracts within their programs, Bailey and his colleagues (Bailey et al., 1990), through an analysis of personnel preparation in eight disciplines including nursing, suggested four priority recommendations pertaining to preservice training. Students need 1) information regarding the legislative mandates, programs, and services in early intervention in order to make them aware of early intervention as a career option; 2) exposure to early intervention programs and services; 3) instructional and clinical experiences in working with families; and 4) instructional and clinical opportunities with other disciplines on teams.

Although these recommendations are consistent with the direction of generalist nursing education, particularly at the bachelor's degree level, two of the four recommendations present major challenges for preservice nursing education programs. First, the need for instruction and opportunities to work with other disciplines on teams is generally recognized as important to prepare nurses for the realities of the work world. However, the challenge is how to expose students to each other through planned interdisciplinary instruction and experience as part of a preservice education program that is clearly directed toward discipline-specific role preparation. Second, exposing students to early intervention programs and services will require that faculty fully appreciate and understand the early intervention system in their state and identify strategies to assist students to create connections among traditional newborn, neonatal, and well-child services common within the nursing curricula and early intervention services. Given the number of students enrolled in generalist nursing, it is unlikely that all students will be able to participate in early intervention programs and services.

Early Intervention Content within Advanced Practice Curriculum

Advanced practice nursing specializations are found most often in programs that prepare clinical nurse specialists and nurse practitioners. As with generalist education, advanced practice graduate nursing education typically is organized by population group. Thus, clinical specialists are prepared in pediatrics (e.g., neonatal, children with special health care needs) and nurse practitioners specialize in family, neonatal, school health, or pediatrics.

Specialization in early intervention falls within the general pediatric or community focus and often occurs in areas in which early intervention clinical sites can be selected for students. Early intervention is not a widely accepted area of specialization in nursing. Some nursing graduate programs offer specialization in children with special health care needs (Brandt & Magyary, 1989; Godfrey, 1991). Other nursing advanced practice programs offer general issues of maternal and child health or prepare nurse practitioners (Urbano, 1990).

Often, clinical supervision is provided by volunteer clinical faculty at the clinical site. These faculty must meet educational and certification requirements commensurate with the role to which the student aspires. Thus, for an early intervention clinical placement to be chosen, the clinical nursing faculty would need to have a master's degree and, in the case of nurse practitioner students, would also need to be a licensed nurse practitioner. Although it is fortunate that there are qualified nursing personnel in some early intervention programs and services, it is often difficult for them to assume the added responsibilities of clinical supervision as a result of time constraints.

Finally, too few advanced practice nursing programs provide the structure and process for linking with other discipline-specific graduate programs to provide formal team learning experiences. The process of socializing professionals to interact effectively and to respect each other's knowledge and skills must be formalized in content and clinical courses and through collaborative research (Brandt & Magyary, 1989).

Continuing Education

Continuing education provides nurses with state-of-the-art knowledge and skills for working with many populations. Continuing professional education is an expectation for licensure renewal in many states. Whether delivered within a discipline-specific context or through planned interdisciplinary workshops or courses, continuing education can be a cost-effective strategy for preparing personnel in early intervention (Hansen, Holaday, & Miles, 1990).

Fortunately, there is a large pool of experienced pediatric and public health nurses, many of whom are already working with children and families in a variety of community settings (Lerner & Ross, 1991). These nurses already possess basic nursing skills as well as knowledge and skills related to observation, developmental screening, assessment, family systems, child rearing, parents, teaching and learning, communication, prevention, advocacy, cultural influences on care, and community health systems. By taking advantage of nurses' sound knowledge and clinical experience backgrounds, it is feasible to develop and implement continuing education programs related to infants and young children with special health care needs within a relatively short time frame (Urbano, 1990).

Given that it will be difficult to increase the amount of early intervention content within existing preservice curricula, continuing education in the form of courses, conferences, workshops, institutes, and symposia is considered educationally sound and a cost-effective solution to expand the knowledge and skills of nurses already working with infants and young children with disabilities and their families. The quality of these early intervention offerings must, however, be monitored and conceptually fit within the requirements of each state participating in Part H and Part B of IDEA.

RECOMMENDED EDUCATIONAL
PRACTICE IN EARLY INTERVENTION FOR NURSES

The move toward interdisciplinary educational preparation for nurses in developmental disabilities began in the late 1960s and early 1970s.

Interdisciplinary Training

Led by the formation of university affiliated preservice training programs that were funded by the U.S. Maternal and Child Health Bureau (MCHB), interdisciplinary educational preparation programs were some of the first integrated learning experiences in collaborative practice for students in health profession disciplines. In 1995, the MCHB funded interdisciplinary leadership training programs in childhood neurodevelopmental and related disabilities at 34 sites nationwide, requiring a complement of 11 disciplines, including nursing (E. Brannon, personal communication, July 1995).

Furthermore, the Administration on Developmental Disabilities provides administrative funds to support interdisciplinary training in developmental disabilities at 55 university affiliated programs in the United States and its territories. The mandate of this agency, however, is that the interdisciplinary training must address all ages and not be limited to children from birth to 6 years old.

Since the 1970s, the interdisciplinary approach to preservice training in developmental disabilities has expanded and, as of 1996, includes university-based training in interdisciplinary centers with a range of specialty areas. For example, since 1989, the U.S. Department of Education, through its Office of Special Education Programs, has funded 37 interdisciplinary personnel preparation programs for related services personnel (Bokee, 1995). Many of these interdisciplinary training programs emphasize preparation in early intervention and early childhood services at the paraprofessional, undergraduate, and graduate levels.

Interdisciplinary Early Intervention Training Model

There are a number of innovative interdisciplinary programs preparing nurse specialists to work with children with special health care needs and their families and with other disciplines (Brandt & Magyary, 1989; Godfrey, 1991; Kilgo, Clarke, Cox, & Carlotti, 1993; Urbano, vonWindeguth, Siderits, & Studenic-Lewis, 1990). These graduate training programs 1) share a commitment to interdisciplinary education for nurses along with other disciplines; 2) involve advanced practice students; and 3) emphasize family-centered services, teamwork, and service coordination. The program summarized below demonstrates how advanced practice nursing students can receive an interdisciplinary early intervention emphasis while completing their graduate degrees.

The Interdisciplinary Related Service Graduate Training Program

The Interdisciplinary Related Service Graduate Training Program in Family-Centered Early Intervention (Cox, 1993) is funded by the U.S. Department of Education. The program was funded in 1993 and is an outgrowth of 8 years of interdisciplinary related service training at the Virginia Institute for Developmental Disabilities, a university affiliated program at Virginia Commonwealth University. The training program is designed for graduate students in nursing, occupational therapy, physical therapy, psychology, and social work.

The foundation of the program is its team approach, which is implemented through coursework, practica, and seminars. Interdisciplinary coursework (three 3-hour graduate-level courses) and supervised interdisciplinary field-based practica (minimum of 150 hours) are required. The courses and practica are designed to enable trainees to meet a comprehensive set of interdisciplinary competencies. A minimum of four interdisciplinary seminars are taken with graduate students in early childhood special education.

The triad of courses provides the central content of the training program. Two of these courses are interdisciplinary in design and delivery, emphasize parent participation in the delivery of content, and are offered in the evening so as not to compete with the discipline-specific curricula. Thus, they are taught by teams and completed by all trainees together. The third course, which is individually chosen (i.e., elective), gives trainees in-depth disciplinary perspectives in a related topic or a greater degree of understanding in an area of perceived weakness. The list of elective courses is approved, and often taught, by the interdisciplinary faculty. This elective course option recognizes the individual needs of trainees, yet provides for quality assurance that the content addresses areas of competency associated with the program.

The courses and seminars are complemented with field-based practica that are individually designed to address the students' learning needs. The interdisciplinary competencies provide the minimal expectations associated with the practica experiences. Field-based practica must meet criteria established by the program.

Nursing students accepted into this program have typically been experienced pediatric nurses returning for advanced practice graduate work for clinical specialty or nurse practitioner roles. They have an expressed desire to focus their graduate nursing program on infants and young children with disabilities and their families. Through the collaboration of the program director, nursing faculty, and student, a clinical practicum experience is designed to meet the competencies and requirements of the early intervention program and the nursing curriculum.

The challenges of an interdisciplinary program such as this require knowledge and acceptance of the unique curricula and level of students in the various graduate programs. The unifying component of this curriculum is the articulation of a set of interdisciplinary competencies in early intervention.

Regional Model of Continuing Education for Nurse Leaders

Continuing education activity for nurses working within the early intervention field has increased significantly. The range of activity includes state-sponsored in-service training (Eggbeer, Latzko, & Pratt, 1993), postprofessional coursework leading to certification (Urbano, 1990), and regional training of nursing leaders (Lee & Pressler, 1989). This later model will serve to illustrate the depth and breadth of a successful continuing education model for nurses.

With 3 years of support from the MCHB, the Leadership Development for Nurses in Early Intervention Project (Lee & Pressler, 1989) targeted nurse leaders from health departments and special health needs programs in 14 southeastern states. The overall goal of the project was to improve community-based systems of care and services for infants and young children and their families. This goal was achieved by preparing nurses in state-level leadership positions and preparing community-based nurses for new roles and expectations in planning and implementing Part H.

The outcome of this 3-year "train-the-trainers" model was that nurse leaders developed plans envisioning the role of nursing to achieve the aims of Part H in their state and identified strategies for preparing nurses for those roles. The selected state nurse leaders received comprehensive in-depth instruction in the mandates and components of Part H and the role of community health nursing as a primary participant in family-centered service provision. The instruction and follow-up monitoring were provided at week-long annual leadership development institutes.

Upon returning to their states, the nurse leaders influenced further training at the state level. In all, more than 3,000 community-based nurses in 14 states received training with the curriculum. An added benefit of this training model was that participants were given the opportunity to receive information and consultation from national leaders in early intervention, thus promoting mutual collaboration and networking. The success of this model is evidenced by its expansion into other regions of the country (Lee & Pressler, 1989).

CONCLUDING REMARKS: FUTURE DIRECTIONS

The profession of nursing is fortunate because it already provides more content related to infants and young children as part of generalist education programs than do many disciplines. However, several themes emerge that have implications for the future direction of nursing education in early intervention. First, although education programs at the generalist level are quite diverse, they do provide foundational learning in early intervention that includes infant and young child growth and development, work with families, knowledge about chronic conditions and disabilities in childhood, and nursing management of these conditions. The education programs, in particular the bachelor's degree, are strengthened by content in interagency collaboration and service coordination. All generalist nursing education content needs to be strengthened and clinical placements in community-based early intervention services need to be developed. The largest percentage of nurses are and will remain educated as generalist nurses. These nurses will require additional learning opportunities after graduation to become fully competent in the delivery of early intervention services.

Second, advanced practice nurses who specialize in childhood disability and chronic illness and pediatric nurse practitioners must begin to receive planned interdisciplinary content and clinical experiences in community-based early intervention programs. Content most lacking in the curriculum includes teamwork, family-centered service coordination, and specific intervention. Movement within the profession regarding designated certification in early intervention will foster more specialization within the profession. Models for early intervention specialization that include interdisciplinary studies and experiences have been developed and can be used to complement traditional graduate programs.

Third, there is a large percentage of nurses who work with infants and young children and their families in the community through public health departments and related programs. The most cost-effective educational approach to prepare these nurses is through continuing education. Of significance is that the continuing education must extend the knowledge and skills of these nurses beyond a disciplinary perspective and engage the larger parent and professional community. Recommended practice would suggest that continuing education activities in early intervention should be coordinated with each state's comprehensive system for personnel development.

REFERENCES

American Nurses' Association. (1990). *Standards of clinical nursing practice.* Washington, DC: Author.

American Nurses' Association. (1991). *Proposal: Council of Nurses in Advanced Practice.* Washington, DC: Author.

American Nurses' Association Council of Clinical Nurse Specialists. (1986). *The role of the clinical nurse specialist.* Kansas City, MO: Author.

American Nurses' Association Early Intervention Consensus Committee. (1993). *National standards of nursing practice for early intervention services.* Lexington: University of Kentucky College of Nursing.

Association of Maternal and Child Health Programs. (1992). *Preliminary summary of key findings: AMCHP survey of Title V programs' participation in early intervention activities.* Washington, DC: Author.

Bailey, D.B., Simeonsson, R.J., Yoder, D.E., & Huntington, G.S. (1990). Preparing professionals to serve infants and toddlers with handicaps and their families: An integrative analysis across eight disciplines. *Exceptional Children, 57,* 26–35.

Bender, K. (1990). Impact of standards on public health nursing and nursing in children with special care needs programs. In University of Kentucky, *Early intervention leadership and curriculum development for nurses* (pp. 32–36). Lexington: University of Kentucky College of Nursing.

Berlin, L.E., & Bednash, G.D. (1995). *Enrollment and graduations in baccalaureate and graduate programs in nursing in 1994–1995.* Washington, DC: American Association of Colleges of Nursing.

Bokee, M.B. (1995). *The training of personnel for the education of individuals with disabilities program preparation of related services personnel.* Washington, DC: U.S. Department of Education.

Brandt, P.A., & Magyary, D.L. (1989). Preparation of clinical nurse specialists for family-centered early intervention. *Infants and Young Children, 1*(3), 51–62.

Carolina Institute for Research on Infant Personnel Preparation. (1993). *Executive summary.* Chapel Hill: Frank Porter Graham Child Development Center, University of North Carolina.

Carpenito, L.J. (1987). *Nursing diagnosis: Application to clinical practice* (2nd ed.). Philadelphia: J.B. Lippincott.

Cox, A.W. (1993). *Interdisciplinary related services training: An expanded approach to inclusive and family-centered early intervention.* Richmond: Virginia Institute for Developmental Disabilities, Virginia Commonwealth University.

Cox, A.W. (1995). Nursing. In B.A. Thayer & N. Kropf (Eds.), *Developmental disabilities: A handbook for interdisciplinary practice.* Cambridge, MA: Brookline.

Education of the Handicapped Act Amendments of 1986, PL 99-457. (October 8, 1986). Title 20, U.S.C. 1400 et seq: *U.S. Statutes at Large, 100,* 1145–1177.

Eggbeer, L., Latzko, T., & Pratt, B. (1993). Establishing statewide systems of inservice training for infant and family personnel. *Infants and Young Children, 5*(3), 49–56.

Federal Register. (1989, June 22). *Early intervention programs for infants and toddlers with handicaps: Final regulations.* Washington, DC: U.S. Government Printing Office.

Fenichel, E.S., & Eggbeer, L. (1991). Preparing practitioners to work with infants, toddlers, and their families: Four essential elements of training. *Infants and Young Children, 4*(2), 56–62.

Ferguson, V.D. (1994). The future of nursing. In O. Strickland & D. Fishman (Eds.), *Nursing issues in the 1990s* (pp. 3–12). Albany, NY: Delmar Publishers.

Ford, L.C. (1979). A nurse for all settings: The nurse practitioner. *Nursing Outlook, 27,* 516–521.

Godfrey, A.C. (1991). Providing health services to facilitate benefit from early intervention: A model. *Infants and Young Children, 4*(2), 47–55.

Hansen, S., Holaday, B., & Miles, M.S. (1990). The role of pediatric nurses in a federal program for infants and young children with handicaps. *Journal of Pediatric Nursing, 5*(4), 246–251.

Hebbeler, K. (1994). *Shortages in professions working with young children with disabilities and their families.* Chapel Hill, NC: National Early Childhood Technical Assistance Program (NEC•TAS).

Holditch-Davis, D. (1989). In light of Public Law 99-457: How well are novice nurses prepared? *In Touch, 7*(2), 5.

Individuals with Disabilities Education Act Amendments of 1991, PL 102-119. (October 7, 1991). Title 20, U.S.C. 1400 et seq: *U.S. Statutes at Large, 105,* 587–608.

Jones, D.A. (1994). Advanced practice: Merging the roles of the nurse practitioner and clinical specialist. In O. Strickland & D. Fishman (Eds.), *Nursing issues in the 1990s* (pp. 133–165). Albany, NY: Delmar Publishers.

Kilgo, J., Clarke, B., Cox, A., & Carlotti, D. (1993). *Interdisciplinary infant and family services training: A professional training model* (2nd ed.). Richmond: Virginia Institute for Developmental Disabilities, Virginia Commonwealth University.

Lee, G., & Pressler, E. (1989). *Leadership development for nurses in early intervention.* Lexington: University of Kentucky College of Nursing.

Lerner, H., & Ross, L. (1991). Community health nurses and high-risk infants: The current role of Public Law 99-457. *Infants and Young Children, 4*(1), 46–53.

Moses, E.B. (1992, July/August). RN shortage seen for 21st century. *American Nurse, 4.*

Redman, B.K. (1994). Nursing's agenda for health care reform: The profession's ability to create a health care system congruent with its philosophy. In O. Strickland & D. Fishman (Eds.), *Nursing issues in the 1990s* (pp. 81–95). Albany, NY: Delmar Publishers.

Shishmanian, E. (1990). Challenges for nursing. In University of Kentucky, *Early intervention leadership and curriculum development for nurses* (pp. 8–18). Lexington: University of Kentucky College of Nursing.

Silvestri, G.T. (1993). Occupational employment: Wide variations in growth. *Monthly Labor Review, 116*(11), 58–86.

Sobsey, D., & Cox, A. (in press). Integrating health care and educational programs. In F. Orelove & D. Sobsey, *Educating children with multiple disabilities: A transdisciplinary approach* (3rd ed.). Baltimore: Paul H. Brookes Publishing Co.

Task Force on Women, Minorities, and the Handicapped in Science and Technology. (1988, September). *Changing America: The new face of science and engineering—Interim report.* Washington, DC: Author.

Urbano, M.T. (1990). Preparing community based nurses for expanded roles in early intervention. In University of Kentucky, *Early intervention leadership and curriculum development for nurses* (pp. 42–47). Lexington: University of Kentucky College of Nursing.

Urbano, M.T., vonWindeguth, B., Siderits, P., & Studenic-Lewis, C. (1990). Developing case managers for chronically ill children: Florida's registered nurse specialist program. *The Journal of Continuing Education in Nursing, 22*(2), 62–66.

U.S. Department of Health and Human Services. (1992). *Health personnel in the United States: Eighth report to Congress, 1991.* Washington, DC: Author.

U.S. Department of Health and Human Services, Public Health Service. (1991). *Health United States 1989 and prevention profile.* Washington, DC: Author.

Wharton, E. (Ed.). (1992). *Credentialing news.* Washington, DC: American Nurses' Association Credentialing Center.

9

PREPARING PEDIATRICIANS

Renee C. Wachtel and Pamela J. Compart

Having a premature baby who weighed only 2 pounds at birth was a nightmare for the Coopers. Their daughter had respiratory problems, infections, feeding difficulties, and an intraventricular hemorrhage (bleeding within the brain). They thought their precious Megan would never survive, but now she weighs 4½ pounds and is ready to go home. The Coopers checked with their family pediatrician. They had a million questions: What are her chances of having developmental problems? What should they look out for? What can they do to help her? Does she need therapy? Is there an early intervention program in their community?

PEDIATRICIANS PRIDE THEMSELVES ON HAVING a child and family focus as a daily part of their practice of medicine. Much of pediatric practice consists of developing and maintaining an ongoing, trusting, and confidential relationship with families about the health, development, and welfare of their children. Many parents consider their pediatrician a trusted advisor because frequently there are few professionals who have the in-depth, longitudinal knowledge about the family that the pediatrician has. Training the pediatrician to assume an appropriate role in the early intervention system should be an easy task, but many factors interfere with the good intentions of well-meaning programs. In addition, pediatricians can misunderstand and therefore become frustrated with their interactions on early intervention teams, which then interferes with their acceptance of feedback from other professionals. The purpose of this chapter is to explore the need for team training, to identify the barriers that have prevented adequate training, and to highlight some effective strategies for preservice and in-service training of pediatricians.

Standards of pediatric practice mandate the identification of developmental delays as part of routine well-child care. Because most children obtain health care on an ongoing basis from birth, health care providers (especially pediatricians) are in an ideal position to identify, evaluate, treat, and refer children with developmental delays and those who might benefit from early intervention. In addition, federal legislation, such as PL 101-476, the Individuals with Disabilities Education Act (IDEA) of 1990, mandates referral of children with suspected delays to the single point of entry into the early intervention system. It is therefore essential for the pediatrician to be able to identify children for referral, to know how the referral system works, and to be able to assist families in gathering information about early intervention. Once a child is referred, the pediatrician may participate as a member of the early intervention team or may

181

primarily support the family as they participate in the process of obtaining early intervention services. The pediatrician also needs to know what services the early intervention system cannot provide, so that other resources for providing these services can be explored. A number of articles have appeared in pediatric journals describing relevant legislation, such as PL 99-457, the Education of the Handicapped Act Amendments of 1986 (since reauthorized as PL 102-119, the Individuals with Disabilities Education Act Amendments of 1991), and opportunities for pediatricians to participate in early intervention services for children with special health care needs (Blackman, Healy, & Ruppert, 1992; Degraw et al., 1988; Downey, 1990). In addition, review articles have been published with the goal of educating pediatricians about their role in identifying children with developmental disorders and in the early intervention process (Bennett, 1982; Solomon, 1995). Although these articles have started the process of providing the relevant information on educating pediatricians, there are still many educational needs and other barriers to overcome.

ROLE OF THE PEDIATRICIAN

Pediatricians who participate on early intervention teams serve a uniquely different purpose from other members of the team. The pediatrician's initial role is to identify, from among the many children in his or her practice, children who have atypical development and require referral for further evaluation or services. Once a child has been so identified, the pediatrician serves a function different from other health professionals on the team, including nurses. An important but often unrecognized and underemphasized responsibility of the pediatrician is to attempt to determine the cause of a child's disability. For example, if a child has mental retardation, the pediatrician needs to assess whether there is an identifiable medical condition that could be causing or contributing to the child's developmental delay. Such conditions include, but are not limited to, chromosomal or other genetic disorders, hypothyroidism, elevated lead levels, and metabolic disorders. Identifying a causative condition is essential because some conditions, such as hypothyroidism and plumbism, are treatable. In addition, for genetic disorders, counseling families regarding risk of recurrence is critical to allow families to make informed decisions about future family planning. Unfortunately, this vital role for the pediatrician is often overlooked, and many children are identified as having developmental delays and are referred for services without an investigation of potential etiologies. Any training program preparing physicians for work in early intervention should include an emphasis on this unique role of pediatricians.

For many children, health-related issues remain an important concern and the pediatrician's management may significantly affect the child's early intervention program (e.g., the supplemental oxygen needs of a child with bronchopulmonary dysplasia, the need for protective isolation of a child with immunodeficiency). In addition, the pediatrician's determination of the presence of a medical condition with a high probability of developmental delay may provide the basis for a child's eligibility for early intervention services. Finally, many parents have questions about the diagnosis and prognosis of their child's developmental disability, which the pediatrician is often the most prepared team member to address.

Interaction with Other Team Members

For the pediatrician to collaborate effectively with the other early intervention team members, it is essential for each person to understand the purpose of the team and the role of each member. Because most early intervention teams are generally consensus driven, the pediatrician will need to assume a different role from the one he or she generally performs in a medical center or hospital setting. This becomes difficult at times for several reasons, including the lack of common terminology, the extremely different levels of training required for different disciplines (ranging from a college degree in some fields to at least 7 years' post-college for pediatrics), the different models for team leadership, and the different expectations for the outcome of the process (a diagnosis versus a family service plan). At times, filling in the communication gaps is indeed challenging. For these reasons, pediatricians need specific training in effective team participation and their role in the early intervention system. Additional barriers to a pediatrician's participation on early intervention teams include limited time availability, lack of financial compensation, and insufficient notice to rearrange schedules. Although many teams can creatively navigate around these barriers, others make little effort to develop the flexibility needed to allow the pediatrician to become an active team participant.

Previous studies (Scott, 1990; Wender, Bijur, & Boyce, 1992) have shown that physicians do not believe they are sufficiently knowledgeable about referral systems in their geographic area or their role in the referral process. Therefore, providing pediatricians with specific knowledge and skills to make appropriate referrals is an important priority in improving the delivery of early intervention services to children.

Knowledge About Early Intervention

Several surveys have been done since the mid-1980s that examine the status of physician knowledge and comfort regarding developmental disabilities and early intervention. In 1988, a survey of chairpersons of state American Academy of Pediatrics Chapter Committees on Disabilities was done (Melmed & Dolins, 1988). Areas in which chairpersons believed their members needed more training included interacting with early intervention personnel, knowing how to refer children to early intervention programs, and working with interdisciplinary teams (Melmed & Dolins, 1988). A 1990 New York American Academy of Pediatrics study found that only 15% of physicians surveyed believed they were well informed about PL 99-457 and many knew nothing about the law (Cohen, Kanthor, Meyer, & O'Hara, 1990). Most pediatricians surveyed desired more information. A 1990 Virginia survey of pediatricians on early identification and early intervention assessed pediatricians' screening methods, referral practices, and training needs (Scott, 1990). The survey found that almost 75% of those surveyed had received formal training in developmental pediatrics, but 42.9% rated their training as insufficient or poor. The majority (94%) of respondents recommended that more training in behavioral and developmental pediatrics was needed. The most frequently requested area of continuing education was developmental screening (65.8%), followed by further education regarding public and private community resources in early intervention (50.7%). Respondents indicated that regional seminars (61.2%) and workshops (53.2%) were the preferred modes of continuing medical education.

The 1978 Task Force on Pediatric Education of the American Academy of Pediatrics recognized underemphasized areas in pediatric residency training (Task Force on Pediatric Education, 1978). The most notable of these areas of deficient training were in biopsychosocial and developmental aspects of pediatrics and adolescent medicine. The report recommended that greater emphasis should be placed on training in these areas. A follow-up survey of graduates who completed their training in or after 1978, conducted 10 years after the Task Force report, found that there was minimal change in pediatricians' perceptions of insufficient training in all the areas of pediatrics described as underemphasized in the Task Force report, including behavioral and developmental disabilities (Wender et al., 1992). However, those residents who received their training during the second half of the 10 years after the Task Force report did note significant improvement in their perceptions of their training in these previously underemphasized areas, including behavioral and developmental pediatrics. Yet, approximately half of those surveyed who had completed their training since 1984 still judged their training in behavioral and developmental disabilities as inadequate.

These surveys clearly indicate the great need perceived by pediatricians for further training in behavioral and developmental pediatrics in general and for working with early intervention teams in particular. Without an appropriate knowledge base, physicians are not able to be fully effective participants on interdisciplinary teams nor will they be able to provide the most appropriate ongoing care for children with special health care needs.

General Training Issues

Training pediatricians for their role in the early intervention process is very different from training other professionals. The educational process of becoming a pediatrician is much more experiential than training in other professions and involves much less formal coursework. In medical school, students spend much of the first 2 of 4 years involved in classroom lecture and laboratory experience in basic sciences. The remaining 2 years are almost exclusively "clinical" and essentially consist of medical apprenticeships in which students learn from "hands-on" experience working and caring for individuals under the supervision of residents and attending physicians. After medical school, physicians interested in specializing in pediatrics must complete a 3-year pediatric residency. The residency primarily involves clinical care of patients with supervision, punctuated by didactic teaching "rounds." These rounds may involve large groups, such as hospital grand rounds; small group teaching regarding specific patients and diagnoses; or daily teaching conferences over the course of the year covering a variety of medical topics. Formal, ongoing courses on an individual topic do not typically occur. Another unique quality of medical training is that clinical care of patients obviously supersedes attendance at rounds or lectures, and, therefore, residents are often not able to attend all didactic teaching sessions. All of these factors make it difficult to simply teach the residents a "course" on what they need to know about early intervention and their role on interdisciplinary teams.

Any effort to train physicians to work with young children and their families should address several issues. First, there is the issue of physician knowledge about behavioral and developmental pediatrics. In order to identify children with developmental delays and/or disabilities appropriately, physicians must be knowledgeable about both typical and atypical behavior and development. In addition, they must be familiar with appropriate screening methods for detecting problems in development (American Academy of Pediatrics, Committee on Children with Disabilities, 1994). Such methods include not only formal screening "tests" but also relevant directed history taking and a physical examination. Second, this knowledge must be applicable to their actual practice behavior. Therefore, training programs must instruct physicians in techniques that are feasible to use in busy primary care settings. Third, a crucial component is addressing physicians' attitudes toward the material being taught and its applicability to their practices. Physicians may be resistant to change for a number of reasons, including 1) beliefs that children will "grow out of" many developmental delays, 2) insufficient time to implement recommended changes in practice, 3) skepticism about the efficacy of early intervention, 4) discomfort in talking to parents about diagnoses that may be chronic and/or lifelong, and 5) a hesitancy to "label" children. Unless physicians are convinced of the value and utility of material being taught, an increase in their knowledge is not likely to be translated into a change in practice behaviors. In addition, physicians' judgment heuristics, or cognitive techniques used to sort relevant from irrelevant information, while often leading to good decisions, may actually interfere with appropriate identification of children with developmental delays (Glascoe & Dworkin, 1993).

It is imperative to incorporate some method of assessing the efficacy of the training program in achieving its objectives. Evaluation allows designers of the training program to make ongoing revisions to the program to improve its effectiveness. In addition, feedback to recipients of the training program regarding changes in their knowledge and behavior may be helpful in reinforcing desired changes.

Training Principles

Instruction in developmental and behavioral pediatrics may occur through both preservice and in-service training. Preservice education can occur at different training levels—during medical school, pediatric or family practice residency, or subspecialty fellowship. Once in practice, pediatricians may update their knowledge and skills through continuing medical education courses. Ideally, sensitizing practitioners to the issues relevant to children with special health care needs should begin in medical school, with increased exposure during residency training. More attention has been paid to preservice training in the years subsequent to the report of the 1978 Task Force on Pediatric Education. Progress has been made since that task force report, but far too many practitioners still believe that their training is insufficient. To this end, approaches to improving preservice training need to be continually evaluated and refined. Determining the content and the process for improving preservice as well as in-service training has been deliberated by many authors and programs, including the Zero to Three/National Center for Clinical Infant Programs (NCCIP). Among other missions, the NCCIP program is very active in promoting training of all disciplines involved in early intervention and has developed a Training Approaches for Skills and Knowledge (TASK) Project (1988–1990), which recommended that four elements of training be available to all infant and family practitioners at each stage of their career preparation and development (Eggbeer, Latzko, & Pratt, 1993; Fenichel & Eggbeer, 1989, 1990). These elements are 1) a knowledge base that includes a conceptual framework common to all disciplines; 2) contact with infants and families through observation, providing respite care, or completing a supervised practicum; 3) individualized clinical supervision; and 4) collegial support, both within and across disciplines. The TASK Project also formulated a number of recommendations for the preservice, in-service, and professional development training of infant and family practitioners.

The following section reviews approaches to preservice and in-service training. Following this, suggestions for a recommended practice approach to developing and implementing training in developmental and behavioral pediatrics is presented, specifically emphasizing training pediatricians for involvement with early intervention teams.

In all fields, physicians are assuming many roles in addition to that of providers of acute care medicine. Physicians are becoming "gatekeepers" and service coordinators or case managers, and therefore must acquire the skills necessary to work with other professionals who may have significantly different training from their own. Physicians have traditionally been prepared to make prompt, independent decisions, especially when dealing with acute care illness. This is strikingly different from the skills necessary to work with children with chronic conditions, for whom, in conjunction with families and other professionals or health care providers, diagnoses may be more complex or slower to evolve and for whom decisions need to be adjusted over time. In addition, these children often have multiple needs, many of which are met outside of the traditional medical setting. Therefore, physicians will increasingly need skills that allow them to interact in a productive manner with professionals from other disciplines (e.g., education, psychology, physical and occupational therapy, speech-language pathology). Physicians will also need to learn to adjust their roles as is needed for a given child. For some children, physicians will be the most appropriate service coordinators; but for others, physicians may function more appropriately as consultants and must be willing and able to give up the team leader role physicians have traditionally been trained to assume. Therefore, educating physicians-in-training about the team process, the variety of possible roles, and the ways for successful team functioning should be started as soon as possible in their medical training. Establishing this core of knowledge and understanding about the team process would be a potentially strong foundation for future work as productive team members, regardless of the ultimate field of specialty chosen by the medical student.

Training Medical Students

A number of programs have been developed to address teaching medical students about developmental pediatrics, early intervention, and family-centered care. At the University of North Carolina at Chapel Hill (Sharp & Lorch, 1988), a program was developed to introduce first-year pediatric residents and fourth-year medical students to community resources available for children and to increase their knowledge of factors affecting children's development. The program was given to the pediatric residents in four 1-month modules over the course of 1 year and to the medical students during a 1-month ambulatory pediatrics elective experience. Two goals relevant to the interdisciplinary early intervention process were included in the program: 1) to increase the trainees' awareness of the availability of nonmedical resources for children, and 2) to increase their ability to communicate with nonmedical personnel and parents to improve service coordination for children. To achieve these goals, residents and students were given educational materials, including journal articles and videotapes. They also visited many community sites, such as child care centers, schools, and a health department clinic, and observed an early intervention team. In addition to providing training in multiple facets of behavioral and developmental pediatrics, this experience also provided exposure to a variety of disciplines in community settings and sensitized the residents and students to the team process.

A community-based educational experience was also provided at the University of Connecticut School of Medicine as part of its Introduction to Clinical Medicine course (Lewis & Greenstein, 1994). This curriculum was designed to teach medical students about family views of chronic and disabling conditions. In this program, first-year students were matched with adults and children with chronic health conditions. A subset of students was matched with children with genetic disorders that resulted in disability. Students made multiple home visits to the family, kept logs of their experiences, and participated in small group discussions with peers and faculty supervisors. Students became well aware of the impact a child with a disability had on numerous areas of family functioning. In addition, many students had their stereotyped views of children with disabilities challenged and often changed by this experience. This type of exposure was valuable for the students' understanding of the effects any chronic health condition has on the individuals with disabilities and their families, regardless of the type of medicine ultimately practiced by the student. An understanding of the role of the family is also vital to any provider involved in early intervention services in which the emphasis is child-focused and family-centered care.

At the University of Wisconsin, in the Department of Family Medicine and Practice, the Physician Education Project on Developmental Disabilities was established in 1986 (Schwab, 1991). The goal of this project was to enhance the health of children and adults with disabilities by improving the awareness and skills of the physicians who provide care for them. The project had a strong emphasis on the concept of family-centered care. The curriculum was required for all medical students and was presented longitudinally over 3 years. In the first year, as part of a semester course entitled "Clinical Medicine and Practice," students were given a lecture on family-centered, community-based, coordinated care. Students also spent time in the homes of families with a child or adult with special health care needs in order to gain firsthand experience on the issues discussed in the lecture. In the second year, as part of a course entitled "Introduction to Clinical Medicine," students were taught an approach to functional assessment that included not only standard history taking but also an appraisal of daily living skills and community supports. Students then practiced these skills by performing a functional assessment interview and examination of an individual with a significant disability, such as cerebral palsy or mental retardation. In the third year, as part of an 8-week required rotation in primary care, students revisited the issues and concepts taught in the first 2 years as related to clinical practice. Students were also assigned to do a "case study" of an individual with a disabling condition who received primary care in the student's practice. This 3-year program offered an opportunity for families to educate students about the realities of individual and family functioning around a chronic disability and ideally improved the care ultimately to be provided by these students.

The University of Vermont College of Medicine collaborated with a parent support group, Parent to Parent of Vermont, and developed a program (the Medical Education Project) designed to allow medical students to learn from families' personal experiences with children with disabilities or chronic illnesses (DiVenere, 1994; DiVenere, Frankowski, & Stifler, 1991). The Medical Education Project is directed to third-year medical students and involves an introductory lecture and discussion, a home visit to a family with a child with a disability or chronic illness, and a follow-up lecture and discussion session. The project has several goals, including 1) helping students recognize their own biases and beliefs about chronic illness and disability, 2) improving knowledge and understanding of family-centered care, and 3) acknowledging the experience and insight of individuals with disabilities and their families. This program provides families with an opportunity to participate in the training of future physicians and gives students valuable exposure to the central role of the family in the care of children with special health care needs.

Training Pediatric Residents

To become board certified in pediatrics, residents must complete 3 years of pediatric specialty training before passing a written certification examination. During these 3 years, residents must be exposed to the wide variety of acute and chronic conditions presented in childhood and must learn to manage these conditions in both inpatient and outpatient settings. This is generally done through a series of "block" rotations, consisting of 1- to 2-month experiences in different clinical settings (e.g., the neonatal intensive care unit [NICU], ambulatory pediatric clinic, inpatient wards). Residents traditionally spend the bulk of their training taking care of patients in a hospital setting, which is in contrast to the settings in which most primary care pediatricians ultimately practice. Although exposure to more outpatient and community settings seems indicated, there is often a conflict between hospital service requirements and what might be viewed as an ideal balance for training. The Residency Review Committee (1993–1994) recommendations regarding developmental-behavioral pediatric training are brief and nonspecific: "The residents must participate in a structured experience in normal and abnormal behavior and development involving didactic and clinical components. The experience must include the care of patients from newborn through young adulthood." These recommendations are being revised and the new guidelines have greater specificity regarding the duration and content of training. However, there is a great deal of flexibility and variety in how this component of pediatric training is designed and implemented. Many programs now recognize the relevance of such training to the general practice of pediatrics and as a result are instituting more comprehensive experiences in behavioral and developmental pediatrics.

A 1993 survey of pediatric residency programs indicated significant improvement in the exposure of residents to rotations in developmental and behavioral pediatrics. Teplin, Kuhn, and Palsha (1993) conducted a survey of the 219 pediatric residency programs in the United States to determine the status of training relevant to infants and toddlers with disabilities and their families. Of the 73% that responded, 89% of the programs offered a specific rotation in child development and behavior, with 73% of these rotations being mandatory. The duration and content of this training was quite variable between programs—ranging from 2 to 13 weeks, with a mean of 5 weeks. Of the responding programs, 39% used or adapted specific curricula or programs for teaching residents about behavioral and developmental pediatrics. Significantly more programs with mandatory rotations used specific curricula for training. It is important to note that only 28% of the programs indicated that parents were involved in the training of residents. Respondents indicated that their programs offered a mean of six didactic conferences per year focusing on infants and toddlers with disabilities and their families. Content areas of typical and atypical infant development and behavior and assessment of infants with disabilities were considered to be strengths in most programs. Areas reported as needing improvement included the physician as advocate, cultural aspects of family functioning, and service coordination. In addition, a few programs (11%) indicated a moderate to high degree of resident exposure to infants with disabilities in community programs or home-based services. Although it is encouraging that the majority of training programs responding did have rotations in place, clearly there is room for improvement in training regarding children with disabilities.

Many investigators have reported assessments of the adequacy and value of different aspects of pediatric training by graduates of residency programs. In an evaluation of a large pediatric residency program by its alumni, 94% of the respondents believed their training was adequate in preparing them for their current position (Liebelt, Daniels, Farrell, & Myers, 1993). However, the alumni believed that too little time was devoted to primary care experiences; the area of training judged lowest in both quality and quantity was behavioral and developmental pediatrics. Survey responses were unaffected by year of training (1974–1990) or type of practice (primary care or academic pediatrics), suggesting to the authors that the results of this survey are generally applicable to many training programs.

A report on 80 graduates of a pediatric residency that *required* training in behavior and development examined graduates' perceptions of their behavioral and developmental training (Breunlin et al., 1990). The aspects of training believed to be of the highest quality and the most useful were child development and counseling and/or anticipatory guidance, with training in school issues, behavior, and discipline receiving the lowest ratings. It is important to note that even those areas rated lowest did not receive scores of less than three on a five-point Likert scale. Most graduates valued and used their behavioral and developmental skills in their clinical work.

Curriculum Development for Pediatric Residents

Efforts have been made to develop specific curricula for training in developmental and behavioral pediatrics. A multidisciplinary committee, appointed by the

Executive Council of the Society for Behavioral Pediatrics, developed a curriculum guide for such training (Yancy et al., 1988). The guide discusses the rationale for inclusion of a structured curriculum during pediatric residency training, describes the interdisciplinary teaching staff recommended, and outlines objectives for different levels of training. Objectives are specifically described for medical students, residents, fellows, and practicing clinicians interested in continuing medical education.

The Task Force on Education in Developmental Pediatrics was established in 1978 to develop a curriculum in developmental pediatrics (Coury, 1990). According to Guralnick, Richardson, and Heiser (1982), the intent of the curriculum was

> to provide pediatric residents with the fundamental clinical skills, knowledge and attitudes to enable them as practicing pediatricians to contribute effectively to the diagnosis, assessment, and management of handicapped children and their families as well as to recognize their role responsibilities in various situations. (p. 340)

The information, to be ideally covered during a 1-month rotation in developmental pediatrics, included topics such as typical and atypical development, screening for and assessment of disabilities, the interdisciplinary process and team functioning, and community resources. The format allowed individual training programs to tailor the curriculum to fit within their resources and constraints. The curriculum included major goals, specific educational objectives, and examples of relevant learning activities (e.g., didactic content outlines; model clinical experiences and protocols; updated, annotated core and supplementary readings).

The effectiveness of this structured curriculum in teaching developmental pediatrics to pediatric residents was examined by Bennett, Guralnick, Richardson, and Heiser (1984). The curriculum was implemented and evaluated in 11 pediatric programs with a developmental pediatrics rotation. Results showed that the clinical decision-making skills of residents working with children who are at risk and/or have disabilities was enhanced significantly through participation in a developmental pediatrics rotation guided by this curriculum. Guralnick, Bennett, Heiser, Richardson, and Shibley (1987) tested the ability of this curriculum to be replicated in multiple training programs, varying in size, scope, and resources. Residents who had participated in the rotation defined by the curriculum scored significantly higher on an objective measure of clinical management skills than those who had not participated in the curriculum.

Residency Training Programs in Behavioral and Developmental Pediatrics

A number of pediatric residency programs have employed specific rotations in behavioral and developmental pediatrics. Some examples of such programs are described below.

The University of Maryland

At the University of Maryland School of Medicine, pediatric residents have two mandatory rotations through the Division of Behavioral and Developmental Pediatrics—1 month in their first year and 2 months in their second year of residency (Wachtel, Grossman, Hyman, & Kappelman, 1992). During these rotations, residents are exposed to a variety of tertiary-care and community-based experiences in order to obtain a broad view of the breadth and depth of the field. Such experiences include didactic lectures, developmental pediatrics rounds on inpatient wards, following patients in a behavioral pediatrics clinic, participating in interdisciplinary assessment teams of children with a variety of developmental disorders, providing general pediatric care to students with multiple disabilities at a school for children who are blind, and observing early intervention teams in the surrounding communities.

Within this program at the University of Maryland, a specific training curriculum for pediatric residents in early intervention has been developed. Goals of this curriculum were to educate residents about four major areas: 1) identification and evaluation of children with developmental delays or disabilities, 2) medical workups of selected developmental disabilities, 3) awareness of community resources in early intervention and how to have access to them, and 4) delivery of difficult diagnoses to parents. The structured curriculum was presented in three 2-hour weekly sessions. Handouts, articles, and videotapes of the children with disabilities and their parents were used to enhance clinical points discussed. The efficacy of the program in meeting its objectives was evaluated by examining changes in knowledge, behavior, and attitudes following the teaching program. Preliminary findings suggested that pediatric residents at both the first- and second-year level of training made significant gains in knowledge following training. Behavioral changes in referral to early intervention programs are being assessed.

Dartmouth-Hitchcock Medical Center

At the Dartmouth-Hitchcock Medical Center in New Hampshire, pediatric residents are exposed to a number of community-based experiences, such as early intervention programs, preschool special education, child care programs, and family support organizations (Cooley, 1994). In addition, each pediatric resident is required to provide respite care at least once for a family of a child with a disability or chronic illness, in order to gain insight into the realities of caring for children with special health care needs.

Michigan State University

At Michigan State University, the Chronic Illness Teaching Program is given to residents during all 3 years of pediatric residency (Cooley, 1994; Desguin, 1988). The goal of the program is to help physicians develop the knowledge, skills, and attitudes needed to care for children with chronic illnesses or disabilities. The major components of this program are 1) family studies, 2) services for children with chronic illness, 3) knowledge and skills, and 4) issues of chronic illness. By participating in a family study, residents can see the effects having a child with a chronic illness has on a family. To learn about services available for these children, residents are exposed to the various models of service delivery through experiences such as accompanying nurses on home visits or observing transdisciplinary teams. Necessary knowledge and skills are transmitted through a combination of didactic lecture and direct clinical experience. Issues of chronic illness are also addressed, such as the value of improving function even if a cure is not possible.

Texas Tech University Health Sciences Center

The Texas Tech University Health Sciences Center School of Medicine collaborated with a special education program for infants and children to develop a training program for pediatric residents focused on early intervention with children with developmental disabilities (Wysocki, Gururaj, Rogers, & Galey, 1987). This program, "Developmental Education Birth Through Two (DEBT)," consisted of 4 half-day weekly sessions. Highlights of these four sessions included 1) observation at a home visit of a special education teacher performing a developmental assessment of a child; 2) review of the child's individualized education program; 3) observation of the child's evaluation by other disciplines, such as occupational therapy or speech-language pathology; 4) observation of a special education teacher discussing results of the assessment and recommendations; and 5) participation in a transdisciplinary conference on ongoing educational planning for the child. Pediatric residents completed assessments of their skills related to early intervention with children who have disabilities before and after this experience that showed significant improvement in all areas.

Fellowship Training

Pediatricians who wish to subspecialize in a particular area of pediatrics must pursue additional training beyond the 3 years of pediatric residency. The length of this additional training varies between 1 and 3 years depending on the field chosen. A number of training programs exist in the field of behavioral and developmental pediatrics (Society for Behavioral Pediatrics, 1992), most of which are 2 or 3 years in length.

The goals of training pediatricians in the pediatric subspecialty of developmental and behavioral pediatrics include having 1) faculty for pediatric residency programs who can convey the knowledge, skills, and attitudes essential for the incorporation of a family-centered approach to caring for children with developmental disabilities; 2) practitioners of developmental and behavioral pediatrics for a variety of clinical settings, such as NICU follow-up programs, early intervention programs, specialty hospitals, and group practices; 3) researchers who can work with colleagues of other disciplines to address critical information needs, such as evaluating treatment alternatives in early intervention; 4) participants in the development of public policy in early intervention incorporating a health-based perspective; and 5) consultants to other providers of health care for children.

Some of the earliest fellowship training programs in developmental pediatrics were established in the 1960s with the development of a major multidisciplinary training initiative affiliated with federally funded (Maternal and Child Health) medical universities—the university affiliated program (UAP). Coordinated through the American Association of University Affiliated Programs, many academic centers developed fellowship programs and curricula for the training of subspecialists in the new field through the 1970s. In the 1980s, federal funding expanded to include training for behavioral pediatricians, and new programs for developmental and behavioral pediatricians began, incorporating critical components of both areas. By the next decade, there were more than 45 fellowship training programs in the field, and subspecialty certification is in the process of being developed (Society for Behavioral Pediatrics, 1992).

Fellowship training programs similar to the one at the University of Maryland train pediatricians by providing a core curriculum that must be mastered by potential practitioners in the field. This training program includes an extensive knowledge base in the following areas:

- Typical and atypical child development
- Medical evaluations, including genetics and neurology
- Treatment of developmental disabilities
- Interdisciplinary management of various disabling conditions
- Working with families
- Advocacy, including rights, responsibilities, and relevant legislation
- Research methodology

Practicum experiences include working in interdisciplinary evaluation centers, NICU follow-up programs, early intervention programs, schools, health department clinics, hospital-based clinics (e.g., children exposed to drugs, children with human immunodeficiency virus), and hospital consultation services. Many training programs require the completion of a relevant research project and provide opportunities for developing teaching skills. A national curriculum and certification examination is being developed, which builds on previously developed curriculum (Coury, Mulick, Eaton, Bruce, & Heron, 1988). This credential is vital to establish academic credibility and appropriate financial reimbursement for developmental and behavioral pediatricians to survive changes in the U.S. health care system.

In-Service Training

Ideally, training in developmental and behavioral pediatrics and early intervention should begin prior to a physician's entry into practice. However, if the physician did not receive such training or perceives his or her training as inadequate, in-service training remains a valuable resource for improving physician knowledge and skills. In addition, physicians need to be updated about changes in programs and community resources. There are multiple auspices under which such training can be provided. For example, programs may be supported by Infants and Toddlers Programs under Part H of IDEA, by the American Academy of Pediatrics, or by individual state or university efforts.

Part H of IDEA mandates that states ensure adequate training of professionals providing services to infants and toddlers and their families. Factors affecting states' abilities to implement such training include the difficulty of establishing comprehensive new programs or revising and updating existing programs and the significant lack of appropriate resource funding for such training services (Eggbeer et al., 1993). According to these authors, key characteristics to consider in establishing a statewide in-service training system include the following:

1. Addressing the training needs of all personnel, regardless of discipline or level of expertise
2. Basing the system on sound and ongoing needs assessments
3. Ensuring both intradisciplinary and multidisciplinary content
4. Making training accessible
5. Ensuring that training is culturally relevant

6. Developing a strong commitment (with funding) among parents, service
    providers, and policy makers to ongoing training of professionals and para-
    professionals and determining who will be responsible for implementation of
    the training plan

Examples of In-Service Training

The American Academy of Pediatrics (1986) developed a program entitled
"Project BRIDGE," which focused on the team approach to decision making for
early intervention services. This workshop was offered to a variety of disciplines
involved in providing services to infants and toddlers and their families and presented the essential components of team decision making and team dynamics.

In Nebraska, the state American Academy of Pediatrics chapter developed
36 hours of training material, which covered two main areas: 1) identification
and treatment of specific disabilities and problems that may compound a disability; and 2) provision of family-centered, community-based, coordinated care to
children with disabilities and their families (Medical Home Training in Nebraska, 1990). To achieve their objectives, pediatricians were educated about
treating disabilities, having access to community resources, discussing developmental diagnoses with parents, and participating in teams, among other topics.
The Nebraska chapter of the American Academy of Pediatrics offered courses to
pediatricians in multiple locations across the state.

Since the mid-1980s, Hawaii has made a dedicated effort to promote physician involvement in the care of children with chronic illnesses or disabilities
(Peter, 1992). As one aspect of this effort, a continuing medical education survey
course entitled "The Pediatrician and the New Morbidity" was developed (Peter,
1992; Peter & Sia, 1994). The 6-hour course is composed of three modules that
focus on the pediatrician's role in family-centered, community-based, coordinated care. The course can be completed in six 1-hour sessions or three 2-hour
sessions. The first 2-hour module addresses the role of the pediatrician in
community-based care and outlines the characteristics of a medical home. Emphasis is placed on developmental surveillance, as well as the use of selected
tools and protocols. The second 2-hour module focuses on the pediatrician's role
on transdisciplinary community-based teams serving children with chronic illnesses or disabilities. In the third module, the focus is on the pediatrician and
family-centered care. Issues discussed include early diagnosis, breaking diagnostic news, and building partnerships with parents. Training is conducted in a
small group format to facilitate active involvement of participants.

In Louisiana, regional programs were developed to specifically target practicing pediatricians (Adams & Sonnier, 1990). A widely known pediatrician with
expertise in early intervention was invited to increase attendance and provide
up-to-date information regarding PL 99-457. A second invited speaker gave an
overview of the state's Part H program. In addition, a local pediatrician who had
been involved in regional pilot programming participated to lend local verifica-
tion of the value of the program. Finally, members of various early intervention
agencies were present to answer questions.

In Arizona, training programs were offered in selected statewide locations
(Melmed, 1991). Prior to the implementation of the training program, 20 interested pediatricians were identified through a statewide survey and were trained

in presentation of the program, ensuring a ready supply of presenters. The course content included an overview of PL 99-457 and the physician's role, issues in early identification, parents' perspectives regarding the importance of the physician to the family and the need for sensitivity when giving difficult diagnoses, and an overview of local resources. The course was conducted by a local physician, a parent, a local developmental disabilities resource person, and a physician "trainer."

The above review represents a sampling of continuing medical education programs initiated nationwide. The number and diversity of the programs offered illustrates the increasing emphasis states are placing on the education of physicians about developmental disorders and the value of early intervention.

GENERAL GUIDELINES FOR DEVELOPING
TRAINING PROGRAMS FOR PEDIATRICIANS

Based on surveys of pediatricians regarding their perceived training needs in behavioral and developmental pediatrics along with the above review of preservice and in-service programs, several suggestions for recommended practice approaches to developing training programs for pediatricians are offered in Tables 1, 2, and 3. The guidelines listed in Table 1 are appropriate for developing pro-

Table 1. Training guidelines for preservice and in-service training

1. Convince pediatricians that the material they are being taught is necessary for them to be able to provide the best care for their patients.
2. Convince pediatricians that the materials and methods they are being taught are practical and feasible for use in a busy primary care setting.
3. Recognize and discuss barriers that exist to the implementation of proposed recommendations, such as time constraints and inadequate financial reimbursement.
4. Provide pragmatic information that physicians can easily use and apply to their practices (e.g., useful screening tests, parent questionnaires, suggestions for implementation, handouts regarding the medical workup for specific disabilities, cards with relevant numbers of intervention resources in their communities).
5. Provide the teaching in small group sessions, if possible. This allows for more interactive sessions with more discussion and questions and provides a more active learning experience.
6. Concentrate on the more mild, common disorders that primary care physicians are more likely to see in greater numbers, although discussion of the greater severity and/or lower incidence disorders is necessary as well.
7. Emphasize the value of the pediatrician's involvement in the care of children with special health care needs, including direct patient care and ongoing support of the child and family.
8. Emphasize the important role of the family in the care of children with special needs, including parents as primary advocates for children. Acknowledge that parents are the most knowledgeable observers of their children.
9. Modify the curriculum as appropriate for the individuals being taught and their level of training (e.g., medical students, pediatric residents, behavioral and developmental fellows, nurse practitioners, community physicians).
10. Develop a method of assessment to determine the efficacy of the program in achieving its objectives.

Table 2.   Guidelines specific to preservice programs

1. Demonstrate support and a commitment to behavioral and developmental pediatrics from medical schools and departments of pediatrics.
2. Use rotations in behavioral and developmental pediatrics as mandatory, not elective, experiences during pediatric residency training. Residents' other commitments, such as coverage for sick residents and night call, should be adjusted so that residents are not "pulled" out of this rotation to cover what have traditionally been viewed as more "important" clinical sites.
3. Use standardized curricula, where available and relevant, to guide training of residents in these areas.
4. Include in this rotation significant exposure to children with special health care needs *outside of* the tertiary care setting, such as in their homes and schools.
5. Expose pediatricians to the "real-life" experiences of families with children with chronic illnesses or disabilities for valuable training experience.
6. View sensitivity to behavioral and developmental issues as an ongoing goal of pediatric residency training, not as limited to the time period of a defined rotation.

grams at both the preservice and in-service level, while those listed in Tables 2 and 3 are appropriate for preservice and in-service training, respectively.

CONCLUDING REMARKS: FUTURE DIRECTIONS

Pediatricians have a valuable role to play in the interdisciplinary care of the child with disabilities. Preservice and in-service training programs are needed to help physicians participate actively in the early intervention system. These programs must provide knowledge about interdisciplinary team function and working with families, in addition to providing pediatricians with information about the identification, evaluation, and service coordination of children with disabilities. A collaborative model between the early intervention system and the medical community is necessary for the child's and family's needs to be adequately addressed. Resources in the community for training include the state chapter of the American Academy of Pediatrics and the developmental pediatrics faculty of the local medical school or hospital.

Table 3.   Guidelines specific to in-service programs

1. Involve local pediatricians in the assessment of their training needs and plans for educational intervention prior to developing and implementing a training program.
2. Have a local, respected pediatrician with an interest in children with special health care needs be a part of providing the training program to provide implicit support that the material being taught is relevant and applicable to the primary care practitioner.
3. Schedule meetings at times that are convenient for community physicians. Seek physician input for the best times for a given community. Examples of settings for such meetings include hospital staff meetings, grand rounds, lunch or dinner meetings, and weekend meetings.
4. Provide food and/or continuing medical education credits along with the training courses to add extra incentive for attendance.

REFERENCES

Adams, R.C., & Sonnier, E. (1990). The pediatrician's role and regional planning for infant screening and evaluation under PL 99-457. *The Medical Home Newsletter, 2*(2), 12–13.

American Academy of Pediatrics. (1986). *Project BRIDGE. Decision-making for early services: A team approach.* Elk Grove Village, IL: Author.

American Academy of Pediatrics, Committee on Children with Disabilities. (1994). Screening infants and young children for developmental disabilities. *Pediatrics, 93,* 863–865.

Bennett, F.C. (1982). The pediatrician and the interdisciplinary process. *Exceptional Children, 48,* 306–314.

Bennett, F.C., Guralnick, M.J., Richardson, H.B., Jr., & Heiser, K.E. (1984). Teaching developmental pediatrics to pediatrics residents: Effectiveness of a structured curriculum. *Pediatrics, 74,* 514–522.

Blackman, J.A., Healy, A., & Ruppert, E.S. (1992). Participation by pediatricians in early intervention: Impetus from Public Law 99-457. *Pediatrics, 89,* 98–102.

Breunlin, D.C., Mann, B.J., Richtsmeier, A., Lillian, Z., Richman, J.S., & Bernotas, T. (1990). Pediatricians' perceptions of their behavioral and developmental training. *Journal of Developmental and Behavioral Pediatrics, 11,* 165–169.

Cohen, H., Kanthor, H., Meyer, M.R., & O'Hara, D. (1990). *American Academy of Pediatrics Survey: District II, Valhalla, New York.* The M.R. Institute, New York Medical College.

Cooley, W.C. (1994). Graduate medical education in pediatrics: Preparing reliable allies for parents of children with special health care needs. In R.B. Darling & M.I. Peter (Eds.), *Families, physicians, and children with special health needs: Collaborative medical education models* (pp. 109–120). Westport, CT: Auburn House.

Coury, D.L. (1990). Training physicians for increased involvement with children with special needs. *Infants and Young Children, 2,* 51–57.

Coury, D.L., Mulick, J.A., Eaton, A.P., Bruce, N.M., & Heron, T.E. (1988). A fellowship curriculum in behavioral-developmental pediatrics. *Journal of Developmental and Behavioral Pediatrics, 9,* 92–95.

Degraw, C., Edell, D., Ellers, B., Hillemeier, M., Liebman, J., Perry, C., & Palfrey, J.S. (1988). Public Law 99-467: New opportunities to serve young children with special needs. *The Journal of Pediatrics, 113,* 971–974.

Desguin, B.W. (1988). Preparing pediatric residents for the primary care of children with chronic illness and their families: The Chronic Illness Teaching Program. *Zero to Three, 8*(3), 7–10.

DiVenere, N.J. (1994). Parents as educators of medical students. In R.B. Darling & M.I. Peter (Eds.), *Families, physicians, and children with special health needs: Collaborative medical education models* (pp. 101–108). Westport, CT: Auburn House.

DiVenere, N., Frankowski, B., & Stifler, D. (1991). The Medical Education Project: A shared learning experience—Incorporating the principles of family centered care in physician education. *The Medical Home Newsletter, 4*(2), 5–8.

Downey, W.S., Jr. (1990). Public Law 99-457 and the clinical pediatrician. Part 2: Implication for the pediatrician. *Clinical Pediatrics, 29,* 223–227.

Education of the Handicapped Act Amendments of 1986, PL 99-457. (October 8, 1986). Title 20, U.S.C. 1400 et seq: *U.S. Statutes at Large, 100,* 1145–1177.

Eggbeer, L.E., Latzko, T., & Pratt, B. (1993). Establishing statewide systems of in-service training for infant and family personnel. *Infants and Young Children, 5,* 49–56.

Fenichel, E.S., & Eggbeer, L. (1989). Educating allies: Issues and recommendations in the training of practitioners to work with infants, toddlers, and their families. *Zero to Three, 10*(1), 1–7.

Fenichel, E.S., & Eggbeer, L. (1990). *Preparing practitioners to work with infants, toddlers, and their families.* Arlington, VA: National Center for Clinical Infant Programs.

Glascoe, F.P., & Dworkin, P.H. (1993). Obstacles to effective developmental surveillance: Errors in clinical reasoning. *Journal of Developmental and Behavioral Pediatrics, 14,* 344–349.

Guralnick, M.J., Bennett, F.C., Heiser, K.E., Richardson, H.B., Jr., & Shibley, R.E. (1987). Training residents in developmental pediatrics: Results from a national replication. *Journal of Developmental and Behavioral Pediatrics, 8,* 260–265.

Guralnick, M.J., Richardson, H.B., Jr., & Heiser, K.E. (1982). A curriculum in handicapping conditions for pediatric residents. *Exceptional Children, 48,* 338–346.

Individuals with Disabilities Education Act (IDEA) of 1990, PL 101-476. (October 30, 1990). Title 20, U.S.C. 1400 et seq: *U.S. Statutes at Large, 104*(Part 2), 1103–1151.

Individuals with Disabilities Education Act Amendments of 1991, PL 102-119. (October 7, 1991). Title 20, U.S.C. 1400 et seq: *U.S. Statutes at Large, 105,* 587–608.

Lewis, J., & Greenstein, R.M. (1994). A first-year medical student curriculum about family views of chronic and disabling conditions. In R.B. Darling & M.I. Peter (Eds.), *Families, physicians, and children with special health needs: Collaborative medical education models* (pp. 77–100). Westport, CT: Auburn House.

Liebelt, E.L., Daniels, S.R., Farrell, M.K., & Myers, M.G. (1993). Evaluation of pediatric training by the alumni of a residency program. *Pediatrics, 91,* 360–364.

Medical home training in Nebraska. (1990). *The Medical Home Newsletter, 2*(4), 7–9.

Melmed, R. (1991). A new world order! Preparing the physicians. *The Medical Home Newsletter, 4*(2), 4–5.

Melmed, R.D., & Dolins, J.C. (1988). *Survey of state chapter committees on children with disabilities on the implementation of Public Law 99-457, Part H.* Elk Grove Village, IL: American Academy of Pediatrics.

Peter, M.I. (1992). Combining continuing medical education and systems change to promote physician involvement. *Infants and Young Children, 4,* 53–62.

Peter, M.I., & Sia, C.C.J. (1994). Preparing physicians through continuing medical education. In R.B. Darling & M.I. Peter (Eds.), *Families, physicians, and children with special health needs: Collaborative medical education models* (pp. 123–134). Westport, CT: Auburn House.

Residency Review Committee. (1993–1994). *Essentials and information items.* The Accreditation Council for Graduate Medical Education.

Schwab, W.E. (1991). Teaching family-centered care to medical students: The University of Wisconsin curriculum. *The Medical Home Newsletter, 5*(2), 4–7.

Scott, F. (1990). *A statewide survey of pediatricians on early identification and early intervention.* Richmond: Virginia Department of Mental Health, Mental Retardation and Substance Abuse Services.

Sharp, M.C., & Lorch, S.C. (1988). A community outreach training program for pediatric residents and medical students. *Journal of Medical Education, 63,* 316–322.

Society for Behavioral Pediatrics. (1992). Fellowship programs in behavioral and/or developmental pediatrics. *Journal of Developmental and Behavioral Pediatrics, 13,* 151–157.

Solomon, R. (1995). Pediatricians and early intervention: Everything you need to know but are too busy to ask. *Infants and Young Children, 7,* 38–51.

Task Force on Pediatric Education. (1978). *The future of pediatric education.* Evanston, IL: American Academy of Pediatrics.

Teplin, S.W., Kuhn, T.H., & Palsha, S.A. (1993). Preparing residents for Public Law 99-457: A survey of pediatric training programs. *American Journal of Diseases of Children, 147,* 175–179.

Wachtel, R.C., Grossman, L., Hyman, S.L., & Kappelman, M. (1992). Helping future pediatricians to know and understand: Preservice education for professionals who care for children with chronic and disabling conditions. In R.B. Darling & M.I. Peter (Eds.), *Creating family-professional partnerships: Educating physicians and other health professionals to care for children with chronic and disabling conditions.* Honolulu: Hawaii Medical Association.

Wender, E.H., Bijur, P.E., & Boyce, W.T. (1992). Pediatric residency training: Ten years after the Task Force report. *Pediatrics, 90,* 876–880.

Wysocki, T., Gururaj, V.J., Rogers, M.A., & Galey, G. (1987). Training pediatric residents in early intervention with handicapped children. *Journal of Medical Education, 62,* 47–52.

Yancy, W.S., Coury, D.L., Drotar, D., Gottlieb, M.I., Kohen, D.P., & Sarles, R.M. (1988). A curriculum guide for developmental-behavioral pediatrics. *Journal of Developmental and Behavioral Pediatrics, 9*(Suppl.), 1–8.

10

PREPARING
PEDIATRIC PSYCHOLOGISTS

Marie Kanne Poulsen

Josie, 4 months old, was brought to the center by her mother, Veronica. Josie was born prenatally exposed to cocaine. Josie's mother was in a drug recovery program, but no one was helping her take care of her infant. Veronica described Josie as "an irritable baby [who] wouldn't always pay attention," and who was "hard to comfort [and] didn't like to cuddle." An assessment process took place weekly for 1½ months. With the trust that began to develop over time, Veronica expressed her concerns about Josie's development and interactions and revealed her own parenting doubts and misgivings.

Josie was easily upset and cried frequently. When her mother approached her too abrubtly, Josie would flail her arms and legs and move her head in excitement. Other times, she calmed herself and focused and engaged her mother with eye contact and an eager smile. At times, when her mother tried to nestle her close to her body, Josie would stiffen and her mother would quickly put her down on her blanket.

Veronica and the psychologist together assessed Josie's developmental and neurodevelopmental competencies and vulnerabilities; her temperament; and her interactions with her mother, the psychologist, and the environment. Together they identified how Josie engaged in interaction when approached by her mother and then a stranger and how she responded differently to her environment when undressed and then when swaddled. Together they observed Josie's capacity for cuddling when handled in different ways. Together they observed for the onset of crying with and without accompanying abrupt movements, bright lights, loud sounds, and commotion. Together they discovered the circumstances that made it more likely for Josie to be soothed, cuddled, responsive, and initiating. Through this parent–professional partnership, caregiving strategies that facilitate infant development and enhance mother–infant interactions were identified and began to be supported.

FAMILY-CENTERED PEDIATRIC INTERNSHIP TRAINING is an essential component of the preparation of psychologists to serve young children from birth to age 5. Psychology programs within universities and professional schools vary in the extent to which pediatric issues and skills are addressed. Programs also differ in their emphasis on culturally sensitive, family-centered experiences and on the provision of training in interdisciplinary team assessment and intervention opportunities. To be responsive to the range of the mental health and developmental needs of very young children and their families, psychologists must be prepared to provide services that 1) contribute to a broad-based, prevention-oriented, child development and family support program; 2) meet the needs of very young children and families exhibiting early signs of distress; and 3) focus on relationship-based interventions for children with identified serious behavioral and emotional difficulties (Piotrkowski, Collins, Knitzer, & Robinson, 1994). In addition, traditional mental health service delivery by psychologists has evolved into new ecocultural service delivery paradigms since the mid-1980s (Knitzer, 1993). Ecocultural service delivery views the emotional, social, and behavioral development of the child in the context of family-system issues, individual family member needs and resources, culture, class, and community circumstances and supports. Therefore, psychologists need an internship program that stresses an array of knowledge and skills that meets the needs of economically, socially, and culturally diverse young children and their families.

This chapter addresses the new directions in infant and child mental health knowledge and service delivery and the related pediatric psychology competencies and experiences needed in a quality personnel pediatric preparation program.

NEW DIRECTIONS IN INFANT AND CHILD MENTAL HEALTH

Since the mid-1970s, findings from mental health and child development research have demonstrated the importance of social and emotional development during infancy and early childhood and the vulnerability of the child to serious emotional and social dysfunction during this time (Lyons-Ruth & Zeanah, 1993).

Importance of Infant Mental Health

Mental health in infants, toddlers, and young children is characterized by emotional growth, attachment to caregivers, emergence of self-confidence, and competency in social relationships. These patterns of emotional and social development are as essential to the child's overall development as are physical growth and maturation and motor and cognitive development (Schrag, 1988). In fact, emotional and mental health is thought to be "the necessary foundation for all further development" (Schrag, 1988, p. 3).

Mental health plays a particularly crucial role in the successful development of children who have or who are at risk for developmental disabilities. Frequently, the very nature of special developmental or health care needs jeopardizes healthy emotional development (Martner, Magrab, Fenichel, Feinberg, & Delago, 1989). Among children with disabilities, those who are emotionally healthy will likely be better equipped to meet the challenges that come with their disabilities. Longitudinal research has suggested that early intervention can promote effective parenting and enhance development in infants and toddlers who are dealing with biological and environmental challenges (Black, 1993). Empirical evidence has suggested that one of the long-term effects of early intervention is increased social competence when children reach school age (Berrueta-Clement, Scheinhart, Barnett, Epstein, & Weikart, 1984).

Legislative Changes

The field of infant and child mental health has experienced critical changes since the mid-1980s because of the passage of significant federal legislation. Federally funded programs now support states in their efforts to develop a comprehensive continuum of care for very young children and their families. PL 99-457, the Education of the Handicapped Act Amendments of 1986 (since updated as PL 102-119, the Individuals with Disabilities Education Act Amendments of 1991); Maternal and Child Health (MCH) Block Grants; Children with Special Health Care Needs (CSHCN); the Early and Periodic Screening, Diagnosis, and Treatment (EPSDT) Programs; and the Child and Adolescent Service System Program (CASSP) all contain mental health initiatives that affect service delivery to infants, toddlers, and young children and their families. These programs focus on interdisciplinary, interagency, family-centered, and community-based services. They require 1) psychologists who have the expertise to work with very young children and their families; and 2) psychology professional preparation programs that specialize in infant, toddler, and young child development, and the formation of family-centered assessment, intervention, and program development competencies.

The changes in federal legislation and policy relating to infant and child mental health were influenced by converging political, economic, and social forces that have given rise to increased numbers of adolescents who are engaging in risk behaviors that have a widespread effect on the quality of their lives. Legislation and policy have also been influenced by new knowledge stemming from research on 1) the psychosocial and biological bases of behavior, 2) the notion of cumulative risks, 3) the constructs of infant and family resilience, and 4) the importance of infant mental health.

Psychosocial and Biological Bases of Behavior and the Notion of Cumulative Risk

Research has confirmed the influence that psychosocial and biological conditions can have on the social, emotional, and behavioral development of infants, toddlers, and young children (Escalona, 1984; Osofsky & Fenichel, 1994; Sameroff, Seifer, Barocas, Lax, & Greenspan, 1987; Werner & Smith, 1992). The escalation of poverty, addiction, unsupported single-parent families, domestic discord, and community violence has led to an increased number of infants and young children who are at risk for emotional, social, and behavior problems (Gabarino, Dubrow, & Kostelny, 1989; National Center for Children in Poverty, 1990). In addition, children who are members of ethnic groups have been found to be at significant risk for experiencing rejection and discrimination and, as a result, are at greater risk for developing psychological and behavior problems than are other children (Dougherty, Saxe, Cross, & Silverman, 1987; Solomon, 1993). Biological data have supported the links between genetics, infectious disease, toxic agents, physical trauma, immunological conditions, metabolic and endocrinologic disorders, and nutritional deficiencies to emotional and behavioral vulnerabilities and disorders in children (Hoffman & Johnson, 1993).

Chronic illness and developmental disabilities can result in difficulties for both infants and young children and their caregivers, which, in turn, may impair their evolving relationships and subsequent emotional well-being. Infants and toddlers with developmental disabilities are found to have a higher rate of behavior problems than children without developmental challenges (Blackman & Cobb, 1988), and the prevalence of significant behavior and emotional problems among children with chronic illness is 2–5 times greater than that of apparently healthy children (Cadman, Boyle, & Szatmari, 1987). Children who have or are at risk for special developmental or health care needs are more likely to have difficulty in social relationships, in the development of a positive self-esteem, in impulse control, in their abilities to distinguish between fantasy and reality, and in their abilities to focus attention, concentrate, and plan (Schrag, 1988).

Neurodevelopmental vulnerabilities or dysfunctions stemming from low birth weight, prematurity, perinatal substance exposure, poor nutrition, maternal infections, and other perinatal insults may affect how the infant and young child respond to people and events. The development of attachment to caregivers, a sense of self-efficacy, and positive social relationships also may be affected (Poulsen, 1992).

The notion of cumulative risk asserts that the greater the number of biological risks, familial psychosocial vulnerabilities, and elements of community discord, the greater the risk for later difficulties (Molfese, 1989; Sameroff et al., 1987). The number of infants and toddlers being referred to pediatric clinics as a result of nonadaptive behaviors has significantly increased over the years. As a result, the pediatric literature has labeled the phenomena as the "new morbidity," and reports that children are referred far more often for psychosocial problems than for infectious diseases (Garmezy, 1991; Molfese, 1989).

Construct of Resilience

Resilience refers to the capacity for successful adjustment and coping in response to a crisis or stressful life event. Resilient individuals and families have the ability to recover from adversity and adjust to change (Patterson, 1991). There has been increased attention to the concept of resilience in the development of infants and young children (Garmezy, 1991; Osofsky & Fenichel, 1994; Patterson, 1991). The construct of resilience, as a counterbalance to the construct of vulnerability (Murphy & Moriarty, 1976), refers to the notion that there is a continuum of potential resilience inherent in all children that allows for adaptation and coping.

A diagnosis of a chronic illness or a developmental disability presents a challenge to the individual and to the family. Resilience can help the growing child and the family cope with biological, psychosocial, and environmental challenges stemming from an illness or disability. Emotional and instrumental family supports can lead to successful adjustment and coping, resulting in a family system that adapts well to the challenges associated with a child who has a chronic illness or disability. Because the family is the primary mediator of the young child's psychosocial well-being, the child's internal resources for coping are also enhanced. There is evidence that infant vulnerability can be reduced by resiliency-enhancing factors that increase the child's capacity to adapt to biological and environmental challenges (Garmezy, 1991; Werner & Smith, 1992). This evidence has provided part of the rationale for the federal legislation mandating early intervention.

Federal Legislative Support for Infant Mental Health Services

There have been several pieces of federal legislation since the mid-1980s that have changed the delivery of developmental services and health care to infants and toddlers with special needs. Policies and regulations stemming from these federal systems-change initiatives have played a critical role in the development and delivery of infant–toddler services and therefore have implications for the training of pediatric psychologists. Significant legislation includes 1) CASSP in 1984, 2) Part H of PL 99-457, and 3) the CSHCN and the EPSDT program amendments of the Omnibus Budget Reconciliation Acts (OBRA) of 1986 (PL 99-509) and 1989 (PL 101-239). Because the mission and philosophies articulated in CASSP, Part H, CSHCN, and EPSDT programs focus on interdisciplinary, interagency, family-centered, and community-based services, the professional preparation needs of psychologists as service providers and program directors are broadened significantly. The most pertinent of these programs are reviewed briefly in this chapter.

Child and Adolescent Service System Program

In 1984 Congress authorized CASSP at the National Institute of Mental Health to provide grants to individual states to improve services to children with serious emotional disorders and their families. CASSP principles articulate changes in mental health service delivery, including the importance of early identification; individualized service plans (ISPs); service delivery within the least restrictive, most normative environment; service coordination; interagency linkages; and family empowerment and full participation in all aspects of the planning and delivery of services.

Part H of PL 99-457, the Early Intervention
Program for Infants and Toddlers with Disabilities

Part H of PL 99-457 includes a number of provisions that delineate the manner in which services are to be delivered to infants and toddlers and that affect the professional training of psychologists as recognized personnel qualified to deliver early intervention services. The purpose of the legislation is "to provide financial assistance to the states to develop and implement a statewide, comprehensive, coordinated, multidisciplinary, interagency program of early intervention services for infants and toddlers with disabilities and their families" (303.16). At the discretion of the individual states, the term *infants and toddlers with disabilities* may also include "children from birth through age two who are at risk of having substantial developmental delays if early intervention services are not provided" (303.16).

Services are to be provided, to the greatest extent possible, in typical environments appropriate to the needs of the children, including the home and community settings in which children without disabilities participate. Parents are to play a central role in the delivery of services, including active collaboration with professionals in the assessment of the child and family needs, in the selection of services, and in the development of individualized family service plans (IFSPs). Family assessments must be voluntary, family directed, and designed to determine the resources, priorities, and concerns of the family related to enhancing the development of the child. Family-centered service delivery is designed to replace the traditional child-focused approach (Dunst, Trivette, & Deal, 1988).

Psychologists are included in the enumeration of personnel qualified to provide early intervention services. Psychological services include

> (i) administering psychological and developmental tests and other assessment procedures; (ii) interpreting assessment results; (iii) obtaining, integrating and interpreting information about child behavior, and child and family conditions related to learning, mental health and development; and (iv) planning and managing a program of psychological services, including psychological counseling for children and parents, family counseling, consultation on child development, parent training and education programs. (Part H, PL 99-457, 303.12)

Omnibus Budget Reconciliation Act Amendments of the Maternal and Child Health and Early and Periodic Screening, Diagnosis, and Treatment Programs

PL 99-509 introduced amendments in MCH programs, including the CSHCN program, to mandate coordinated, comprehensive, family-centered systems of care for all children from low-income families served by these programs. PL 101-239 strengthened an earlier mandate that required states to make the Medicaid EPSDT program services available *whenever* a child is suspected of having a physical, mental health, or developmental problem or condition that requires an assessment and further diagnosis and treatment.

The federal CSHCN program provided the impetus for specialized services for children to be organized at the state level and introduced the concept of multidisciplinary and interdisciplinary teams as an intervention strategy to state CSHCN programs (Association of Maternal and Child Health Programs, 1993).

The EPSDT program is a potential source of funding for more than 126 million children with family incomes less than 200% of the federal poverty level (Orloff, Rivera, Harris, & Rosenbaum, 1992). To ensure funding for services for infants and toddlers whose families lack financial resources, Congress specifically included a Part H program requirement that Medicaid, and other third-party insurers covering costs for individuals with disabilities, pay for the needed therapy for infants and toddlers. In Medicaid's case, services to infants and toddlers potentially are covered through the EPSDT program.

PL 101-239 mandated that cognitive and mental health screening be provided as part of the EPSDT medical screening program. The U.S. Department of Health and Human Services has issued guidance to state Medicaid programs specifying that for younger children, medical screening should include social-emotional development. It should focus on the child's ability to engage in social interaction with other children, parents, and other adults, and on the child's cognitive skills, focusing on problem solving.

CASSP, MCH, EPSDT, and Part H programs offer new models of service delivery to children and families in the United States. The EPSDT program and Part H of the Individuals with Disabilities Education Act (IDEA) of 1990, PL 101-476, are two federal programs that directly play a significant role in building comprehensive health service programs for infants and toddlers at the low-income level with, or at risk for, disabilities and developmental delays (Orloff, Rivera, Harris, & Rosenbaum, 1992). The two programs form the structural and financial foundation for early intervention services. By bringing these two programs together, infants and toddlers from low-income families have access to and the means to pay for a specialty health care delivery system (Orloff, Rivera, & Rosenbaum, 1992).

New Models of Family-Centered Service Delivery

Mental health service delivery has expanded from a traditional psychological model focusing on intra- and interpersonal phenomena to more complex models that reflect biopsychosocial and ecological theoretical perspectives (Friesen, 1993). These changes are noted in Table 1, which delineates the modifications in service delivery to infants, toddlers, and young children that have been reflected in the provisions of the CASSP, the Part H program, and PL 99-509 and PL 101-239.

The new directions in infant and child mental health service delivery discussed in this section require that the following dimensions are included in the preservice pediatric psychology personnel preparation:

1. Family-centered care
2. Culturally competent service delivery
3. Promotion of wellness and recognition of family resources, as well as risk factors
4. Parent–professional partnerships
5. Interdisciplinary and interagency approaches to service delivery

These are discussed in the following section.

PROFESSIONAL PREPARATION OF PEDIATRIC PSYCHOLOGISTS

The professional preparation of psychologists to work with infants, toddlers, and young children must reflect the important changes that have occurred since the mid-1980s, including the broadened knowledge base, expanded theoretical frameworks, new service delivery models, and practice roles (Friesen, 1993). Personnel preparation must focus on the knowledge, attitudes, and skills that lead to interdisciplinary, interagency, family-centered, culturally competent, community-based care.

General licensure granted by the states allows the psychologist to practice in any one of a number of specialties. The American Psychological Association (APA) sees the practitioner as a psychologist first and a specialist second (Committee on Accreditation, APA, 1980). Thus, psychology programs are geared to provide training in the fundamentals of theory and methodology, which are shared by all psychologists regardless of area of specialization. The basic psychology training programs include the following:

• Material on life-span approach to human development
• Individual differences and the bases of behavior, generic skills of assessment, diagnosis and treatment, scientific and professional ethics, and standards
• Research design and methodology
• Psychological measurement and statistics
• History and systems of psychology
• Program evaluation (Roberts, Fanurik, & Elkins, 1987)

Table 1.   Comparison of traditional and ecologically based service delivery models

Traditional psychology service delivery model	Ecologically-based service delivery model
Child-centered services	**Family-centered services**
Focus on supporting the health and development of infants, toddlers, and young children; emphasis on developing child competencies	Focus on supporting family capacity to meet special needs of young children; emphasis on enhancement of child–caregiver relationships
Focus on intervention to eliminate identified deficits	Focus on the promotion of wellness, the recognition of family strengths and resources
Families seen as recipients of intervention services from "experts"	Focus on families as partners in the development and implementation of child service plans
Program-centered services	**Child- and family-centered services**
Focus on match of child to services offered to determine appropriateness of referral	Focus on matching practice to needs, values, and preferences of families; culturally competent practice
Unidisciplinary focus on child social, emotional, behavioral development, and on family dynamics, leading to fragmented service delivery plans	Transdisciplinary focus as part of a comprehensive service plan that addresses a full range of child and family needs, leading to coordinated service delivery plans
Focus on formal services	Focus on informal supports (e.g., friends, churches, social clubs) as well as formal services
Focus on services primarily offered in center and/or clinic based programs	Focus on services also offered in homes, infant–toddler programs, preschools, and other usual environments

In a 1988 survey of 41 universities with clinical psychology programs, only 12% reported actually having a separate track in pediatric psychology (Routh & La Greca, 1990). Most pediatric training offered throughout the country is a track concentration of training embedded within a general clinical psychology program (Tuma, 1990). Because the general preparation is so broad, the pediatric psychology specialty requires significant additional training in knowledge and skills that focus on the developmental needs of infants, toddlers, and young children and their families (Fenichel & Eggbeer, 1990). The application of the psychology discipline to infants and young children is a specialty that is offered in several different university training programs, including school psychology, applied developmental psychology, pediatric psychology, child health psychology, and clinical child psychology (Roberts, Erickson, & Tuma, 1985). Great variability exists in training program curricula among and within specialty areas. There is not a clearly defined set of standards or competencies for psychologists who work with infants and young children. Psychology training programs that offer a child specialty program may have fundamentally different perspectives in terms of areas of emphases, theoretical frameworks, and applications in the delivery of services.

The emphasis placed on infancy, child, and adolescent issues in the curriculum may differ in several respects. Coursework and training experience may provide varying degrees of exposure to typical and atypical infants and young children; cultural and linguistic diversity; normal developmental processes; the impact biological, psychological, and sociological influences have on developmental and behavioral risk and resilience; promotion of mental health; and the prevention and intervention for emotional disorders.

Licensed psychologists, however, are bound by the APA *Standards for Providers of Psychological Services* to "limit their practice to their demonstrated areas of professional competence" (APA, 1977). Thus, pediatric psychology, as a subspecialty, requires additional coursework and experience focused on developing therapeutic alliances with family members and assisting them in meeting their infants' and/or children's physical, developmental, emotional, and behavioral needs in the context of positive caregiver–child relationships.

The CAASP and the National Center for Clinical Infant Programs collaborated on the development of an issues paper that addresses mental health roles in the implementation of Part H of PL 99-457 (Schrag, 1988) and provides guidelines for personnel preparation. These guidelines suggest that knowledge and skills needed by professionals in order to provide family-centered, coordinated, community-based services to infants and young children include the following:

- Knowledge of physical, cognitive, motor, sensory, social, and emotional typical and atypical development of infants and toddlers
- Ability to form and maintain effective partnerships with parents, family members, and other caregivers
- Ability to coordinate early intervention services for very young children and their families
- Ability to function as a member of an interdisciplinary team

In addition, psychologists contribute to the interdisciplinary team a set of specific skills that includes mental health and developmental screening, assessment, diagnosis, intervention, and program evaluation. These skills should be used to collaborate with the interdisciplinary team and with parents and/or caregivers in direct clinical services, in consultation, in program development, and in training and technical assistance (Schrag, 1988).

In order to work effectively with infants, toddlers, and young children and their families, psychologists must not only acquire the knowledge and skills of their own discipline but also must be able to work effectively with an interdisciplinary team that includes both parents and/or caregivers and professionals from other disciplines.

The shortage of trained psychologists to work with infants and very young children, which became apparent after the passage of PL 99-457 (Meisels, Harbin, Modigliani, & Olson, 1988), must be addressed by increased pediatric professional training of high quality. The changes in service delivery to infants, toddlers, and young children, which call for modifications in the skills and attitudes of professionals, should be reflected in the content of the university-based or professional school core curricula and internship training.

UNIVERSITY-AFFILIATED INTERDISCIPLINARY PEDIATRIC PSYCHOLOGY INTERNSHIP PROGRAMS

Internship and practicum experiences constitute the field-based phase of the professional development of psychologists and allow for the application of the knowledge, skills, and attitudes acquired in the university or professional school setting. Because the core curriculum of most academic psychology training programs is geared toward teaching the general fundamentals shared by all psychologists, pediatric internship programs typically offer in-depth didactic and experiential curriculum that focuses specifically on the development of the knowledge, skills, and attitudes needed for quality service delivery to infants, toddlers, and young children and their families. Faculty liaisons between university psychology departments and/or professional schools and university-affiliated internship programs provide ongoing feedback to each other. Mutual discourse between academic and internship program faculty can result in modification of curriculum and/or internship experience, and thus influence the quality of each. University-affiliated internship experiences differ from many community-based internship programs. When the internship program is in a center where the mission includes intern training as well as service delivery, more resources are available to enhance the training experience, including the availability of faculty to accompany interns on home visits and field experiences, a core curriculum of workshops and seminars, research support, and extended supervision and mentoring.

Interdisciplinary pediatric internship programs should be offered within centers that serve infants, toddlers, and young children who represent a population of economically and culturally diverse individuals who are at risk and/or have developmental delays, disabilities, or special health care needs. The mission of the center should include 1) the promotion of the developmental, health, and mental health well-being of very young children; 2) the provision of preventive intervention services for children and families exhibiting early signs of distress; and 3) the provision of family-centered intervention services for young children with identified serious health, developmental, and mental health care needs. Interns should have the opportunity to participate in the interdisciplinary delivery of health, mental health, and developmental services, including assessment, diagnosis, treatment, and family support offered in the home, at the center, and/or in the community. Service coordination, parent advocacy, and interagency collaboration are important training experiences.

Values-based training emphasizes the training of compassionate, caring, and culturally competent interdisciplinary professionals who, in collaboration with parents and other caregivers, will become leaders in the development and delivery of services to infants and young children and their families. A year-long internship program should include experiential, mentor, and didactic training models and be offered to a variety of trainees from the health, education, and social services disciplines, which may include communication disorders, education, nursing, nutrition, occupational therapy, physical therapy, psychiatry, psychology, and social work.

The interdisciplinary framework integrates psychology with other health, education, and social services disciplines, emphasizing family-centered, community-based, coordinated care. Parents and other caregivers are included in the training process, both in the selection and delivery of didactic and experiential content. The psychology curriculum addresses child development, parent–child relationships, family systems, and mental health issues that are needed by the psychologist "to derive a comprehensive picture of child and family functioning and to identify, implement and/or evaluate psychological interventions" (Bailey et al., 1988, p. 14).

Pediatric Psychology Internship Program Goals

The goals of the pediatric psychology internship training program are to result in compassionate, caring psychologists who have the values, attitudes, knowledge, and skills that will enable them to provide sensitive family-centered, culturally competent, coordinated, community-based care. Internship training components are selected to develop values, attitudes, knowledge, and skills that lead to recommended practices in early intervention program development and service delivery. To accomplish these goals, the internship program components must include an interdisciplinary core curriculum, pediatric psychology seminars, practica (e.g., disciplinary assessment clinics, infant–child program visits, home visits, parent conferences, consultation, direct developmental and psychological services to children and families), exchanges with parents and an interdisciplinary faculty, family service community program and/or agency visits, program development, supervision, and mentoring.

Discussed below are the basic components that should be included in pediatric psychology internship programs:

1. Development of family-centered and interdisciplinary values and attitudes
2. Development of knowledge relating to child development—family-centered service delivery; prevention, assessment, and intervention strategies; and community programs and resources
3. Development of skills
4. Opportunity for mentoring and supervision

Development of Family-Centered and Interdisciplinary Values and Attitudes

The quality of communication among professionals and between professionals and families is basic to the delivery of quality services. Attitudes about disabilities, cultural differences, the team process, and parent–professional partnerships need to be carefully explored by individual professionals. Values and attitudes develop from one's own background experiences and can be modified by 1) an accurate knowledge base; 2) direct experience with culturally, economically, professionally, and philosophically diverse individuals; 3) self-exploration; 4) honest discussion; and 5) feedback. Appropriate family-centered and interdisciplinary values and attitudes are evidenced by the following competencies:

1. The intern demonstrates respect and empathy for young children with disabilities and their families.
2. The intern demonstrates respect and an understanding of socially and culturally diverse beliefs, values, child-rearing practices, priorities, and lifestyles of families.
3. The intern demonstrates a willingness to develop collaborative, supportive partnerships with parents in the development and implementation of assessment and child and/or family service plans, as well as program development and evaluation.

4. The intern explores personal beliefs and feelings about disabilities, economic and cultural diversity of values and lifestyles, the interdisciplinary process, and parent–professional partnerships and recognizes the impact of one's own belief system on service delivery.

5. The intern demonstrates 1) respect for disciplines other than his or her own; 2) an interest in working with others on an interdisciplinary team; 3) an interest in adopting and adapting appropriate techniques of other disciplines and the willingness to share techniques with others; and 4) the realization that, depending on the needs of the infant, toddler, very young child, and/or the family, a member of another discipline may have a more primary role in service delivery to the family (i.e., role release).

Training Experiences that Develop Family-Centered Values and Attitudes   Direct experience, readings, self-exploration, discussion, and feedback are the principal ways that appropriate attitudes and values can evolve. Most critical is the modeling that is provided by the internship program faculty. Interns can only be expected to develop family-centered and interdisciplinary values and attitudes if the center is imbued with an atmosphere of respect for individuals with disabilities, for economically and culturally diverse families, and for parent–professional collaborative partnerships.

In addition, interns can only confront their own attitudes and values if they have been provided with direct experiences with economically and culturally diverse individuals with disabilities in a variety of natural environments and clinical situations. Readings of parents' and first-person accounts of individuals with disabilities and selected literature relating to health, disabling conditions, and cultural diversity can be catalysts for self-exploration and discussion. It is important that interns participate in group discussions relating to family dynamics and family systems with faculty, other interns, individuals with disabilities, and parents. Discussion should be designed to ensure the understanding of economically and culturally diverse families of children with disabilities: their similarities, differences, challenges, resources, and partnership roles as collaborators with professionals.

Pediatric psychology training programs provide weekly individual supervision with an assigned licensed psychologist. Relationship-based supervision provides the intern with an important opportunity for the exploration of personal beliefs and feelings regarding disabilities, working with children with disabilities and their families, culturally diverse beliefs, values, child-rearing practices and priorities, and parent–professional partnerships.

Training Experiences that Develop Interdisciplinary Values and Attitudes   The most effective way for interns to learn to value the team approach is through observation and participation in joint service delivery, professional presentations, and program development with members of other disciplines. Cross-disciplinary instruction, cross-disciplinary supervision in clinical techniques, informal cross-disciplinary contacts, role plays, seminars, and interdisciplinary case conferences can demonstrate the activities, knowledge base, training background, technical skills, jargon, and terminology of different disciplines.

It is important that interns participate in faculty-conducted frank discussions of the interdisciplinary process, its evolution, contribution, challenges, and barriers and in group evaluations of the interdisciplinary process following team assessments, interdisciplinary intervention services, and team presentations.

Development of Knowledge

A sound foundation of knowledge regarding the development of children; the needs of infants, toddlers, and young children and their families; prevention and intervention strategies; and community resources that can provide services and supports will help the psychologist enhance family capacity to maximize the development of their children. A sound foundation of knowledge is evidenced by the following competencies:

1. The intern demonstrates a basic understanding of the growth, development, and needs of infants, toddlers, and young children—physical, psychological, social, cultural, and spiritual aspects, including basic theoretical frameworks; typical and atypical patterns of development; and biological, psychosocial, familial, and community conditions contributing to the disability, risk, and resilience.
2. The intern demonstrates a basic understanding of families and methods of family-centered service delivery issues in developmental assessment, diagnosis, intervention models, and program planning, including family dynamics and family systems, and parents as individuals and as partners in the interdisciplinary process.
3. The intern demonstrates knowledge of a continuum of care service and support resources available for infants, toddlers, and young children and their families and the eligibility criteria and methods of referral.

Training Experiences that Develop Knowledge Relating to Child Development and Family-Centered Service Delivery Knowledge is acquired in the most meaningful way when theory and research are coupled with extensive opportunities to observe and interact with infants, toddlers, and young children without delays and with disabilities, behavioral and emotional disturbances, chronic illnesses, and histories of abuse or neglect. Observations and interactions should take place in homes, child care centers, Head Start classrooms, preschools, and other early intervention settings.

Interns are provided with the opportunity to observe and participate as members of interdisciplinary infant, toddler, and young child assessment and intervention teams with follow-up group discussion on child health and development, assessment, diagnostic, intervention, and program planning issues.

One day a week should be set aside for the acquisition and observed application of knowledge and skills. Assigned readings and interdisciplinary and pediatric psychology presentations and discussions play an important role in the core curriculum. Acquired knowledge should be discussed and applied weekly at interdisciplinary child development assessment conferences. Interdisciplinary and pediatric psychology topics that should be a part of the pediatric psychology training curriculum are included in Table 2.

Training Experiences that Develop Knowledge Relating to Resources and Service Coordination The interns participate in core curriculum seminars that focus on community resources and informal family support networks, which can provide emotional support and developmental guidance. In addition, core curriculum seminars address legislative initiatives pertaining to family-centered service delivery to infants, toddlers, and young children, including Part H and Part B of PL 99-457, PL 99-509 and PL 101-239, EPSDT and CSHCN programs, and the CASSP.

Table 2.   Pediatric psychology curriculum seminar and/or course topics

Research and theory related to infant, toddler, and child health, behavior, and
  development
Biological and psychosocial factors contributing to risk and resilience
Impact of disabling conditions on development, cognition, and parent–infant
  interactions
Resilience-building infant–caregiver strategies
Standardized and play-based assessment
Utilization of diagnostic classification systems: Part H, the *Diagnostic and
  Statistical Manual of Mental Disorders* (4th ed.) (American Psychiatric
  Association, 1994), the *International Classification of Diseases* (ICD 9 or ICD 10)
  (Public Health Services Health Care, Health Care Financing Administration,
  US/DHHS, 1991; World Health Organization, 1992), and the *Diagnostic
  Classification of Mental Health and Developmental Disorders of Infancy and
  Early Childhood* (Zero to Three/National Center for Clinical Infant Programs,
  1994).
Treatment and intervention models
Infant mental health continuum of care models
Transdisciplinary team: Development, barriers, group process, problem-solving
  strategies

Community services and supports include child care; Part H programs; CSHCN programs; MCH High Risk Infant programs; Parent and Child Centers of Head Start; EPSDT programs; Mommy and Me classes; public and private preschool programs; Head Start; child guidance clinics; community mental health and family services; infant–parent psychotherapy services; and parent counseling, support, and education programs. Interns should visit community programs and agencies that provide family-centered developmental, therapeutic, and mental health services to infants, toddlers, and young children and their families. Interns should also participate in informal and formal program planning for infants, toddlers, and young children, including the preparation of IFSPs and individualized education programs and Head Start consultations.

Development of Skills
The focus of the internship is to develop attitudes and knowledge that can be applied to the acquisition of interdisciplinary skills and to the refinement of the psychologists' family-centered skills. Critical competencies include

1. The intern demonstrates the ability to provide interdisciplinary, family-centered psychological and developmental assessment, intervention, and service coordination for infants, toddlers, and young children. Tables 3 and 4 have specific assessment and intervention competency areas.
2. The intern demonstrates an ability to adopt and adapt appropriate techniques of other disciplines.
3. The intern demonstrates an ability to give and receive consultation.

   Training Experiences that Develop Skills Relating to Family-Centered Interdisciplinary Service Delivery Competencies   Interns should observe and participate in unidisciplinary and/or interdisciplinary family interviews, parent–child interactions, infant and/or child play, child–peer situations, home visits, infant and/or child program visits, family-centered child assessments, service coordina-

Table 3.   Pediatric psychology competency areas: Infant and young child assessment

Developmental assessment
Cognitive assessment
Assessment of emotional and social styles
Visual-motor assessment
Neuropsychological assessment
Assessment of parent and child interaction
Play-based assessment
Temperament and personality assessment
Assessment of family needs and supports
Synthesis of data and diagnosis
Generation of specific goals for intervention
Oral and written communication skills

tion, parent counseling, parent support, parent education, infant–family service plans, child–parent psychotherapy, and child play therapy. In addition, sustained contact with infants and families over time leads to an appreciation of family member roles, dynamics and systems, and an understanding of parent and family development.

Interns should participate in seminars and role plays that address principles of service delivery skills from interdisciplinary and family-centered perspectives. Weekly group observation of skills and discussion with faculty and individual time with psychology supervisors should allow the students to evaluate their disciplinary and interdisciplinary skills development. Interns should attend service coordination conferences for infants, toddlers, and young children, including transition-planning conferences. They should visit other programs to observe infant and young child assessment and service coordination, and they should observe and receive direct instruction and supervision from other disciplines in order to adapt and adopt appropriate service delivery strategies.

Training Experiences that Develop Consultation Skills   In order to develop consultation skills, the interns will engage in discussions regarding consultation, including the consultation process and the role of the consultant. They should observe and participate in infant, toddler, and young children service coordination conferences utilizing the consultative process. A critical element in

Table 4.   Pediatric psychology competency areas: Infant and young child intervention

Anticipatory guidance
Parent–infant psychotherapy
Play therapy
Child behavior therapy
Family therapy
Parent support
Parent counseling
Parent education
Service coordination

the development of skills is the discussion of consultation experiences with supervisors for feedback and refinement.

Opportunity for Mentoring and Supervision

Close supervision, feedback, and mentoring are the hallmarks of a quality internship program. Observation of service delivery that allows for modeling by faculty and close supervision opportunities should be available. Initially, faculty should model service delivery for the interns, followed by the development of faculty–intern service delivery teams that continue to work closely throughout the year. Faculty accompany and/or directly supervise home and program visits, team assessment, and intervention. Audiotape and videotape recordings can also be used if faculty are not actually present. Service delivery by interns should be critiqued and evaluated on a regular basis regarding the quality of demonstrated family-centered knowledge, attitudes, and skills and the quality of the interdisciplinary team process. Interns can pair up as teams, allowing for peer feedback. Psychology interns should meet weekly with interns from other disciplines for group interdisciplinary discussion and for psychology group supervision. In addition, each psychology intern should receive 1–2 hours of individual supervision and/or mentoring weekly. Individualized supervision allows the intern to reflect upon all facets of work with infants, toddlers, and young children and their families.

CONCLUDING REMARKS: FUTURE DIRECTIONS

A quality pediatric psychology interdisciplinary internship program endeavors to respond to the four elements identified by the National Center for Clinical Infant Programs as critical to the preparation of practitioners to work with infants and toddlers and their families. The four elements are 1) a knowledge base built on a framework of concepts common to all disciplines concerning infants and young children and their families; 2) opportunities for direct observation and interaction with a variety of infants and young children and their families; 3) individualized supervision that allows the trainee to reflect upon all aspects of work with young children, families, and colleagues from a range of disciplines; and 4) collegial support, both within and across disciplines, that begins early in training and should continue throughout the practitioner's professional life (Fenichel & Eggbeer, 1990). These four elements enable the pediatric psychologist to develop the attitudes, knowledge, and skills needed to provide quality family-centered, interdisciplinary, interagency, culturally competent care to infants, toddlers, and young children and their families.

REFERENCES

American Psychiatric Association (APA). (1994). *Diagnostic and statistical manual of mental disorders* (4th ed.). Washington, DC: Author.

American Psychological Association (APA). (1977). *Standards for providers of psychological services.* Washington, DC: Author.

Association of Maternal and Child Health Programs. (1993). *Building systems: A report on Title V programs' collaboration with the Part H early intervention initiative.* McLean, VA: Author.

Bailey, D., Simeonsson, R., Huntington, G., Cochrane, C., Crais, E., & Humphrey, R. (1988). *Preparing professionals from multiple disciplines to work with handicapped infants, toddlers and their families: Current status and future directions.* Chapel Hill, NC: Carolina Institute for Research on Infant Personnel Preparation.

Berrueta-Clement, J.R., Scheinhart, L.J., Barnett, W.S., Epstein, A.S., & Weikart, D.P. (1984). Changed lives: The effects of the Perry preschool program on youth through 19. *Monograph of the High Scope Educational Research Foundation, 8.* Ypsilanti, MI: High Scope Educational Research Foundation.

Black, M. (1993). Strategies to promote healthy child development and parenting. *Quarterly, 16,* 1–2.

Blackman, J.A., & Cobb, L.S. (1988). A comparison of parents' perceptions of common behavioral problems in developmentally at-risk and normal children. *Child Health Care, 18,* 108–113.

Cadman, D., Boyle, M., & Szatmari, P. (1987). Chronic illness, disability and mental and social well-being. *Pediatrics, 79,* 805–813.

Committee on Accreditation, American Psychological Association (APA). (1980). *Accreditation handbook.* Washington, DC: Author.

Dougherty, D.H., Saxe, L.M., Cross, T., & Silverman, N. (1987). *Children's mental health: Problems and services.* Durham, NC: Duke University.

Dunst, C.J., Trivette, C.M., & Deal, A.G. (1988). *Enabling and empowering families: Principles and guidelines for practice.* Cambridge, MA: Brookline Books.

Education of the Handicapped Act Amendments of 1986, PL 99-457. (October 8, 1986). Title 20, U.S.C. 1400 et seq: *U.S. Statutes at Large, 100,* 1145–1177.

Escalona, S. (1984). Social and other environmental influences on the cognitive and personality development of low birth weight infants. *American Journal of Mental Deficiency, 88,* 508–512.

Fenichel, E.S., & Eggbeer, L. (1990). *Preparing practitioners to work with infants, toddlers and their families: Issues and recommendations for the professions.* Arlington, VA: National Center for Clinical Infant Programs.

Friesen, B. (1993). Overview: Advances in child mental health. In H.C. Johnson (Ed.), *Child mental health in the 1990s* (pp. 12–19). Rockville, MD: U.S. Department of Health and Human Services.

Gabarino, J., Dubrow, N., & Kostelny, K. (1989). *Progress report.* Chicago, IL: Erikson Institute.

Garmezy, N. (1991). Resilience in children's adaptation to negative life events and stresses environments. *Pediatric Annals, 20,* 459–466.

Hoffman, K., & Johnson, H.C. (1993). Biological factors in child mental health. In H.C. Johnson (Ed.), *Child mental health in the 1990s* (pp. 47–61). Rockville, MD: U.S. Department of Health and Human Services.

Individuals with Disabilities Education Act (IDEA) of 1990, PL 101-476. (October 30, 1990). Title 20, U.S.C. 1400 et seq: *U.S. Statutes at Large, 104* (Part 2), 1103–1151.

Individuals with Disabilities Education Act Amendments of 1991, PL 102-119. (October 7, 1991). Title 20, U.S.C. 1400 et seq: *U.S. Statutes at Large, 105,* 587–608.

Knitzer, J. (1993). Children's mental health policy: Challenging the future. *Journal of Emotional and Behavioral Disorders, 1*(1), 8–16.

Lyons-Ruth, K., & Zeanah, C.H. (1993). The family context of infant mental health: I. Affective development in the primary caregiving relationship. In C.H. Zeanah (Ed.), *Handbook of infant mental health* (pp. 14–37). New York: Guilford Press.

Martner, J., Magrab, P., Fenichel, E., Feinberg, E., & Delago, G. (1989). *Mental health services for infants and toddlers: A three state perspective on the implementation of Part H of PL 99-457, the Education of the Handicapped Act Amendments of 1986.* Washington, DC: National Institute of Mental Health, Child and Adolescent Service System Program.

Meisels, S.J., Harbin, G., Modigliani, K., & Olson, K. (1988). Formulating optimal state early childhood intervention policies. *Exceptional Children, 55,* 159–165.

Molfese, V.J. (1989). *Perinatal risk and infant development: Assessment and prediction.* New York: Guilford Press.

Murphy, L.B., & Moriarty, A.E. (1976). *Vulnerability, coping and growth.* New Haven, CT: Yale University Press.

National Center for Children in Poverty. (1990). *Five million children: A statistical profile of our poorest young citizens.* New York: Columbia University School of Public Health.

Omnibus Budget Reconciliation Act (OBRA) of 1986, PL 99-509. (October 21, 1986). Title 42, U.S.C. 679 et seq: *U.S. Statutes at Large, 100,* 1874–2078.

Omnibus Budget Reconciliation Act (OBRA) of 1989, PL 101-239. (December 19, 1989). Title 42, U.S.C. 1396 et seq: *U.S. Statutes at Large, 103,* 2253–2273.

Orloff, T.M., Rivera, L., Harris, P., & Rosenbaum, S. (1992). *Medicaid and early intervention services: Building comprehensive programs for poor infants and toddlers.* Washington, DC: U.S. Children's Defense Fund.

Orloff, T.M., Rivera, L.A., & Rosenbaum, S. (1992). *Medicaid reforms for children: An EPSDT chartbook.* Washington, DC: U.S. Children's Defense Fund.

Osofsky, J.O., & Fenichel, E. (1994). *Caring for infants and toddlers in violent environments: Hurt, healing and hope.* Arlington, VA: National Center for Clinical Infant Programs.

Patterson, J. (1991). Family resilience to the challenge of a child's disability. *Pediatric Annals, 20,* 491–499.

Piotrkowski, C., Collins, R., Knitzer, J., & Robinson, R. (1994). Strengthening mental health services in Head Start: A challenge for the 1990's. *American Psychologist, 57*(2), 220–223.

Poulsen, M.K. (1992). *Schools meet the challenge: Educational needs of children at risk due to prenatal substance exposure.* Sacramento, CA: Resources in Special Education.

Public Health Services Health Care, Health Care Financing Administration, US/DHHS. (1991). *International classification of Diseases (ICD9).* Washington, DC: Author.

Roberts, M.C., Erickson, M., & Tuma, J. (1985). Addressing the needs: Guidelines for training psychologists to work with children, youth and families. *Journal of Clinical Child Psychology, 14,* 70–79.

Roberts, M.C., Fanurik, D.B., & Elkins, P.D. (1987). Training the child health psychologist. In P. Karoly & C. Mays (Eds.), *Handbook of child health assessment: Biopsychosocial perspectives* (pp. 611–632). New York: Wiley Interscience.

Routh, D.K., & La Greca, A.M. (1990). Current status of graduate training in pediatric psychology: Results of a survey. In P.R. Magrab & P. Wohlford (Eds.), *Improving psychological services for children and adolescents with severe mental disorders: Clinical training in psychology* (pp. 139–144). Washington, DC: American Psychological Association.

Sameroff, A., Seifer, R., Barocas, R., Lax, M., & Greenspan, S. (1987). Intelligence quotient scores of 4 year old children: Social environmental risk factors. *Pediatrics, 79,* 343–350.

Schrag, E. (1988). *Sensitivities, skills and services: Mental health roles in the implementation of Part H of PL 99-457, the Education of the Handicapped Act Amendments of 1986.* Washington, DC: National Institute of Mental Health, Child and Adolescent Service System Program.

Solomon, B. (1993). Ethnocultural issues in child mental health. In H.C. Johnson (Ed.), *Child mental health in the 1990s* (pp. 27–46). Rockville, MD: U.S. Department of Health and Human Services.

Tuma, J.M. (1990). Standards for training psychologists to provide mental health services to children and adolescents. In P.R. Magrab & P. Wohlford (Eds.), *Improving psychological services for children and adolescents with severe mental disorders: Clinical training in psychology* (pp. 51–55). Washington, DC: American Psychological Association.

Werner, E., & Smith, S. (1992). *Overcoming the odds.* New York: Cornell University Press.

World Health Organization. (1992). *International statistical classification of diseases and related health problems (ICD 10).* Geneva: Author.

Zero to Three/National Center for Clinical Infant Programs. (1994). *Diagnostic classification of mental health and developmental disorders of infancy and early childhood.* Arlington, VA: Author.

11

PREPARING SCHOOL PSYCHOLOGISTS

Barbara A. Mowder

Not long after I moved to New York State in the late-1980s, I was invited to attend a meeting for training personnel on facilitating early intervention professional preparation. All of the attendees were asked to introduce themselves, present their institutional affiliations, and describe their specialty areas. I was one of the last to introduce myself and it was clear to me that I was most likely the only school psychologist at this meeting. What I was unprepared for, however, was the vituperative response to my introduction I received from one of the participants.

This early childhood program administrator angrily demanded to know what a school psychologist was doing at this meeting and, furthermore, what school psychology had to do with early intervention anyway. It took me a moment to calm down from this attack and tactfully offer a synopsis of school psychology, a description of how early intervention for children and their families benefits from the contributions of many professions, and, indeed, how early intervention does not "belong" to any one field.

SCHOOL PSYCHOLOGISTS HAVE AN IMPORTANT role in providing services to young children who are at risk and/or have disabilities and their families. They have assessment, consultation, and intervention skills and, moreover, expertise in facilitating the movement of children with disabilities from diverse community service settings into public schools (Mowder, 1994). They understand children in the context of their families and appreciate the importance of family–school collaboration (Conoley, 1987). They are also the professionals within the educational milieu who focus on family, psychoeducational, and psychosocial issues frequently associated with children who are at risk and/or have disabilities. Finally, they are in a special position, unlike other infant interventionists, to track children throughout their educational careers (Mowder, 1994).

Although it may seem obvious that school psychologists should be providing early intervention services, they have only just begun to be included as members of the early intervention team. Elardo (1979) pointed to the need for services targeting the early childhood population; and Mowder (1979) suggested that training in this area would be necessary for school psychologists to meet the mandates of PL 94-142, the Education for All Handicapped Children Act of 1975 (reauthorized as PL 101-476, the Individuals with Disabilities Education Act [IDEA] of 1990). Yet, relatively few school psychology training programs provide the didactic and field training necessary to prepare school psychologists to work in early intervention (Epps & Jackson, 1991; McLinden & Prasse, 1991). Although training efforts have not kept pace with personnel preparation needs, there are a number of school psychologists with backgrounds in early intervention who are serving children who are at risk and/or have disabilities. Increasing numbers of training programs and professional organizations (e.g., National Association of School Psychologists [NASP], School Psychology Educators Council of New York State) are developing curricula and field-training guidelines to prepare school psychologists for effective participation in early intervention programs.

THE SCHOOL PSYCHOLOGIST'S ROLE IN EARLY INTERVENTION

Because school psychologists have special training and expertise, they are able to perform a variety of early intervention roles. Assessment is one of the obvious and relatively well-established skills of school psychologists. Although the assessment role is familiar to school psychologists, the assessment issues and application to young children are qualitatively different from those associated with elementary and secondary school populations (McLinden & Prasse, 1991; Mowder, Widerstrom, & Sandall, 1989). Assessments with young children focus on measuring developmental progress in cognitive, language, motor, adaptive behavior, sensory, and social-emotional domains in a relatively balanced manner, whereas with elementary and secondary students assessments are more frequently oriented toward cognitive and social-emotional issues. Furthermore, early childhood assessments are (or should be) family focused rather than focused on the individual child because of the recognition of the primary role parents play in their young children's growth and development (Mcloughlin, 1988). In addition, assessments conducted on young children occur in more diverse early intervention settings, employing more varieties of service delivery models, which include an array of service delivery professionals (Hanson & Brekken, 1991), than are usually present in a kindergarten-to-12th-grade setting.

Another important role filled by school psychologists is consultation. As with early childhood assessment, early childhood psychological consultation is qualitatively different from psychological consultation focused on elementary and secondary school populations. One difference is that when school psychologists are consulting with professionals in the elementary and secondary school setting, they are working primarily with teachers who are certified within their state, who are trained in education, who work in an educational setting, and who provide services from an educational perspective primarily to children rather than to families.

In early intervention, the range of professionals providing services is wider than is the case in elementary and secondary education. The typical early intervention team may include infant and/or early childhood special educators, speech-language therapists, occupational and physical therapists, nurses, social workers, pediatricians, and nutritionists. With the exception of the infant and/or early childhood special educators, early intervention professionals do not necessarily share the educators' training or perspectives.

Consultees in early intervention include parents as well as professional service providers. Although school psychologists frequently consult with parents of school-age children, psychological consultation takes a different focus in early intervention. Parents of young children must make decisions for the children, themselves, and their families. Parents of young children who are at risk and/or have disabilities often are coping with children who have chronic illnesses and find themselves balancing work and other family commitments with their children's needs, which might include a variety of therapies. Parents of older children often have had more time to adjust to their children's special needs, have had their children enrolled in school longer, and are in better positions to understand and utilize the array of professionals and services available to assist them and their families.

When working with young children, school psychologists must expect to spend considerable time with the children's parents. Indeed, consultation with parents is a crucial aspect of early childhood psychological services (Berger, 1991; Conoley, 1987; Mahoney, O'Sullivan, & Dennebaum, 1990) because it can assist parents in becoming better communicators and developing advocacy skills for their children (Dunst & Trivette, 1988; Dunst, Trivette, & Deal, 1988). Parent education and consultation on young children's social-emotional development and mental health needs are other aspects of psychological consultation (Mowder, 1994).

Not only are the range of consultees different in early intervention from elementary and secondary education, but their use of psychological consultation is unique as well. Although the research in this area is far from extensive, there are data that suggest that early childhood special educators seek the school psychologist's help primarily concerning young children's social-emotional development (O'Sullivan, 1991; Widerstrom, Mowder, & Willis, 1989). They prefer the mental health consultation model over the behavioral model, with the medical model considered the least desirable consultation service delivery model (Mowder, Widerstrom, & Willis, 1986). While supporting prior early childhood consultation research, Mowder, Unterspan, Knuter, Goode, and Pedro (1991) found that Head Start consultation services focus on preschoolers' behavior, with social-emotional development a major issue.

Intervention skills are also part of the school psychologist's role. Typical early childhood psychological interventions include 1) providing parental guidance and support, including counseling and psychotherapeutic services; 2) developing behavior management programs; and 3) planning, with other professionals, interventions that take advantage of community resources (Drotar & Sturm, 1989). Because the child who is at risk and/or has a disability may have significant health risks, crisis intervention may also be involved (Mowder et al., 1989). Research, program development, and program evaluation are also among the many service activities school psychologists may provide.

Epps and Jackson (1991) have argued that the role of the psychologist serving young children who are at risk and/or have disabilities is extremely complex and that a full range of direct and indirect school psychological services is necessary. Advocacy and coordination with other disciplines and agencies are necessary complements to psychological services for these children. Coordinated, interdisciplinary intervention team services are essential for providing quality services for infants and their families (Anastasiow, 1981; Mcloughlin, 1988).

However, many professionals have not been trained to deliver services in an interdisciplinary manner due to their separate professional preparation programs (Bricker, 1976; Mcloughlin, 1988).

Early childhood school psychology is qualitatively different from services offered to older school-age children. Targeting a younger age group of children who are at risk and/or have disabilities, appreciating parents and incorporating a family orientation, and working with a range of service providers require an expanded set of service delivery skills for the school psychologist working in early intervention. An appreciation of service coordination models and sensitivity to diverse cultures and values also are required. These requirements affect the interdisciplinary training of early childhood school psychologists.

INTERDISCIPLINARY TRAINING IN
EARLY CHILDHOOD SCHOOL PSYCHOLOGY

Interdisciplinary training usually refers to training that includes both discipline-specific skills and specific strategies that enable professionals from several disciplines to work together. There are a variety of models (e.g., consultant, transdisciplinary, interdisciplinary) (Klein & Campbell, 1990), but the overall goal of early childhood interdisciplinary training is to help professionals from various disciplines collaborate to effectively address the interdisciplinary requirements of PL 99-457, the Education of the Handicapped Act Amendments of 1986 (since updated as PL 102-119, the Individuals with Disabilities Education Act Amendments of 1991).

To some people, the term *interdisciplinary* lies somewhere between multidisciplinary and transdisciplinary training (LaRoche, 1992). The multidisciplinary training model implies that a diverse set of professionals each provides services relative to a particular referred client, while the interdisciplinary team represents a group of professionals who perform their tasks independently but who actively share information and coordinate their efforts toward a common goal. The transdisciplinary team has maximal interaction (McCollum & Hughes, 1988) with team members sharing not only information but roles as well. Regardless of the specific model, Christenson, Abery, and Weinberg (1986) stated that the goal is the integration of data from each discipline or specialty and the formulation of a set of conclusions leading to appropriate recommendations.

A key feature in personnel preparation is to provide team training designed to ensure that professionals from different disciplines collaborate on the assessment, intervention, and evaluation of early intervention services for young children and their families (Harbin & McNulty, 1990; Klein & Campbell, 1990). Indeed, team training may assist professionals in overcoming barriers to effective team functioning. Those barriers include the use of discipline-specific jargon, a lack of understanding and appreciation of other professionals' skills, and ineffective interpersonal communication (Bray, Coleman, & Gotts, 1981; Golin & Ducanis, 1981). In addition, Harbin and McNulty (1990) recommended that staff of training programs for individual disciplines should examine their approach to parent–professional partnerships. These authors suggested that service programs often rely on the philosophy of finding pathology or deficiency in both the child and the family. A shift in philosophy to recognizing, assessing, and enhancing families' strengths is required in early intervention services (Simeonsson & Bailey, 1990).

Most training approaches do not prepare professionals to work effectively in teams (Bailey, 1984; Graham & Bryant, 1993; Magrab, Flynn, & Pelosi, 1985). Harbin and McNulty (1990) wrote that training should assist professionals in understanding and working with professionals from other disciplines. They suggested models and strategies for training professionals across disciplines and joint training programs.

MAJOR BARRIERS TO INTERDISCIPLINARY TRAINING

There are many barriers to interdisciplinary training that need to be addressed in early intervention training of school psychologists. The following are some major barriers, including the location of the training programs, the differing philosophies of service delivery, and limited training materials.

Physical Location of Training Programs

One barrier to training school psychologists in an interdisciplinary framework is that school psychology training programs typically are housed organizationally within academic departments located in schools of education or colleges of arts and sciences. In these cases, school psychologists may be trained with other educators, or, at the very least, curriculum materials should address the context of educational practice and field training should occur with other education practitioners.

However, it is more challenging for trainees in school psychology to receive professional preparation with other early interventionists (e.g., nurses, occupational and physical therapists). Although they may be trained with special educators for infants and toddlers in the same classroom, it is doubtful their training will include preparation with the other early intervention service providers. Nurses, for example, are usually trained in schools of medicine. Likewise, occupational and physical therapists, nutritionists, and social workers are also more likely to be trained in medically oriented or clinical settings.

Therefore, the question is "How can early interventionists, in general, and school psychologists, in particular, be exposed to interdisciplinary training?" One approach is to provide extensive curriculum materials that sensitize school psychologists to the other professionals with whom they may work. The reading materials and lectures should provide adequate coverage of other early intervention disciplines, the roles of other professionals, and the interdisciplinary model of service provision so that students are able to generalize this form of service delivery to field training and ultimately to practice. Another approach is to rely heavily on field training to provide opportunities for interdisciplinary training; this method assumes the availability of such field-training sites. A third approach is to combine curriculum and instruction with professional field training so that the coursework matches and enhances field-training practice. The third approach is preferred because it combines knowledge and practice. Trainees learn about the team members with whom they will be working and their specific roles. In addition, students have the opportunity to observe other early intervention professionals at work. The combination should enhance learning, in the classroom and the field, about other team members in conjunction with myriad modeling opportunities provided by school psychologists and other professionals who are providing services in the field.

Taking this training model one step further, early interventionists should participate together in some of the same courses. For example, a variety of students being trained in early intervention (e.g., early childhood special educators, occupational and physical therapists, speech-language therapists, school psychologists) should enroll in the same course on developmental disabilities. This approach would allow early intervention professionals not only to learn a body of knowledge, but in addition it would allow them to interact and engage with one another, share points of view, and learn from other disciplines and perspectives about early intervention (Klein & Campbell, 1990).

Although there is substantial logic to training early interventionists together, the physical location of the various training programs creates a number of problems. There may be concerns about the physical location of coursework, for example. Because programs are housed within schools of education, schools of medicine, and schools of social work—usually with their own separate physical location, sometimes miles apart—the class location is bound to inconvenience students who must travel to another location. Other concerns involve who is going to teach a course (e.g., a psychologist, speech-language therapist, nurse) that enrolls a variety of professionals, and which academic department will receive student credit and associated tuition and student fees for the course. Is it the unit in which the student is enrolled or is it the unit in which the course is offered?

Not only are there the practical concerns about where the course is to be offered; who is going to teach it; and how the credit, fees, and tuition will be distributed, but additional concerns arise regarding faculty preparation to teach from an interdisciplinary framework. Although many believe in an interdisciplinary focus, few professors are trained to provide or even conceptualize services from this point of view. Old boundaries, professional prejudices, and methods of thinking and performing must be surmounted.

Other Barriers

Another major barrier is that not all early interventionists share a common theoretical model or philosophy of service delivery. For instance, one approach is the diagnostic-prescriptive or pathology-seeking model (Harbin & McNulty, 1990) in which service provision does not include families in any meaningful manner and, furthermore, perpetuates the notion that the child and the families are *patients* who are sick and need the help of professionals to solve their problems. Other approaches to service delivery, such as empowerment, stress children's and families' strengths. This perspective allows parents to be fully involved and to utilize their decision-making skills to the betterment of their child and family.

Although the diagnostic-prescriptive model does not accommodate and appreciate families, neither do consultation models necessarily. As Mowder (1994) suggested, there is much that school psychologists do not know about working with parents. There are many recommendations for professionals to create an open, hospitable atmosphere conducive to problem solving (Fine, 1989), but there is not a great deal of material about how to do this in terms of understanding who the parent is, what the role of the parent is, and how early interventionists can or should make a difference in what individuals do as parents. In essence, it is known that working with parents is desirable and good, but it is not known exactly what to do with parents or how to do it (Mowder, 1994). This is awkward for professionals working with parents because interactions stem, in part, from an assumed knowledge base regarding parenting that simply does not exist.

In addition, ethical guidelines for professional practice from the American Psychological Association and NASP are not necessarily sensitive to the interdisciplinary service delivery approach. In school psychology, for example, ethical guidelines are meant to ensure that psychological services are delivered in a manner that fully respects the rights of the individual receiving services. In general, the ethical guidelines assume psychological services are delivered to individuals or families by individual psychologists, and, thus, ethical guidelines favor and assist those working within a discipline-specific or multidisciplinary framework. The interdisciplinary and transdisciplinary models, however, require more sharing and collaboration among professionals and parents than is directly addressed by psychologists' ethical guidelines. For example, there is the issue of confidentiality. Early childhood school psychologists must specifically ensure that parents agree to have potentially confidential information made available to other members of the team. Psychologists should be sensitive to parents who may not wish to have some information shared with others and may have conflicts or other difficulties with individual team members; thus, issues may arise about the "need to know" information. Psychologists' ethical guidelines may be stretched and challenged by attempting to provide services in an interdisciplinary framework.

Specific Training Issues

Only limited curriculum and instructional materials are available to assist in interdisciplinary personnel preparation. Written materials similar to this book are beginning to be produced, and interdisciplinary models are beginning to be disseminated. For example, McWilliam and Strain (1993) suggested that the various disciplines, with input from the family, coordinate their objectives into the child's daily routine. Indeed, guidelines for interdisciplinary work are beginning to be available, but there is still a lack of research supporting various team-training approaches.

Furthermore, field-training sites that embrace an interdisciplinary model are not always available. If a training program is located in a major urban area, there may be many opportunities to develop interdisciplinary training sites. However, if a program is located in a more isolated or rural location, the opportunities for interdisciplinary training may be more limited.

A final set of issues involves the time at which early childhood school psychology is introduced in the preservice training sequence. Should this specialty training be introduced after the general school psychology preparation? Should early childhood specialty coursework take the place of program electives? Should the specialty course sequence be added to the typical 60 graduate credit hour (minimum) preparation? Should this specialty be available as part of doctoral training or might it represent postdoctoral preparation? Should early childhood specialization training represent preservice training only, or are there elements that might be offered through in-service or continuing professional development workshops?

Most of the writing in this area speaks of early childhood preparation as a preservice issue that should be provided in the context of existing graduate school psychology training programs. This is not to say, however, that effective methods of providing in-service and postgraduate training should not be explored. The need and interest exist among practicing school psychologists to receive additional training but in formats other than the traditional college or university course offerings (Mowder & DeMartino, 1979).

Many issues still exist in the interdisciplinary preparation of school psychologists to provide early intervention services. They include the location of training programs, the diverse service delivery models and ethical guidelines, the lack of appropriate curriculum and instructional materials, and questions about the level of training at which to teach early intervention skills. Although each of these issues must be kept in mind when interdisciplinary, early childhood school psychology training opportunities are developed, there is an emerging consensus about what represents recommended practice.

RECOMMENDED PRACTICES IN INTERDISCIPLINARY EARLY CHILDHOOD SCHOOL PSYCHOLOGY TRAINING

In general, early childhood training has received substantial attention in the professional literature. For instance, the National Association for the Education of Young Children (1994) presented the common knowledge base necessary for all those providing early childhood services. Its outline included the following:

- The understanding and application of child development knowledge
- Observing and assessing children's behavior to plan and individualize curriculum and instruction
- Establishing and maintaining safe and healthy environments for children
- Planning and implementing developmentally appropriate curriculum
- Establishing supportive relationships with children and utilizing developmentally appropriate guidance and group management techniques
- Establishing and maintaining positive and productive professional relationships with families
- Supporting and appreciating the development and learning of individual children within their family, culture, and society
- Demonstrating an understanding of the early childhood profession and making a commitment to professionalism

Fenichel and Eggbeer (1990) presented similar domains of knowledge necessary to provide quality early intervention services. In particular, these authors highlighted knowledge in child development, an appreciation of human relationships, transactions between young children and their environment, parenting, and the *helping* relationship. Fenichel and Eggbeer (1990) stressed the need for training in direct observation and interaction with a variety of children as well as individualized supervision and collegial support within and across disciplines. Finally, the Division for Early Childhood of the Council for Exceptional Children (DEC) (1992) compiled professional competencies for early intervention personnel. The competency areas include 1) educational foundations, 2) foundations of early childhood special education, and 3) methods in early childhood special education.

The DEC (1992) also developed lists of competencies for each early intervention service provider, including psychologists. For psychologists, the DEC outlined the following knowledge base:

- Social and philosophical foundations
- Life-span human development and learning
- Professional orientation and development
- Historical and philosophical bases of early childhood special education
- Child development
- Development of young children with special needs
- Survey of exceptionalities
- Families of young children with special needs
- Assessment of the young child
- Curriculum and methods: birth to 5 years old
- Physical and medical management, including health management
- Interdisciplinary and interagency teaming
- Organizational environments for early intervention

Bailey (1989), too, discussed the specialized knowledge and skills the psychologist brings to the early intervention team. He wrote that psychologists must be trained to assess the psychological and behavioral characteristics of children and families, identify psychological needs and resources, plan and provide psychological and developmental interventions, coordinate interdisciplinary efforts, consult with families and other professionals, serve as service coordinators, and design and implement program evaluations.

From the early childhood school psychology literature, it is clear that 1) early childhood school psychology includes special knowledge and skills that traditionally trained school psychologists do not have available to them (Mowder et al., 1989); 2) the best way to train school psychologists in early childhood education is to provide specialized training (McLinden & Prasse, 1991; Mcloughlin, 1988); 3) the knowledge base needed includes specific preparation in assessment and intervention in early childhood, developmental disabilities, early childhood consultation, family systems, interdisciplinary teaming, multicultural issues, and typical and atypical child development; 4) there are many curriculum and instruction avenues to provide training in early childhood school psychology, with the preferable mode to include training with other early interventionists; and 5) there are different levels at which to provide training in early intervention (e.g., continuing professional development, in-service training, postgraduate training, preservice training).

Specific Course- and Fieldwork in Early Childhood School Psychology

The curriculum and instruction needed to train school psychologists in early intervention services should include the special knowledge and skills that traditionally trained school psychologists do not have available to them. This training should come in the form of specialty coursework and field-training experiences and not simply be added on or infused with existing course offerings. Furthermore, to the extent possible, school psychologists' training in early intervention should be offered with other early intervention trainees. Training programs should initially direct their efforts toward preservice training, particularly because many states (e.g., Kansas, New York) are changing their certification guidelines to include services from birth to 21 years old or offering a separate endorsement for early intervention. As early childhood school psychology coursework and field-training opportunities are developed, they should be made available to practicing professionals needing this additional preparation. Some institutions, for example, are offering a series of courses in conjunction with field-training opportunities in order to meet this need.

The early intervention coursework offered to school psychologists should include preparation in assessment and intervention for children birth through age 5. Frequently, information is presented in two courses: 1) infant and/or toddler assessment and intervention, and 2) preschool assessment and intervention. As the material is presented, it is often coordinated with the history and philosophy of early intervention, multicultural issues, family dynamics, and interdisciplinary teaming (Bracken, 1991; Nuttall, Romero, & Kalesnik, 1992; Widerstrom, Mowder, & Sandall, 1991).

Typical and atypical child development, focusing in particular on children birth to 5 years of age, also needs to be taught. All areas of child development, including the domains of cognitive, language, motor, adaptive behavior, and personal and/or social functions should be included, with emphasis placed on factors that might place a child at risk for later developmental problems (McLinden & Prasse, 1991). A separate course (different from the child development course) in developmental disabilities and disabling conditions is usually included in early intervention preparation. This material includes discussions of low incidence as well as the more prevalent disabling conditions.

Many school psychology training programs with an early childhood specialization include a separate course in family dynamics, family systems, or family therapy. The primary focus of the course is to sensitize trainees about how young children are part of a larger social unit and that the family affects, supports, and encourages growth and development of young children. The understanding of families, individual family roles, and multicultural issues is included in these courses, as well as family assessments, interventions, and interdisciplinary family-focused service delivery models.

Thus, at a minimum, early childhood school psychology coursework must include courses in assessment and intervention in early childhood, early childhood development (including typical and atypical development), developmental disabilities, and family dynamics and systems. Additional courses may be developed in multicultural issues and interdisciplinary teaming, or these issues may be infused in other courses.

Field-training experiences are part of early childhood preparation. Experiences in a variety of settings (e.g., early intervention classrooms and medical facilities) are typical. School psychology trainees often participate in parent and family interviews, develop assessment plans, coordinate program planning with the other early interventionists, and conduct research. Early intervention settings should have a variety of components to facilitate early intervention training, including children birth to 5 years old, diverse disabling conditions, family involvement, a number of early intervention professionals working within a team model, and representation of diverse cultural and value backgrounds.

TRANSLATING TRAINING INTO PRACTICE IN EARLY CHILDHOOD SCHOOL PSYCHOLOGY

The key point in translating training into practice in early childhood school psychology is the recognition among practitioners, students, and trainers that early intervention service provision is distinct and qualitatively different from the services that school psychologists traditionally provide to older children and their families. Early childhood school psychology requires specialty training and specific preparation in early childhood assessment and intervention services, developmental disabilities, early childhood development, and family systems. Beyond specific knowledge needs, early childhood school psychologists need opportunities to learn and appreciate interdisciplinary service delivery and the provision of culturally sensitive services in classroom and in field-based internships.

School psychologists practicing in early childhood education need to appreciate the special role parents play in the lives of their children and welcome parents as full participants in the early intervention enterprise. For this to happen, practitioners, trainees, and trainers need to embrace an empowerment model for service delivery (Dunst & Trivette, 1988). An empowerment or any other equally powerful, facilitative, service delivery model ensures that parents enter the early intervention arena on equal footing with the service professionals who are assisting them.

CONCLUDING REMARKS: FUTURE DIRECTIONS

Early childhood school psychology represents an important subspecialty in school psychology (Bagnato, Neisworth, Paget, & Kovaleski, 1987; Barnett, 1986). To realize the potential benefit of school psychological services in early intervention, however, specific high-quality training opportunities need to be offered to practitioners and trainees (Bennett, Watson, & Raab, 1991). Training includes not only knowledge but also field-training experiences. And, finally, although there is a relative explosion of material available on early intervention services (e.g., Bryant & Graham, 1993; Meisels & Shonkoff, 1990; Zeanah, 1993), there is a striking need for more research in this area, research not only in the field of early childhood school psychology but also research on training itself.

REFERENCES

Anastasiow, N. (1981). Early childhood education for the handicapped in the 1980s: Recommendations. *Exceptional Children, 47*, 276–284.

Bagnato, S.J., Neisworth, J.T., Paget, K.D., & Kovaleski, J. (1987). The developmental school psychologist: Professional profile of an emerging early childhood specialist. *Topics in Early Childhood Special Education, 7*(3), 75–89.

Bailey, D.B. (1984). A triaxial model of the interdisciplinary team and group process. *Exceptional Children, 51*, 17–25.

Bailey, D.B. (1989). Issues and directions in preparing professionals to work with young handicapped children and their families. In J.J. Gallagher, P.L. Trohanis, & R.M. Clifford (Eds.), *Policy implementation and PL 99-457: Planning for young children with special needs*. Baltimore: Paul H. Brookes Publishing Co.

Barnett, D.W. (1986). School psychology in preschool settings: A review of training and practice issues. *Professional Psychology Research and Practice, 17*(1), 58–64.

Bennett, T., Watson, A.L., & Raab, M. (1991). Ensuring competence in early intervention personnel through personnel standards and high-quality training. *Infants and Young Children, 3*(3), 49–58.

Berger, E.H. (1991). *Parents as partners in education: The school and home working together*. New York: Charles E. Merrill.

Bracken, B. (Ed.). (1991). *The psychoeducational assessment of preschool children* (2nd ed.). Needham, MA: Allyn & Bacon.

Bray, N., Coleman, J., & Gotts, E. (1981). The interdisciplinary team: Challenges to effective functioning. *Teacher Education and Special Education, 4*, 44–49.

Bricker, D. (1976). Educational synthesizer. In M.A. Thomas (Ed.), *Hey, don't forget about me* (pp. 84–97). Reston, VA: Council for Exceptional Children.

Bryant, D.M., & Graham, M.A. (1993). *Implementing early intervention: From research to effective practice*. New York: Guilford Press.

Christenson, S., Abery, B., & Weinberg, R.A. (1986). An alternative model for the delivery of psychological services in the school community. In S. Elliot & J. Witt (Eds.), *The delivery of psychological services in schools* (pp. 349–391). Hillsdale, NJ: Lawrence Erlbaum Associates.

Conoley, J.C. (1987). Schools and families: Theoretical and practical bridges. *Professional School Psychology, 2*, 191–204.

Division for Early Childhood of the Council for Exceptional Children (DEC). (1992). *Compilation of professional competencies for early intervention personnel*. Reston, VA: Author.

Drotar, D., & Sturm, L. (1989). Training psychologists as infant specialists. *Infants and Young Children, 2*(2), 58–66.

Dunst, C.J., & Trivette, C.M. (1988). Enabling and empowering families: Conceptual and intervention issues. *School Psychology Review, 16*, 443–456.

Dunst, C.J., Trivette, C.M., & Deal, A.G. (1988). *Enabling and empowering families: Principles and guidelines for practice*. Cambridge, MA: Brookline.

Education for All Handicapped Children Act of 1975, PL 94-142. (August 23, 1977). Title 20, U.S.C. 1400 et seq: *U.S. Statutes at Large, 89*, 773–796.

Education of the Handicapped Act Amendments of 1986, PL 99-457. (October 8, 1986). Title 20, U.S.C. 1400 et seq: *U.S. Statutes at Large, 100*, 1145–1177.

Elardo, R. (1979). Preschool psychology: A personal view. *School Psychology Review, 8*, 311–318.

Epps, S., & Jackson, B.J. (1991). Professional preparation of psychologists for family-centered service delivery to at-risk infants and toddlers. *School Psychology Review, 20*(4), 489–509.

Fenichel, E.S., & Eggbeer, L. (1990). *Preparing practitioners to work with infants, toddlers and their families: Issues and recommendations for the professions*. Washington, DC: National Center for Clinical Infant Programs.

Fine, M. (1989). *The second handbook on parent education: Contemporary perspectives*. San Diego: Academic Press.

Golin, A.K., & Ducanis, A.J. (1981). *The interdisciplinary team: A handbook for the education of exceptional children*. Rockville, MD: Aspen Publishers, Inc.

Graham, M.A., & Bryant, D.M. (1993). Characteristics of quality, effective service delivery systems for children with special needs. In D.A. Bryant & M.A. Graham (Eds.), *Implementing early intervention: From research to effective practice* (pp. 233–252). New York: Guilford Press.

Hanson, M.J., & Brekken, L.J. (1991). Early intervention personnel model and standards: An interdisciplinary field-developed approach. *Infants and Young Children, 1*(1), 54–61.

Harbin, G.L., & McNulty, B.A. (1990). Policy implementation: Perspectives on service coordination and interagency cooperation. In S.J. Meisels & J.P. Shonkoff (Eds.), *Handbook of early childhood intervention* (pp. 700–721). Cambridge, MA: Cambridge University Press.

Individuals with Disabilities Education Act (IDEA) of 1990, PL 101-476. (October 30, 1990). Title 20, U.S.C. 1400 et seq: *U.S. Statutes at Large, 104* (Part 2), 1103–1151.

Individuals with Disabilities Education Act Amendments of 1991, PL 102–119. (October 7, 1991). Title 20, U.S.C. 1400 et seq: *U.S. Statutes at Large, 105*, 587–608.

Klein, N.K., & Campbell, P. (1990). Preparing personnel to serve at-risk and disabled infants, toddlers, and preschoolers. In S.J. Meisels & J.P. Shonkoff (Eds.), *Handbook of early childhood intervention* (pp. 679–699). Cambridge, MA: Cambridge University Press.

LaRoche, M. (1992). Implementing the results of preschool assessments: Transforming data and recommendations into action. In E.V. Nuttall, I. Romero, & J. Kalesnik (Eds.), *Assessing and screening preschoolers: Psychological and educational dimensions* (pp. 395–405). Needham, MA: Allyn & Bacon.

Magrab, P., Flynn, C., & Pelosi, J. (1985). *Assessing interagency coordination through process evaluation*. Chapel Hill, NC: National Early Childhood Technical Assistance System.

Mahoney, G., O'Sullivan, P., & Dennebaum, J. (1990). Maternal perceptions of early intervention services: A scale for assessing family focused intervention. *Topics in Early Childhood Special Education, 10*(1), 1–15.

McCollum, J.A., & Hughes, M. (1988). Staffing patterns and team models in infancy programs. In J. Jordan, J. Gallagher, P. Hutinger, & M. Karnes (Eds.), *Early childhood special education: Birth to three* (pp. 129–146). Reston, VA: Council for Exceptional Children.

McLinden, S.E., & Prasse, D.P. (1991). Providing services to infants and toddlers under PL 99-457: Training needs of school psychologists. *School Psychology Review, 20*(1), 37–48.

Mcloughlin, C.S. (1988). Provision of psychological services to very young children and their families. In J.L. Graden, J.E. Zins, & M.J. Curtis (Eds.), *Alternative educational delivery systems: Enhancing instructional options for all students* (pp. 269–290). Washington, DC: National Association of School Psychologists.

McWilliam, R.A., & Strain, P.S. (1993). Service delivery models. *DEC Task Force on Recommended Practices: Indicators of quality in programs for infants and young children with special needs and their families* (pp. 39–48). Reston, VA: Council for Exceptional Children.

Meisels, S.J., & Shonkoff, J.P. (Eds.). (1990). *Handbook of early childhood intervention*. Cambridge, MA: Cambridge University Press.

Mowder, B.A. (1979). Legislative mandates: Implications for changes for school psychology training programs. *Professional Psychology, 10*, 681–686.

Mowder, B.A. (1994). Consultation with families of young at-risk and handicapped children. *Journal of Educational and Psychological Consultation, 5*(4), 309–320.

Mowder, B.A., & DeMartino, R.A. (1979). Continuing education needs in school psychology. *Professional Psychology, 10*, 827–833.

Mowder, B.A., Unterspan, D., Knuter, L., Goode, C., & Pedro, M. (1991). Psychological consultation and Head Start: Data, issues, and implications. *Journal of Early Intervention, 17*, 1–7.

Mowder, B.A., Widerstrom, A.H., & Sandall, S. (1989). School psychologists serving at-risk and handicapped infants, toddlers, and their families. *Professional School Psychology, 4*(3), 159–171.

Mowder, B.A., Widerstrom, A.H., & Willis, W.G. (1986). Early childhood special educators' perceptions of psychological consultation. *Psychology in the Schools, 23*, 373–379.

National Association for the Education of Young Children. (1994). Position statement: A conceptual framework for early childhood professional development. *Young Children, 49*(3), 68–77.

Nuttall, E.V., Romero, I., & Kalesnik, J. (Eds.). (1992). *Assessing and screening preschoolers: Psychological and educational dimensions.* Needham, MA: Allyn & Bacon.

O'Sullivan, J. (1991). *Consultation with parents of preschool children with special needs.* Unpublished doctoral project, Pace University, New York City.

Simeonsson, R.J., & Bailey, D.B. (1990). Family dimensions in early intervention. In S.J. Meisels & J.P. Shonkoff (Eds.), *Handbook of early childhood intervention.* Cambridge, MA: Cambridge University Press.

Widerstrom, A.H., Mowder, B.A., & Sandall, S. (1991). *Newborns and infants at risk: A multidisciplinary approach to assessment and intervention.* Englewood Cliffs, NJ: Prentice Hall.

Widerstrom, A.H., Mowder, B.A., & Willis, W.G. (1989). The school psychologist's role in the early childhood special education program. *Journal of Early Intervention, 13*, 239–248.

Zeanah, C.H. (Ed.). (1993). *Handbook of infant mental health.* New York: Guilford Press.

12

THE PARAPROFESSIONAL'S ROLE

Nancy Striffler

"Sometimes I feel like I work in a vacuum. Because I'm a teacher assistant, I don't have anyone to share ideas with. I work hard with the infants and toddlers with disabilities at my center but sometimes I don't understand why I'm told to do the things the teacher asks me to do. I wish I could attend some of the team meetings and the in-service programs. Another thing—my annual evaluation is conducted by the administrator of our center. The administrator has no idea what I do in my work with the children; she only knows if I come to work every day." This strict demarcation between teacher assistants (often referred to as paraprofessionals) and teachers, administrators, and other service providers discourages any collaboration and cross learning.

Today in the 1990s, children with disabilities are best served by a team of individuals who work collaboratively to meet the needs of children with disabilities and their families. Policies and procedures that recognize and support paraprofessionals as integral partners in providing early intervention and preschool services reflect commitment to providing services that fully meet the diverse needs of children and families.

"I never understood why Bobby was so stiff until I attended the workshop on children with motor difficulties. It also helped me to understand Bobby's feeding difficulties when I finally attended an IFSP meeting during which we discussed techniques to use during lunch time." Paraprofessionals with adequate training and supervision can be an integral part of the team. Preservice and in-service training programs compatible with the setting in which the paraprofessional practices enable the paraprofessional to understand the service delivery environment and expectations.

As THE AVAILABILITY OF SERVICES for infants, toddlers, and preschoolers with disabilities and their families increased nationally, the demand for qualified personnel to perform these services also increased. The capacity to meet the needs of all children eligible to receive services is dependent largely upon the availability of sufficient numbers of personnel who are qualified to provide the services. The employment of paraprofessionals is one strategy that has been adopted by some states and communities to ensure the availability of quality personnel. The need for preservice and in-service training programs for paraprofessionals has been recognized (Lorenz, 1995; Morgan, 1995; Steckelberg & Vasa, 1995).

The purpose of this chapter is to examine the role and function of paraprofessionals in early intervention (birth through 2) and preschool services (ages 3–5) and to identify some promising service delivery practices and training approaches. Understanding the roles of paraprofessionals is critical before considering the training needs and approaches appropriate for these personnel. Specifically, this chapter discusses 1) the extent to which paraprofessionals comprise the work force in early intervention and preschool service delivery, 2) the role function of paraprofessionals, 3) service delivery challenges and promising practices, and 4) considerations for paraprofessional training.

THE WORK FORCE

Across the United States, states and jurisdictions are in various stages of development of their service systems for infants, toddlers, and preschoolers with disabilities and their families. The extent of the available work force is difficult to determine because of the evolving nature of these service delivery systems. Valid data on personnel providing infant–toddler services will be difficult to obtain on a large scale until states finalize the qualifications for the various service providers and develop mechanisms for collecting data across multiple service agencies and providers. Personnel data from 1991, as shown in Table 1, suggest that early intervention services in the United States are being provided primarily by paraprofessionals and special educators, with paraprofessionals constituting one fifth of those involved in providing services. Preschool special education data do not reflect the number of paraprofessionals or related services personnel working with the nation's 3- to 5-year-olds with disabilities (U.S. Department of Education, 1993). When considering the full age spectrum (3–21 years), however, there is a national trend toward the increased use of paraprofessionals in special education. Pickett (1990) reported the number of paraprofessionals in special education to be in excess of 155,000. This number increased from 140,000 in 1983 and 27,000 in 1973. Given this trend, there is a need to understand the various roles and responsibilities that paraprofessionals are asked to assume and to ensure that quality training programs are available.

Table 1. Personnel employed or contracted in infant–toddler services in 47 states and jurisdictions

Category of personnel	Number	Percent[a]
Paraprofessionals	5,950	20.0
Special educators	4,509	15.2
Other professional staff	3,487	11.8
Nurses	3,248	10.9
Speech-language pathologists	3,239	8.8
Occupational therapists	1,734	5.9
Physical therapists	1,616	5.5
Physicians	1,332	4.5
Psychologists	1,059	3.6
Audiologists	530	1.8
Nutritionists	313	1.1
Total employed	**29,610**	

Source: U.S. Department of Education (1991).

[a]Percentage of the total full-time equivalent (FTE) workers employed and contracted across all categories.

ROLE FUNCTION

The term *paraprofessional* has a variety of meanings within differing contexts. In some states, paraprofessional may refer to someone with a high school diploma. In other states, it may be used to describe someone with a 2- or 4-year college degree who lacks all the qualifications for licensure. There is much dissatisfaction with the term *paraprofessional*. To many, it does not foster the respectful rapport that is essential among all members of the service team. Yet there is need for a generic term, just as the term *professional* refers to individuals representing various disciplines and personnel categories. Perhaps *paraprofessional* would be acceptable as an umbrella term referring to the many service providers who work together with and in support of professionals. *Paramedic*, a subcategory of paraprofessional, is an accepted term connoting an individual who works alongside a medical specialist. So too, an early intervention assistant or *paraeducator* are part of the term *paraprofessional*, referring to individuals who work in support of certified or licensed professionals. Some states are using the term *paraeducator* to refer to an individual providing services under the supervision of a licensed educator or special educator (Pickett, 1994). The term *paratherapist* has begun to emerge as one designation for an individual working in allied health or related services under the supervision of a certified therapist (Longhurst, personal communication, 1994). More typically, in the area of allied health and related services, those states that employ certified occupational therapy assistants (COTAs), physical therapy assistants (PTAs), and speech-language pathology assistants (SLPAs) tend to classify these providers as paraprofessionals (Striffler, 1993). In contrast, the American Occupational Therapy Association (1993) considers COTAs to be technical-level practitioners; the American Physical Therapy Association identifies PTAs as paraprofessionals (1993); and the American Speech-Language-Hearing Association (ASHA) (1994) uses the term *support personnel* to classify SLPAs.

Regardless of the specific term, the role and function of paraprofessionals in early intervention and preschool services must be considered with care. Paraprofessionals perform a range of functions within many employment settings. Paraprofessionals provide direct services to children and support and education to families. The substantive roles and contributions of these providers need to be recognized through adequate role definition and clear role assignments. All too often outdated job descriptions remain intact, while paraprofessionals are asked to assume responsibilities for which they may be ill prepared.

Throughout the United States, paraprofessionals have moved from performing routine clerical and housekeeping tasks to having systematic involvement in the delivery of services to individuals with disabilities. It used to be the paraprofessional who ran the photocopy machine before the start of a classroom activity and washed the toys or cleaned up after snack time. These tasks still may be the responsibility of some paraprofessionals, but increasingly the paraprofessional is involved in direct service delivery related to addressing a specific objective or outcome on individualized family service plans (IFSPs). The paraprofessional in early intervention does not function in isolation and, therefore, the role and function of a paraprofessional must not be determined separate from the state's or community's total service system. Specific selection criteria, job descriptions, responsibilities, service settings, and supervision requirements should be outlined and clarified to all team members. The role function of paraprofessionals needs to be made clear before training needs can be identified and paraprofessional training programs developed.

CHALLENGES AND PROMISING PRACTICES

A number of challenges signify the need to examine how paraprofessionals provide early intervention and preschool services. The first challenge is the movement toward more family-centered approaches to service delivery. Next, the need for inclusion demands the movement beyond traditional service delivery models and settings. The third challenge is the demand for increased service delivery in rural settings. These three challenges and related promising practices are discussed in this section.

Family-Centered Care

The needs of a child and family can be met most appropriately by skilled individuals who are familiar with the social, ethnic, and economic aspects of that family's culture. Often, a paraprofessional who is familiar with the family receiving services has the potential for unique insights and empathy. His or her firsthand knowledge of the family's culture combined with an understanding of the specialized needs of young children with disabilities may enable paraprofessionals to provide quality services and supports as a member of an early intervention team.

Examples of the use of paraprofessionals as members of early intervention teams are found in several states. Hawaii's commitment to the provision of culturally competent, family-centered, community-based, coordinated systems of services for children with disabilities led to the establishment of parent involvement assistants (PIAs) as an occupational category in early intervention. PIAs are responsible for the provision of culturally appropriate service coordination and family support services for infants and toddlers with disabilities. PIAs assist families in developing and implementing IFSPs and proactively work with family members and service providers to develop and promote family–professional partnerships. Embracing the philosophy of family-centered care, Hawaii is committed to using the expertise of paraprofessionals who understand the cultural variations and the unique needs of families with children with disabilities (Striffler, 1993).

The Massachusetts early intervention program established the paraprofessional position of community outreach worker. The community outreach worker, familiar with the community culture, joins the team with substantial prior knowledge of the physical and social conditions in which families live. Often, the community outreach worker is the bridge between the neighborhood and the larger community in which child and family services are available. There is a strong belief in Massachusetts that, because the children and their families are members of the community receiving services, community outreach workers are essential to the provision of culturally competent services in a manner most relevant and appropriate to meet the needs of families (Striffler, 1993).

Inclusion

The concept of inclusion is a challenge for service delivery personnel concerned with integration opportunities for young children with disabilities. Traditional school-based delivery models offer few opportunities for including infants, toddlers, and preschoolers because local educational agencies are not routinely required to serve this age group. As a result, publicly and privately funded child care programs are often the primary options for including young children with disabilities.

As the concept of inclusion is embraced more fully, it is anticipated that a variety of child care settings will be considered the most appropriate for many infants, toddlers, and preschoolers with disabilities. Many individuals provide quality care in child care settings, yet they lack the formal education or credentials recognized by the state. The Early Childhood Mentor Teacher Program of the Child Care Employee Project in California represents promising practice in this area. Begun in 1988, the program trains experienced child care teachers to become mentors to students in community college training programs for child care providers, creates a career ladder, rewards increased responsibilities with additional income, and provides an incentive to remain in the child care field. The program offers students the opportunity to observe model infant and toddler caregiving and to receive individualized supervision (Pemberton, 1990).

Partnerships between Head Start programs and university affiliated programs (UAPs) were designed to support inclusion of children with developmental disabilities in Head Start programs. One such program was developed by the Tri-County Special Education Cooperative in southeast Kansas, the Southeast Kansas Community Action Program's Head Start program, and the UAP at the University of Kansas. The program was built around the Head Start classroom and general curriculum by placing an early childhood special education teacher together with the Head Start teacher and paraprofessional teacher assistant. By doing this, children with disabilities are integrated into the instructional activities and are provided with opportunities for social interaction. Specific individualized education program objectives are embedded within these learning opportunities. This dynamic team-training process blends discussion workshops with experiential learning in a natural setting. Program outcomes measured at the end of the project indicated that the paraprofessional trainee learned specific strategies for bringing about positive behavior changes in children with disabilities and that the children were afforded social opportunities both within and outside of school that they might not have otherwise been afforded (Buchman, 1993).

Rural Service Delivery

Distance and travel time constraints, most acutely felt in rural communities, have led some state planners to examine the use of paraprofessionals to meet service demands. Often professionals (e.g., occupational and physical therapists) are unable to provide adequate service to remote areas. As an alternative, an early intervention aide or provider can conduct an intervention program several times a week, with direct supervision from a licensed or certified professional on a periodic basis. For example, rural Eagle Pass, Texas, has no occupational therapist, physical therapist, or speech-language pathologist located within 100 miles of the town. Here, paraprofessionals under the supervision of certified early intervention teachers provide activities to foster infant development in a variety of service settings. To ensure that paraprofessionals provide quality motor and language services, state licensing standards for occupational therapy, physical therapy, and speech-language pathology address the credentials and supervision of paraprofessionals in these fields. Table 2 lists these licensing standards. The IFSPs for the infants living in Eagle Pass are developed by their families, teachers, and the paraprofessional in collaboration with an itinerant transdisciplinary team of licensed professionals. This same team travels to Eagle Pass once a month to provide consultation to the family and early intervention staff (Samuelson, personal communication, 1993).

The employment of paraprofessionals in rural areas has many advantages. These include a decrease in travel time on the part of the family or service provider, provision of services close to the family's home, and the extension of services of professionals, including allied health professionals. With appropriate training and supervision, paraprofessionals can ensure consistency and continuity in service delivery in professions and geographic areas where personnel shortages abound.

CONSIDERATIONS FOR PARAPROFESSIONAL TRAINING

Paraprofessional personnel development issues include defining personnel standards and competencies, career ladders, training approaches and supervision, and curricula. These four issues and selected practices in addressing them are discussed in this section.

Personnel Standards and Competencies

In the field of personnel development, the terms *standards* and *competencies* often are used interchangeably. For the purpose of discussion, a distinction between the two will be made. *Standards* is used as a set of policy guidelines that

Table 2. State of Texas—Personnel standards

Occupational category	Educational requirements	Examination requirements
Physical therapist assistant	Completion of an accredited physical therapy assistant program	Texas State Board of Physical Therapy Examiners
Occupational therapist assistant	Associate degree in occupational therapy (COTA)	Texas Advisory Board of Occupational Therapists
Licensed aide in speech-language pathology	Bachelor's degree with minimum of 24 hours in speech-language from a state with reciprocity or that holds national certification of clinical competence (CCC)	Examination may be waived if candidate holds valid license

Adapted from Texas Early Childhood Intervention Program (1990).

reflect the system's support of and commitment to key components articulated in the standards. *Competencies* is used as a statement of core knowledge and skills necessary for personnel who work with young children with disabilities and their families.

There is growing interest nationwide in developing standards and procedures for improving the status, performance, and effective inclusion of paraprofessionals in education and related services fields (Hanson & Brekken, 1991; Likins, 1994; Pickett, 1994). State-level personnel standards developed by an interagency collaborative group, including policy makers, administrators, providers, and consumers, can serve as a guide for the development of personnel competencies and certification and credentialing procedures. Standards built on a shared vision and service delivery philosophy can support the effective involvement of personnel in a service system. Following are four standards that specifically address the training of paraprofessionals:

1. *The entire team shall participate within clearly defined roles to provide appropriate services for young children with disabilities and their families.* Such role definition is essential and often overlooked. An up-to-date written individualized job description needs to be provided to each paraprofessional and supervisor. In most cases, due to the complexity of services and settings, a generic job description will be inappropriate.
2. *Administrators shall assume a central role in the support and recognition of paraprofessionals as integral partners in providing services.* Administrators need to understand the roles and responsibilities of paraprofessionals and assume a central role in the administration of an effective paraprofessional program. Program administrators at the community level should provide support for paraprofessionals in the form of newsletters, in-service training, and other staff development activities.
3. *Paraprofessionals shall receive career development support and supervision consistent with their assigned responsibilities.* Effective preservice and in-service training programs, as well as consistent supervision, are essential. Paraprofessionals need opportunities for career development and pay commensurate with their responsibilities, experience, and training. Higher education institutions cooperating with the state and local districts should be encouraged to develop and maintain associate degree programs for paraprofessionals in early intervention and preschool services.
4. *An advisory committee consisting of all key stakeholders, including paraprofessionals and consumers, shall regularly review the implementation of the paraprofessional standards and make recommendations for change.* An information-sharing system can ensure that the paraprofessional standards reflect the service delivery philosophy and the extent to which paraprofessionals are supported for their contributions.

States must develop their own standards, reflecting their unique needs, philosophies, and values. Once developed, personnel standards can serve as a valuable resource for those involved at administrative, university, and policy-making levels with services to young children and their families. State agencies might use the standards as a basis for developing competencies or for establishing in-service activities or other staff development programs. Universities, community colleges, or other institutions of higher education may use them as the basis for their curricula. Direct services programs may use them as a basis for role clarification among team members or for the development of supervisory guidelines.

A number of states (Alabama, Colorado, Idaho, Iowa, Kentucky, Texas, and others) and projects (Longhurst & Witmer, 1994; Pickett, 1994) have developed paraprofessional personnel competencies. In each case, competencies represent a scope of practice and delineate the knowledge and skills that an individual will possess in order to practice in his or her assigned role. Table 3 identifies some common competency areas specifically for paraprofessionals in early intervention and preschool services. Although paraprofessional competencies across states may contain some common core elements, the competencies for a single state or specific program should reflect the unique nature, strengths, and limitations of that state or program. Personnel competencies should flow directly from the articulated service mission and guidelines and reflect family-centered philosophy and approaches. Personnel competencies can serve as a basis for establishing preservice and in-service training programs and for developing a competency-based curriculum.

Prior to the development of competencies, some project staff found it beneficial to outline job tasks and responsibilities. These responsibilities may include delivering services to infants and toddlers and their families, assisting in observation and assessment activities, working as a team member, and assisting in service coordination components. In some cases, the service setting was a consideration in determining job responsibilities and degree of supervision. Several experts have suggested that the paraprofessional should perform independent home visits only after extensive program experience and training preparation and only with frequent and direct supervision (Hanson & Brekken, 1991).

Career Ladders

Establishing career ladders as a mechanism for recruitment and retention of

Table 3. Paraprofessional competency areas

Core competency areas	Additional competencies for home programs
Characteristics of children with disabilities	Ability to participate as a member of the IFSP team
Roles and responsibilities	Ability to listen to and communicate with caregivers
Legal and ethical issues	
Cultural diversity	Knowledge of community resources and support services
Typical and atypical growth and development	Ability to demonstrate effective techniques to family members
Health, safety, and emergency procedures	
Interpersonnel skills	
Problem-solving skills	
Team skills	
Developmentally appropriate practice	
Inclusion issues and practices	
Translation of assessment information into learning objectives	

paraprofessionals for the provision of care in early intervention and preschool services is essential. A study (Passaro, Pickett, Latham, & Wang, 1991) of paraprofessionals in three of the nation's most sparsely populated states (North Dakota, South Dakota, and Wyoming) reported that the greatest contributing factor to their decision to leave the field was the lack of opportunity to advance. A career ladder not only prepares paraprofessionals for a particular role but also helps them obtain further education and reduces exiting from the field. Several states, including Florida, Idaho, Kansas, North Dakota, and Utah, have taken the initiative to establish career ladders for paraprofessionals. A well-conceived career ladder begins with recruitment and initial training in high school and leads to progressively higher levels of certification and potential for employment advancement.

The National Association for the Education of Young Children (NAEYC) (1994) identified six levels of professional development, beginning with those individuals just starting on a professional path. This system is designed to reflect a continuum of career development and includes three levels typically considered to be in the paraprofessional category and three levels traditionally in the professional category. Level I designates individuals "who are employed in an early childhood professional role working under supervision . . . and participating in training designed to lead to the assessment of individual competencies or acquisition of a degree" (p. 4); Level VI designates an individual who has successfully completed a doctoral or master's program conforming to NAEYC guidelines.

Career ladders can be a powerful tool for enhancing the quality and quantity of personnel available for the provision of services to children with disabilities and their families. The low pay and status of many individuals working with young children can undermine practitioners' self-esteem, which in turn can have negative effects on their interactions with young children and their families. Career ladders build on existing strengths and provide opportunities for career advancement.

Training Approaches and Supervision

All practitioners who work with young children and their families need specialized training to address the children's unique needs. Paraprofessionals, as well as professionals, require specialized knowledge and skills to provide quality services. The quality of training, support, and supervision provided to paraprofessionals will influence their successes in supporting the development of children and the effectiveness of interaction with parents and professionals. Both preservice and in-service training approaches are useful.

Training Approaches

Early intervention for children with disabilities is a relatively new field, and therefore the number of preservice programs designed to prepare paraprofessionals to work with young children and their families is limited. The majority of available preservice programs are designed for those intending to work with school-age children. These programs have valuable structures, content, and formats for consideration in the field of early intervention. For example, the state of Kansas has a well-developed system of training through junior college courses, established and run directly by the state department of education. The curriculum is a 2-year associate program consisting of didactic and practicum requirements. Course content includes human growth and development, an overview of individuals with disabilities, behavior and classroom management, instructional competencies, and first aid (Kansas State Board of Education, 1993).

Another preservice training program, the Child Development Associate (CDA) Credential Award System, is designed for employed, precredentialed child care workers and those who lack child care experiences or formal child care education. The CDA credential is awarded for three child care settings: center-based programs for which age level endorsements (birth to 3 years and 3–5 years) are available; home visitor programs; and family child care programs. The training standards and competency-based curriculum were developed and validated by the early childhood profession for the purpose of preparing workers in the care of typically developing young children and their families. However, the well-developed curriculum, training strategies, and evaluation tools can serve as valuable resources in the training of individuals preparing to work with young children with disabilities and their families. Table 4 shows the CDA training content areas that should be considered core competency areas for any professional or paraprofessional providing early intervention services. The CDA credentialing process is administered by the Council for Early Childhood Professional Recognition, and the training is available throughout the country in community colleges and other institutions of higher education (Council for Early Childhood Professional Recognition, 1993).

Although there is a strong demand in educational agencies and the health care field for paraprofessionals in physical therapy, occupational therapy, and speech-language pathology (Longhurst & Witmer, 1994; National Early Childhood Technical Assistance System, personal communication, 1994), until the early 1990s there were no preservice training programs designed specifically for those preparing to work in the area of speech-language services. In 1994, the Idaho Division of Vocational Education, through a grant from the Idaho Infant–Toddler Interagency Coordination Council, developed training programs for aides and assistants in speech-language pathology, as well as for occupational and physical therapist assistants (Idaho State Board of Vocational Education, 1994). The content of the curricula for preparing *aides* includes communication skills, leadership skills, human relations, and employability skills, as well as safe and efficient work practices. Upon completion of the training program, the aide is prepared to assist the certified speech-language pathologist in individual and group therapy activities and clerical duties. The *assistant* training program includes specialized content related to speech-language development and disabilities, as well as screening and treatment approaches. Upon completion of the

Table 4. Child Development Associate (CDA) training content areas

Planning a safe, healthy environment to invite learning
Steps to advance children's physical and intellectual development
Positive ways to support children's social and emotional development
Strategies to establish productive relationships with families
Maintaining a commitment to professionalism
Observing and recording children's behavior
Principles of child growth and development

training program, the assistant is prepared to perform services for the children and offer family support with supervision from a certified professional. Curriculum guides for both the aide and assistant include performance competencies and the scope of practice. The training programs are designed to work in conjunction with a variety of postsecondary level training programs when they are offered in a transdisciplinary training program at the community college and vocational/technical school. Other states and programs seeking to develop preservice paraprofessional training programs with an emphasis in motor or language should consider the curriculum guides developed in Idaho (Idaho State Board of Vocational Education, 1993a, 1993b, 1994).

Quality in-service training can enable paraprofessionals to acquire knowledge and skills needed to carry out their responsibilities (Linder, 1983). The possibilities for in-service training approaches are limited only by the imaginations of individuals responsible for the development and implementation of in-service training programs. As of 1996, people's ideas suggest that the traditional workshop approach to in-service training aimed at discipline-specific audiences is insufficient. Instead, active participation and team approaches have been stressed as especially appropriate for paraprofessional training (Wasik, Bryant, & Lyons, 1990). Training that focuses on a change process and includes interdisciplinary community-based teams, including administrators and families, is needed (Winton, McWilliam, Harrison, Owens, & Bailey, 1992). Such community-based team training not only has the potential of increasing the knowledge and skills of the service providers but also has the potential to build team collaboration and coordinated service delivery. Team training reduces the possibility of role confusion, unclear job expectations, and conflict over selection of strategies and techniques for intervention, while at the same time acknowledges the paraprofessional as a team member.

Team in-service training presents a challenge because of the diverse backgrounds and levels of expertise of the members. An effective in-service plan can be developed by carefully assessing the level of staff needs and then working with staff to determine what combinations of activities will lead to the achievement of individualized training objectives. Collaborative presentations across personnel, together with the case study method of instruction (McWilliam, 1992) that uses realistic, clinical situations as a training tool, provide opportunities for learning key concepts as well as opportunities for problem solving, decision making, and reflection. These approaches also enable personnel to learn from each other and to better understand the skills and personal qualities of their team members.

Action-oriented workshops with follow-up assignments, specific to an individual's skill and learning objective provide opportunities for application of new knowledge and skills. The trainee's worksite and other community-based service programs and family settings can be used by both paraprofessional and professional staff to expand knowledge and skills. Child care, nursery programs, respite care, and other programs serving infants, toddlers, and preschoolers and their families provide rich opportunities for learning.

Observation of and interaction with young children and families is an essential ingredient in the process of translating theory into effective practice. Opportunities to view video presentations that depict typically and atypically developing infants, toddlers, and preschoolers and their families are valuable.

Observations of young children at home on a typical morning, getting a well-child checkup, or working with a therapist enable paraprofessionals to gain a full picture of children and families. These experiences also enable the trainee to develop keen observation skills, not only of children and families but also of a range of personnel and work settings.

Following these observations there should be time for discussing what is observed. Such process discussions with other team members provide opportunities to clarify and validate one's ideas, gain new insights, and learn from team members. Such discussions can serve to highlight the tremendous individual variations in typical and atypical development and cultural differences in child-rearing practices and family life. This is especially important for paraprofessionals as they begin to understand what makes them respond to and work differently with various children and families.

Hawaii's Healthy Start program established an in-service training system that incorporates many of the training approaches described above. The Healthy Start program is a comprehensive child abuse prevention program that serves children at risk through a home visit program. Two key elements have been critical to the success of the program. First, the program is well developed and well documented, and second, it offers a training and technical assistance system that provides standardized training and regular technical assistance to all paraprofessional and professional program staff (Breakey & Pratt, 1991). The orientation course includes an overview and introduction to the Healthy Start program and focuses on personal values, job responsibilities, and program philosophy and approach. Other topics include skills for working with families who are at risk, the importance of cultural sensitivity, ways to support families, and guidelines for making referrals. Typical and atypical infant and toddler development and health and safety issues are also included. Throughout the training, the trainees are given the opportunity to follow an experienced worker and visit community resources. Weekly supervision as well as weekly team meetings and monthly agency-wide staff meetings are recommended for all personnel. After orientation (4–6 months), 6 days of advanced training are provided. This training reinforces key concepts and introduces other topics to supplement the orientation training. In addition, each Healthy Start program annually chooses four topics for ongoing in-service training. Training sessions for these are provided on site, which permits each program team to learn and share together. Learning is a process that takes place over time. Hawaii's in-service training system responds to the continuing and long-term needs of the paraprofessionals who serve infants and toddlers and their families.

Supervision

Ongoing and sensitive supervision during preservice and in-service training is necessary to respond to the needs of individual trainees and to improve program effectiveness. Working with very young children and their families is an intense and challenging experience. The provider requires a confidante, someone with whom to focus, investigate, and brainstorm and with whom to share experiences and reactions.

All paraprofessionals should have a person whom they can trust, with whom they can discuss their experiences, and from whom they can receive feedback and support. The format and intensity of supervision depend on many factors, including the characteristics of the people receiving services; the type of service provision; the service setting; the combination of knowledge, skills, and experience of the paraprofessional; and the program's place within the larger service delivery system.

The most commonly reported type of supervision in family-focused home visiting programs in which paraprofessionals provide services is weekly individual supervision. Weekly group supervision is the second most common type (Roberts & Wasik, 1990). On-site or field-based supervision is the least frequently used supervision format, possibly because it is the most time consuming, and, hence, expensive. Home visiting programs should consider using all three supervision formats because each has advantages (Wasik et al., 1990). For example, weekly individual supervision, monthly group supervision, and bimonthly on-site supervision may respond not only to the program needs for careful monitoring but to the providers' needs for feedback and support.

Definitive supervision requirements are prescribed for speech-language pathology (SLP) aides and assistants practicing in Idaho (Idaho State Board of Vocational Education, 1994). SLP aides and assistants "must not practice unless supervised, at least on a weekly basis, by an ASHA certified speech-language pathologist" (p. 24). Documented direct, on-site supervision of care for children with disabilities is required no less than 10% of the time for each SLP aide and 5% for each SLP assistant. This allows the speech-language pathologist to model techniques and to monitor and change therapy approaches as needed. Consultation and feedback regarding the aide's or assistant's performance can be provided during this on-site supervision time. Additional documented indirect supervision is required no less than 10% of the time for an aide and 5% for an assistant. This may include record review, prescription clarification, review and evaluation of audiotaped or videotaped sessions, and/or supervisory conferences that may be conducted by telephone.

Frequent on-site supervision may not be feasible in some service settings. Physical distance presents unique challenges to adequate supervisory experiences. In some rural communities in Alaska, it is not uncommon for a therapist to visit a community only once a year. Training needs of isolated community-based programs may be addressed by identifying and supporting the development of innovative approaches to supervision. Telecommunication technologies can be used to surmount distance barriers by connecting service providers with sources of expert guidance. Lesson plans are transmitted by facsimile to supervisors, who then transmit comments back by facsimile. An expert trainer receives videotapes made by paraprofessionals and comments on these in regularly scheduled supervision via telephone conference calls. Audiotapes might be used to record comments and questions, particularly in programs in which workers travel long distances to provide services. Additional approaches might include reading specific and self-study materials and maintaining service provision journals. Such strategies provide opportunities for ongoing interchange and feedback between supervisor and supervisee in remote geographic locations or otherwise isolated work settings.

An example of a project that used several supervisory formats is South Carolina's Resource Mothers Program. The goal of the program is to support the development of maternal and infant health through home visits by paraprofessionals known as resource mothers. Supervision of the paraprofessionals includes monthly group conferences to review caseloads, solve problems, and provide continuing education. In addition, the supervisor makes one supervisory home visit monthly with each resource mother. Individual conferences are held at least monthly to guide work with selected cases and to examine relationships and to resolve specific problems. The various supervisory options in this project match the purpose of supervision with the needs of the paraprofessional and the goals of the program.

Peer teaching has gained increased acceptance and is used in many training settings (Fenichel & Eggbeer, 1990). This is the process of having more experienced individuals assist and teach newcomers in the field. Group conferences are a common supervisory vehicle that provide an opportunity for individuals to give feedback and encouragement to their peers. As the group matures, members can try out new ideas and reflect attitudes and personal beliefs. Role playing between peers in a group conference allows supervisors to gain information about strengths and limitations that can be used to individualize additional training.

Mentorship as a supervisory approach has largely been confined to the professional (Eggbeer, Latzko, & Pratt, 1993; Fenichel & Eggbeer, 1990). A faculty member or experienced professional serves as a model and guide to a young professional, teaching ways of approaching and solving problems. Mentorships are valuable in improving the skills of new personnel entering programs as well as providing new challenges and opportunities for expanding roles of more experienced professionals. Mentoring holds promise as a supervisory mechanism and ongoing continuing education tool for the paraprofessional. A program supervisor, team member, or a seasoned paraprofessional might serve as a mentor and provide a nurturing relationship. Paraprofessionals new to the field receive help on issues such as program policies, health and safety, and role clarification; more experienced paraprofessionals learn intervention approaches and techniques to support families. Although the goals of each partnership will vary, mutual respect is essential to the success of the mentorship (Hurley, 1988).

Supervision can take place individually, in a group, and in the field. Each format has its advantages and limitations. Individual supervision can be more intensive and, at times, respond more fully to an individual's needs. Group or team supervision provides opportunities for group problem solving and peer teaching. On-site or field-based supervision provides firsthand knowledge of the child and family situation and allows observation and feedback on the paraprofessional's actual performance.

Training Curriculum and Materials

Although paraprofessionals have provided services to children and families since the 1960s, training materials developed prior to the 1980s are insufficient to meet the training needs of paraprofessionals in the 1990s. The knowledge and skills required to perform assigned responsibilities are diverse and complex. Paraprofessionals serving young children with disabilities and their families must know and be able to support the development of children, and recognizing that children are best understood in the context of the family, they must also be able to establish and maintain partnerships with the families. Table 5 lists training curricula and materials that may be valuable for use in preservice and inservice training programs for paraprofessionals.

Table 5.   Training resources

Title/author/date	Content and format	Target audience	Source
AGH Associates. (1992). *Supporting children in the regular education classroom: A handbook for integrating aides.* Hampton, NH: Author.	This three-ring bound reference book includes philosophy of inclusion, child development, caregiving and emergency procedures, equipment and adaptive devices, working with consultants, and understanding therapists. It can serve as a resource to the practicing paraprofessional.	Paraprofessionals responsible for integrating children with severe disabilities into the typical classroom	AGH Associates, Inc. Box 130 Hampton, NH 03842
Baird, S. (1994). *Preparing paraprofessional early interventionists.* Tucson, AZ: Communication Skill Builders.	This curriculum consists of a trainer's manual and seven training modules. Modules can be modified and supplemented to address needs of particular service and training programs.	Paraprofessionals serving infants and toddlers with disabilities in home-based, center-based, or community-based early intervention programs	Communication Skill Builders 3830 East Bellevue Avenue Post Office Box 42050 Tucson, AZ 85733
Davis, K. (1993). *Beyond the sandbox: Teaching assistants in early childhood education.* Bloomington, IN: Center for Innovative Practices for Young Children.	A videotape that provides an overview of the changing and expanding roles of teaching assistants in early childhood settings that include children with and without disabilities.	Teachers, teaching assistants, related services personnel, parents, and administrators	Center for Innovative Practices for Young Children ISDD, Attention CeDIR 2853 East Tenth Street Bloomington, IN 47408-2601
Deer, M. (1994). *Strategies for instruction in natural environments (SINE).* Logan: Center for Persons with Disabilities, Utah State University.	SINE is a videodisc-assisted program that includes 10 units of study, an instructor's manual, and a participant's manual. Naturalistic teaching methods for young children with disabilities are stressed.	Early childhood personnel and caregivers working with young children with disabilities	Center for Persons with Disabilities Utah State University Logan, UT 84322-6805

(*continued*)

Table 5. (continued)

Title/author/date	Content and format	Target audience	Source
Haviland, N. (1993). *Stand by me: Self instruction for paraprofessionals.* Columbia: Missouri Education Center.	This manual covers the role of the para-professional in the school setting, the special education process, disability issues, behavior management, and confidentiality and family rights.	Paraprofessionals working in school settings	Missouri Education Center 1206 East Walnut Street Columbia, MO 65201
Long, C. (1994). *Piecing together the paraprofessional puzzle.* Columbia: Instructional Materials Laboratory, University of Missouri–Columbia.	This is a handbook of 24 chapters cover-ing a range of topics, including policies and pro-cedures, role expectations, con-fidentiality, team skills, characteristics of various disabili-ties, and instruc-tional strategies. Each chapter could be adapted to a variety of training formats.	First-year para-professionals working in class-room settings	Instructional Materials Laboratory University of Missouri–Columbia 2316 Industrial Drive Columbia, MO 65202
Mueller, P. (1993). *Certificate of study program for instruc-tional assistants.* Burlington: University Affiliated Program of Vermont, University of Vermont.	This program consists of an 8-credit di-dactic and practical curriculum covering role functions; accommodations for inclusion; managing behavior; disabili-ties; and federal, state, and local policies.	Instructional assistants working with school-age children with disabilities (components of the program could be adapted for use in training those work-ing in early intervention)	University Affiliated Program of Vermont 499C Waterman Building University of Ver-mont Burlington, VT 05405
National Resource Center. (1994). *The training program to prepare para-educators to work in center and home visitor programs that service children ages birth to five.* New York: Author.	This training program consists of seven competency-based modules. Each mod-ule includes objec-tives, trainer guidelines, hand-outs, and overhead transparencies. Modules can be modified and supplemented to address needs of par-ticular service and training programs.	Paraprofessionals working with children with disabilities and their families in inclusive education and community-based programs	The National Resource Center for Parapro-fessionals CASE/CUNY, Room 620 New York, NY 10036

(continued)

Table 5. (*continued*)

Title/author/date	Content and format	Target audience	Source
Partnership for Inclusion. (1993). *Can I play too?* Chapel Hill: Frank Porter Graham Child Development Center, University of North Carolina.	These three videotapes are about the inclusion of young children and their families in community child care programs. Content includes the legal, social, and educational rationale for inclusion. These videotapes have been used effectively in in-service and preservice training formats.	Child care teachers and assistants	Partnership for Inclusion Frank Porter Graham Child Development Center University of North Carolina 300 NationsBank Plaza 137 East Franklin Street, CB 8040 Chapel Hill, NC 27514
Shelton, G. (1994). *Sourcebook for teaching assistants in early childhood education.* Bloomington, IN: Center for Innovative Practices for Young Children.	This book includes fact sheets on disabilities, a glossary, and discussion questions. A companion *Teacher's Guide* is included. It is appropriate for preservice and in-service training and as an on-site resource to help address specific issues as they arise.	Paraprofessionals working with children with disabilities in early childhood inclusive environments	Center for Innovative Practices for Young Children ISDD, Attention CeDIR 2853 East Tenth Street Bloomington, IN 47408-2601
University of Colorado Health Sciences Center, School of Nursing. (1992). *First start.* Denver, CO: Author.	This combines a seminar approach with hands-on clinical experiences. It offers general knowledge about developmental disabilities, methods of providing direct care, emergency procedures, skills in communication with professionals and parents, and community resources. It is designed as a trainer-of-trainers program.	Child care providers and aides serving infants and toddlers with disabilities in child care centers, nurseries, and family care homes	University of Colorado Health Sciences Center School of Nursing Denver, CO 80262

(*continued*)

Table 5. *(continued)*

Title/author/date	Content and format	Target audience	Source
Wesley, P. (1992). *Mainstreaming young children: A training series for child care providers.* Chapel Hill: Partnerships for Inclusion, Frank Porter Graham Child Development Center, University of North Carolina.	This 44-hour curriculum consists of eight modules designed to be offered sequentially or as freestanding sessions. An instructor manual and student handbook are available. It is designed to assist child care providers in including children with disabilities in child care programs.	Teachers, teaching assistants, and child care providers	Partnerships for Inclusion Frank Porter Graham Child Development Center University of North Carolina 300 NationsBank Plaza 137 East Franklin Street, CB 8040 Chapel Hill, NC 27514

The recurrent theme of the materials included in Table 5 is that of preparing paraprofessionals to work with children with disabilities by providing them with the necessary skills and knowledge to work with children in inclusive environments. This emphasis reflects both the changing roles of paraprofessionals, to include skills previously considered the exclusive domain of the professional, and the movement toward service delivery in natural environments. The most frequently occurring content areas were characteristics of disabilities, managing behavior, instructional strategies, paraprofessional roles and responsibilities, and team skills. The inclusion of team skills reflects the growing trend for paraprofessionals to be considered an integral part of the service delivery team. The resources offer a picture of practice in the 1990s and give insight into the variety of training that is being made available to paraprofessionals who work with young children with disabilities and their families.

CONCLUDING REMARKS: FUTURE DIRECTIONS

Fulfilling the challenges of effective implementation of early intervention services depends to a great extent on the availability of qualified professionals to provide services to young children with disabilities and their families. Paraprofessionals have a vital role to play in the provision of family-centered, culturally relevant service delivery. Specific job descriptions, including clear role definitions and responsibilities, can help identify individuals who would be effective as paraprofessionals. Paraprofessionals can extend the impact of the professional team; assist with direct programming in community-based, inclusive environments; provide ongoing support to families; assist families with gaining access to needed resources; and provide respite care.

Carefully defined personnel standards and competencies can guide the training and supervision of paraprofessionals. Competency and mastery are evolving processes that are facilitated by ongoing training, support, supervision, and experience. A number of training programs, including competency-based curricula, have been developed and can serve as valuable resources for personnel development.

As the need for services continues to grow, the United States must have the capacity to accommodate eligible children who require services and to ensure that programs are of high quality and are affordable. This cannot be accomplished until personnel development issues are addressed. A number of assumptions should underlie any system of staff development that seeks to ensure qualified providers for services to young children with disabilities and their families. First, a career development system must be dynamic. The system needs to link entry-level skills and work experience with training, credentialing, and degree programs. There must be bridges between life experience and competencies, noncredit training, and community colleges and university training programs. Second, in order to attract and retain individuals in this field, all personnel must be compensated fairly for their work. Everyone needs to earn a living wage and receive benefits. A system of incentives that addresses salary, benefits, and status must be established. Third, a system of training must be available, accessible, and affordable; and a system of ongoing supervision that supports and enhances the effectiveness of the practitioner must be established. Fourth, to ensure the availability of high-quality supervision, preservice and in-service training programs must take seriously the need to train future supervisors. Finally, any system of personnel development must reflect the diversity of service models and types of personnel working in early intervention and preschool service delivery. With careful planning, comprehensive systems of personnel development can be established to incorporate the effective utilization of paraprofessionals in the provision of services for infants, toddlers, and preschoolers with disabilities and their families.

REFERENCES

AGH Associates. (1992). *Supporting children in the regular education classroom: A handbook for integrating aides.* Hampton, NH: Author.

American Occupational Therapy Association. (1993). *Occupational therapy roles.* Rockville, MD: Author.

American Physical Therapy Association, Commission on Accreditation in Physical Therapy Education. (1993, February 24). *Evaluation criteria for accreditation of education programs for the preparation of physical therapy assistants.* Alexandria, VA: Author.

American Speech-Language-Hearing Association (ASHA). (1994, August). *Proposed position statement and guidelines for the education/training, use and supervision of support personnel in speech-language pathology and audiology.* Rockville, MD: Author.

Baird, S. (1994). *Preparing paraprofessional early interventionists.* Tucson, AZ: Communication Skill Builders.

Breakey, G., & Pratt, B. (1991). Healthy growth for Hawaii's "Healthy Start": Toward a systematic statewide approach to the prevention of child abuse and neglect. *Zero to Three, 11*(4), 15–22.

Buchman, N. (1993). Providing educational options for children with disabilities and their families within Head Start programs. *National Head Start Bulletin, 45,* 1–3.

Council for Early Childhood Professional Recognition. (1993). *The child development associate national credential.* Washington, DC: Author.

Davis, K. (1993). *Beyond the sandbox: Teaching assistants in early childhood education.* Bloomington, IN: Center for Innovative Practices for Young Children.

Deer, M. (1994). *Strategies for instruction in natural environments (SINE).* Logan: Center for Persons with Disabilities, Utah State University.

Eggbeer, L., Latzko, T., & Pratt, B. (1993). Establishing statewide systems of inservice training for infant and family personnel. *Infants and Young Children, 5*(3), 49–56.

Fenichel, E., & Eggbeer, L. (1990). *Preparing practitioners to work with infants, toddlers, and their families: Issues and recommendations for policymakers.* Arlington, VA: National Center for Clinical Infant Programs.

Hanson, M., & Brekken, L. (1991). Early intervention personnel model and standards: An interdisciplinary field-developed approach. *Infants and Young Children, 4*(1), 54–61.

Haviland, N. (1993). *Stand by me: Self-instruction for paraprofessionals.* Columbia: Missouri Education Center.

Hurley, D. (1988, May). The mentor mystique. *Psychology Today,* 36–39.

Idaho State Board of Vocational Education. (1993a). *Technical committee report and curriculum guide for occupational aide (Vol. Ed. 282) and certified occupational therapy assistant (Vol. Ed. 284).* Boise, ID: Author.

Idaho State Board of Vocational Education. (1993b). *Technical committee report and curriculum guide for physical therapy aide (Vol. Ed. 283) and certified physical therapy assistant (Vol. Ed. 285).* Boise, ID: Author.

Idaho State Board of Vocational Education. (1994). *Technical committee report and curriculum guide for speech-language aide (Vol. Ed. 293) and certified speech-language assistant (Vol. Ed. 292).* Boise, ID: Author.

Kansas State Board of Education. (1993, June). *Kansas state regulations for special education.* Topeka, KS: Author.

Likins, M. (1994). *Utah state standards for paraeducators in special education.* Salt Lake City: Utah State University.

Linder, T.W. (1983). *Early childhood special education: Program development and administration.* Baltimore: Paul H. Brookes Publishing Co.

Long, C. (1994). *Piecing together the paraprofessional puzzle.* Columbia: Instructional Materials Laboratory, University of Missouri–Columbia.

Longhurst, T., & Witmer, D. (1994). *Initiating therapy aide/assistant training in a rural state.* Paper presented at the 13th Annual Conference on the Training and Employment of Paraeducators, Albuquerque, NM.

Lorenz, G. (1995). The 1994 Minnesota paraprofessional survey: Who, where, what, and why. *Para Link,* Spring, 1–4.

McWilliam, P.J. (1992). The case method of instruction: Teaching applications and problem-solving skills to early interventions. *Journal of Early Intervention, 16*(4), 360–373.

Morgan, B. (1995). Distance learners: Utah paraeducators participate in two-way interactive training. *New Directions, 16*(1), 3–5.

Mueller, P. (1993). *Certificate of study program for instructional assistants.* Burlington: University Affiliated Program of Vermont, University of Vermont.

National Association for the Education of Young Children (NAEYC). (1994). NAEYC position statement: A conceptional framework for early childhood professional development. *Young Children, 49*(3). Washington, DC: Author.

National Resource Center. (1994). *The training program to prepare paraeducators to work in center and home visitor programs that service children ages birth to five.* New York: Author.

Partnership for Inclusion. (1993). *Can I play too?* Chapel Hill: Frank Porter Graham Child Development Center, University of North Carolina.

Passaro, P.D., Pickett, A.L., Latham, G., & Wang, H.B. (1991). Training and support needs of paraprofessionals in rural special education settings. *Exceptional News, 15*(1), 3–11.

Pemberton, C. (1990). *Child care mentor teacher pilot program: Final report.* Oakland, CA: Child Care Employee Project.

Pickett, A.L. (1990). *Paraprofessionals in education. The state of the art.* New York: National Resource Center for Paraprofessionals, Center for Advanced Study in Education, Graduate School, City University of New York.

Pickett, A.L. (1994). *A core curriculum and career ladders for paraeducators.* Paper presented at the 13th Annual Conference on the Training and Employment of Paraeducators, Albuquerque, NM.

Roberts, R., & Wasik, B. (1990). Home visiting programs for families with children birth to three: Results of a national survey. *Journal of Early Intervention, 14*(3), 220–231.

Shelton, G. (1994). *Sourcebook for teaching assistants in early childhood education.* Bloomington, IN: Center for Innovative Practices for Young Children.

Steckelberg, A., & Vasa, S. (1995). *Establishing paraeducator preservice training programs through cooperative efforts with local educational agencies.* Paper presented at the

14th Annual Conference on the Training and Employment of Paraprofessionals, St. Paul, MN.

Striffler, N. (1993). *Current trends in the use of paraprofessionals in early intervention and preschool services.* Chapel Hill, NC: National Early Childhood Technical Assistance System.

Texas Early Childhood Intervention Program. (1990). *Texas licensure/certification/registration standards for ECI personnel.* Austin, TX: Author.

University of Colorado Health Sciences Center, School of Nursing. (1992). *First start.* Denver, CO: Author.

U.S. Department of Education. (1991, December). *Office of Special Education Programs, Data System Analysis System.* Washington, DC: Author.

U.S. Department of Education. (1993). *Fifteenth annual report to Congress on the implementation of the Education of the Handicapped Act.* Washington, DC: Author.

Wasik, B., Bryant, D., & Lyons, C. (1990). *Home visiting: Procedures for helping families.* Beverly Hills, CA: Sage Publications.

Wesley, P. (1992). *Mainstreaming young children: A training series for child care providers.* Chapel Hill: Partnerships for Inclusion, Frank Porter Graham Child Development Center, University of North Carolina.

Winton, P., McWilliam, P., Harrison, T., Owens, A., & Bailey, D. (1992). Lessons learned from implementing a team-based model of change. *Infants and Young Children, 5*(1), 13–21.

13

PREPARING PERSONNEL IN RURAL AREAS

Jane Squires

It was always June's dream to move to the country and have a house with acres of land for farm animals and a vegetable garden. That dream began to unravel after June's third year in rural Pleasant Valley.

June was suddenly faced with losing her job after the local school district took over administration of the early intervention program. June had been working with young children with special needs and their families for more than 10 years, but she had no formal coursework, training, or teaching license. She was given 2 years in which to earn the early childhood teaching specialty license required by the school district for all instructional employees.

The state university, 4 hours away by car, offered summer-only programs leading to the early childhood teaching specialty license and a master's degree. Leaving her family for three summers, however, would be a great hardship for June. The only other option, moving to the campus and completing the program in 1 year, was not possible for financial reasons. Suddenly, the very reasons that had brought June and her family to the country—isolation, distance from big cities, and lack of large institutions—were about to force her to leave.

DELIVERY OF EARLY INTERVENTION SERVICES in rural areas poses great challenges and offers great rewards. In rural areas, strains such as a sense of isolation, lack of supports, and inadequate resources are among the challenges, and a more relaxing working atmosphere and slower pace are among the rewards (Carlson, 1992). Rural areas can be defined as those areas with fewer than 150 inhabitants per square mile or counties with 60% or more of the population living in communities with no more than 5,000 inhabitants (Helge, 1984).

Delivery of training to personnel living and working in rural areas poses great challenges because of geographic isolation, travel distances, and conflicting work schedules. Because of these challenges, early intervention personnel may be less well trained than their urban counterparts (Royce, Cummings, & Cheney, 1990; Smith, Fasser, Wallace, Richards, & Potter, 1990) and less likely to be certified (Rule, Fiechtl, & Huntington, 1993).

Although many imagine a calm, bucolic life that is devoid of urban dangers and pressures, the social and economic pressures on children in rural areas often

Support for the preparation of this chapter was provided in part by the U.S. Department of Education, Office of Special Education Programs, Grant #H02903006. The views expressed herein do not necessarily reflect those of the funders.

rival those of the inner city (Helge, 1990). School administrators from rural settings identified a higher percentage of children (with and without developmental delays) to be at risk because of factors such as poverty, illiteracy, involvement with crime, and depression than did urban administrators (Helge, 1990). Thus, rural early intervention personnel may be faced with complex problems related to the needs of children and families yet may have less training and fewer resources than their urban counterparts.

Severe shortages of adequately trained early intervention personnel are reported in many rural locales (Hebbeler, 1994; Reid & Bross, 1993; Royce et al., 1990; Shaeffer & Shaeffer, 1993). As part of the implementation of PL 99-457, the Education of the Handicapped Act Amendments of 1986 (since updated by PL 102-119, the Individuals with Disabilities Education Act Amendments of 1991), most states are in the final phases of developing a comprehensive system of personnel development (CSPD) to help alleviate these shortages (Gallagher, Trohanis, & Clifford, 1989; McCollum & Bailey, 1991). State planners will need to consider the barriers posed by demographics and geography, as well as the inherent challenges of rural service delivery, when devising systems that will adequately serve early intervention personnel in rural areas as well as those in large urban centers.

The purpose of this chapter is to describe and discuss the training of early intervention personnel in rural areas. First, issues such as personnel recruitment and retention, quality of personnel, and service delivery are discussed. Second, selected training strategies are described. Finally, recommendations for effective early intervention training in rural areas are given.

ISSUES IN EARLY INTERVENTION TRAINING

The recruitment and retainment of qualified personnel are two of the most important issues in early intervention training in rural areas.

Personnel Recruitment and Retention

Attracting and retaining qualified education personnel in rural areas has long been an issue in personnel recruitment. In a survey of 19 states, Helge (1981) reported that 94% listed recruiting and retaining qualified staff as the major barriers to full implementation of services to school-age children with disabilities. Prior to the passage of PL 99-457 and PL 102-119, 28 of the nation's 54 states, territories, and jurisdictions predicted significant shortages of early intervention personnel—estimating 88% more staff would be needed to provide services to children from birth to 3 years old and 81% would be needed for children from birth to 6 years old (Meisels, Harbin, Modigliani, & Olson, 1988). As states are now undertaking the implementation of PL 99-457 requirements for preschool children, rural program planners and administrators are facing significant challenges of recruitment and retention of personnel (Watson & Bennett, 1993).

Several factors contribute to increased stresses and high turnover rates for rural personnel. A sense of professional isolation is one such factor (Carlson, 1992). Practitioners may work without other colleagues and with few resources while at the same time covering vast land areas and scattered populations (Carlson, 1992; Helge, 1981). Lack of diverse contacts, scarcity of information, a less stimulating work environment than that found in urban areas, and having to provide more services with fewer resources are reasons frequently given for these feelings of isolation (Carlson, 1992).

A second factor leading to high turnover rates is that recent graduates from training programs are often the only personnel who can be recruited for positions in rural areas, as experienced professionals are preferred for positions in more desirable urban and suburban settings (Watson & Bennett, 1993). Young and inexperienced graduates are not well equipped for rural living nor are they equipped for the difficulties encountered in rural service delivery systems. As a result, they often quit their jobs after short periods of time; an attrition rate of 30%–50% is reported for this group (Helge, 1983).

Other stresses include lack of anonymity and difficulty with effecting change. In rural areas, service providers believe that their work is more closely observed than it would be in metropolitan areas and that urban anonymity is not possible in the "fishbowl" of the rural workplace (Carlson, 1992). In addition, some providers and administrators believe that it is difficult to effect change because the families they serve are suspicious of outside interference and generally resist change; such characteristics are reported to be typical of many rural areas (Helge, 1981).

As a solution to these problems, many programs prefer to train people who live in a given rural locale for jobs in that area (Hutinger, 1981; Watson & Bennett, 1993). Personnel who are already living and working in rural areas may be satisfied with their jobs and able to implement program change because of their knowledge of, and connections to, the rural community. Extending training to individuals who already reside in the target community and are likely to remain there may result in better staff stability, a better capacity for long-range program development, and a higher quality of services.

Educational Backgrounds of Existing Personnel

Early intervention personnel often are not adequately educated for their positions (Bricker & Slentz, 1988; Smith, 1988). In a survey conducted in Utah prior to the implementation of PL 99-457, 23% of early intervention providers had only a high school diploma or associate degree (Huntington, 1988). Of those with bachelor's or master's degrees, less than 55% had a teaching certificate or endorsement. In Oregon, 78% of early intervention teachers surveyed did not hold any form of certification ("Need for Early Intervention," 1985). Rule et al. (1993) reported that only 33% of rural early intervention programs in Utah required certification for employment, while 90% of urban directors made certification mandatory. Of the rural early intervention programs in Utah, 47% reported that certification was either unnecessary or that they were unsure of its necessity (Rule et al., 1993).

Preservice and in-service training opportunities to upgrade skills are less available in rural areas (Reid & Bross, 1993; Widerstrom, Domyslawski, & McNulty, 1986). Few professional resources (e.g., libraries, resource centers, training programs) are available for consultation as well. Rural service providers, therefore, may be less well trained than those in urban settings, while at the same time they may be less able to obtain training and resources to improve their job performance.

Delivery of Services

Coupled with fewer educational opportunities, having fewer professional resources may cause problems unique to rural areas. For example, an infant with acquired immunodeficiency syndrome (AIDS) may present challenges to service providers because there are no health care practitioners available in the area to consult about the baby's medical status. In addition, the prevalence of disabling conditions is somewhat higher in less populated areas than in metropolitan areas (Smith et al., 1990). Families with diverse needs, and their infants and young children with a variety of disabling conditions, are part of the typical rural caseload (Mills, Vadasy, & Fewell, 1987). In the same week, providers may be called upon to intervene with children who have sensory impairments, motor disabilities, genetic syndromes, and language delays. Meanwhile, therapeutic services (e.g., physical and occupational therapy) and specialists (e.g., nutritionists, rehabilitation teachers for people with visual impairments) may be unavailable (Parsons, 1990; Shaw & Nye, 1993). Technological advances such as computer simulation for wheelchair training and ultrasound equipment for the monitoring of heart defects may be unavailable (Smith et al., 1990; Sontag, Schacht, Horn, & Lenz, 1993). Difficult terrain—snowy mountain passes, poor roads, and long distances between communities—may further compound service delivery problems (Helge, 1981).

Racial, ethnic, and cultural differences prevalent in early intervention programs are also found in rural communities, often with an accompanying lack of resources to meet these diverse needs. For example, there may be no interpreters for a Bosnian family who recently immigrated to the area and no resources for interventionists to consult about the family's cultural traditions. Language barriers and cultural differences were reported as major problems for rural schools in the implementation of PL 94-142, the Education for All Handicapped Children Act of 1975 (Helge, 1984). Cultural and language differences may be even greater barriers to programs with a family-centered focus.

Resources for families of children with disabilities may be limited in rural areas. Because of large, widely scattered caseloads, early intervention practitioners may visit families only once or twice a month. Health care may be the only additional service received, and the health care professionals may not have had specialized training in pediatric care and/or developmental disabilities. Limited service networks for children with disabilities may exist with few people with any knowledge of disability-related services (e.g., independent living) available (Smith et al., 1990). In addition to lack of family supports, there may be few appropriate role models in the community for children with disabilities and their families.

PERSONNEL DEVELOPMENT APPROACHES

To meet the training needs of early intervention personnel in rural settings, several training approaches and associated strategies have been developed. These approaches include *rural on-site training* in which university personnel travel to the student in the rural area; *telecommunications-based distance training*, such as interactive television via satellite and audio teleconferencing; *university-based training* specifically designed for access by rural personnel; and *statewide combined training* jointly sponsored by school districts, state agencies, and colleges or universities. These training approaches and associated strategies are listed in Table 1.

Rural On-Site Training

Several strategies have been used in early intervention personnel preparation to bring preservice and in-service opportunities to rural areas. One strategy is to teach short, intensive courses and seminars to practitioners in rural areas. This is the strategy used by a University of Colorado early intervention project in which 1- to 2-week, all-day courses were offered at rural sites around the state by full-time faculty from the university (Widerstrom et al., 1986). Project staff found that interventionists were more able to attend short, intensive courses for a few days during the school year than courses offered over an extended time period. A needs assessment determined topics to be covered in the offered courses. For supervision of practicum experiences, a microteaching model was devised using videotaped lessons of students delivering services and returned by mail to program instructors for review. In reviewing evaluation data, 80% of the teachers ($N = 113$) who showed an initial interest in the project received their early childhood special education certification and most earned their master's degrees. This program was well accepted by rural communities and an increase in com-

Table 1. Approaches and associated strategies for rural early intervention personnel training

Approach	Associated strategies
1. Rural on-site training with university collaboration or sponsorship (preservice and in-service)	1. Short-term seminars and intensive courses 2. Year-long series of courses lead to certification or degree 3. Centralized summer courses on university campus or at rural site
2. Telecommunications-based distance training (preservice and in-service)	1. Courses use interactive television via satellite 2. Courses use interactive slow-scan television 3. Courses use interactive audio teleconferencing 4. Packaged courses use mixed media (videotape, audiotape, printed materials)
3. University-based training (preservice)	1. Weekend only "fly-in" courses on campus 2. Traditional year-long courses on campus
4. Statewide combined training (in-service)	1. Large school district or local education agency-sponsored workshops, courses 2. Regional education district or collaboratively sponsored workshops, courses 3. Courses conducted by interagency, trans-disciplinary technical assistance teams

munication and a sense of collegiality were developed statewide among university faculty, service providers, and state education administrators (Widerstrom et al., 1986).

Another approach offering short intensive courses is the Family Specialist Training Program in North Carolina. Instructors for this project traveled to rural sites to deliver seminars to clusters of students from several programs and agencies in a designated geographic area (Watson & Bennett, 1993). Topics were identified through a needs assessment and were followed by an application phase during which the instructor worked directly with students on site, either individually or in small groups. During this application phase, students prepared learning activities or portfolios to meet individual learning objectives. During the follow-up phase, students met in small groups to share their experiences and evaluate their progress toward learning objectives and outcomes. The goal of the follow-up phase was to facilitate generalization of the knowledge and skills learned in the seminars and portfolio preparation into the daily work environment. An analysis of evaluation data suggested that portfolio assignments did assist with generalization and that training that was responsive to individual needs and provided choices was optimal.

Rather than short, intensive courses, the University of Oregon developed a rural model in which a year-long course of studies leading to a master's degree was offered to rural practitioners. The Rural Early Intervention Training Project (Squires & Ryan-Vincek, 1994) brought coursework and practicum instruction to 8–10 students in rural sites in Oregon. Each year a different region of the state consisting of four or five counties was targeted. Instructors traveled monthly to that region to provide intensive coursework and instruction for 2 days. Twice monthly, supervisors traveled to individual worksites to observe students and provide feedback on identified intervention competencies. During the summer, students traveled to the University of Oregon's campus to take foundations courses and specialized practica leading to a master's degree. Increased competence as reflected in student self-ratings, and supervisor observations was reported during the academic year (Squires & Ryan-Vincek, 1994). The students' ratings of coursework, supervisors, and practicum opportunities were consistently in a "good" to "excellent" range. In addition, follow-up survey data indicated continued high satisfaction (> 80%) with practica, coursework, and faculty and/or staff (Squires & Ryan-Vincek, 1994).

Another strategy for rural on-site training is a model using centralized summer trainings for practitioners. For example, each year the Office of Public Instruction, nine educational service districts, and various professional organizations sponsor the Washington State Summer Institutes. These institutes offer 2 weeks of intensive coursework in early childhood special education, usually at a central site away from population centers. Topics are determined through a needs assessment developed by each educational service district and coordinated through Washington's CSPD. Through this process, training needed statewide for certification as well as topics of regional interest, such as those pertaining to rural service delivery, can be addressed.

One advantage of rural on-site training is economic—that is, rural practitioners can keep their current jobs while receiving training. In addition, students can meet family commitments and responsibilities by staying within their communities. Last, by clustering students or offering training to a group of students within a rural locale, networks may be formed among early intervention personnel from different programs and agencies. These networks may provide personal and professional support for rural service providers, which may counteract feelings of isolation and may continue to provide support after the training project has ended. However, on-site programs offered by universities tend to strain university resources because of personnel time and travel necessary for rural training and may require additional financial resources. Programs, such as the Oregon Rural Early Intervention Training Project and the North Carolina Family Specialist Training Program, were supported through federal funds, while projects such as the rural Colorado project (Widerstrom et al., 1986) were jointly supported through state and federal funds.

Telecommunications-Based Distance Training

The telecommunications-based distance training approach involves coursework brought to rural locations through the use of telecommunications technologies (Barker, Frisbie, & Patrick, 1993). Interactive television broadcast via satellite, computer networks, and audio teleconferences are examples of strategies that can be used with this approach.

The Early Intervention Special Education Program at West Virginia University (Ludlow, 1994) used satellite telecourses broadcast to local sites and on-the-job supervision of practicum experiences by doctoral-level graduate assistants to provide graduate-level training in rural sites. Eight interactive telecourses were offered throughout the state, each augmented with simulation and discussion activities, an audio call-in segment, applied intervention projects, and essay examinations. Trainees were required to complete at least six credits of practicum experience in an early intervention site; graduate assistants traveled to the trainees' sites to observe intervention skills and to evaluate acquisition of competencies. This program led to a master's degree and teaching certification for services to young children from birth to 6 years with at-risk conditions, developmental delays, and disabilities.

Project NETWORC Distance Learning in Nevada (Royce et al., 1990) offered a four-course teleseries leading to a master's degree and teaching credential to early intervention students throughout Nevada. Audio teleconferencing via a convener box allowed students to interact with the instructor and other students while text and photographs were relayed to the students via facsimile, which allowed the students and staff to have immediate access to written materials. Supporting materials included a curriculum guide with objectives, lecture notes, and a glossary of terms. Preliminary data reported moderate to high satisfaction with both the technical and course content components of the teleseries.

In addition to interactive television courses, a second strategy for telecommunications-based distance training is slow-scan television in which the television monitor is filled with serial still frames, like slides. This technology is less expensive than satellite technology, while it allows for interactive voice communication. In Utah, Rule et al. (1993) used slow-scan television courses to deliver training to early intervention personnel scattered in rural areas. Eleven sites across the state were equipped with studio classrooms that had slow-scan television equipment. Students and the instructor communicated through a microphone, supplementing the slow-scan television images. In addition to the text and photographs exchanged through facsimiles, videotapes and films were used with this technology. This method provided an economic means of accommodating small numbers of participants in rural and remote areas (Rule et al., 1993).

A third telecommunications-based distance training strategy is the use of audio teleconferencing, which was employed in Wyoming where interactive television systems were not feasible for geographic and economic reasons (Shaeffer & Shaeffer, 1993). Although the lack of face-to-face contact between student and instructor may have been a disadvantage, specific adaptations such as slowing down the presentation, adding more repetition and summaries, and frequent discussion and question sessions helped to compensate (Shaeffer & Shaeffer, 1993). Although students could not see the instructor or other students, speaker telephones allowed the students and teachers to interact. Student feedback indicated displeasure with some limitations of the audio-teleconferencing technology (e.g., not being able to see other students, having to use a microphone), but also indicated that courses were relevant in content and fulfilled a variety of training needs at convenient locations.

A fourth strategy combines telecommunications-based distance education with traditional correspondence courses. For this approach, university personnel mailed prepared multimedia materials to students in rural areas, and the use of these materials was combined with telecommunications technologies. The Alternative Education Program developed by the University of Alaska in Anchorage offered videotapes, audiotapes, printed modules, and exams for special education courses (Starlings, Wheeler, Ryan-Vincek, Schnoor, & Barrett, 1993). Because a correspondence strategy, which is noninteractive, may be less effective (Knowles, 1980), program developers at the University of Alaska sought to include a variety of interactive telecommunications-based strategies (e.g., telephone conferencing, electronic mail, U.S. postal service) with video- and audiotaped instruction and faculty-developed printed materials (Starlings et al., 1993). To encourage peer-supported learning, participants met as a group at designated sites to view videotapes and discuss assignments. Statewide conferences and individual contacts supplemented written correspondence and telephone advising. For the University of Alaska Alternative Education Program, students spent 6–12 weeks on campus during the summer for a supervised field practicum. Although this strategy is flexible in terms of the students' whereabouts and the course arrangements, individual organizational skills and self-reliance may be needed for students to complete the program (Starlings et al., 1993).

University-Based Training

A third approach for training personnel in rural areas is for universities to prepare and teach courses on campus, tailoring them for rural service providers in terms of scheduling and content areas. Some campuses offer a summers-only sequence of courses, leading to master's degrees and early intervention certification (Early Intervention Program, 1994). Others offer weekend or condensed 1- or 2-week courses that are taught on the university campus.

One example of the on-campus training approach is the "fly-in" program for occupational therapists offered by Texas Woman's University. Classes are taught over an entire semester on weekends at once-a-month intervals to accommodate participants living in rural areas. This model is effective for trainees in rural areas who seek specialized advanced training.

A second example of the on-campus approach is for universities to offer traditional year-round programs for students who can leave their rural location and employment to receive training. The Wisconsin TRAIN (Training Rural Area Interventionists to meet Needs) project (Reid & Bross, 1993) offered early intervention preservice training focused on service delivery in rural areas. Coping with issues such as lack of resources, professional isolation, and difficulty in gaining access to specialized services in rural areas was part of the course content. Although students received financial assistance through a grant to participate in the TRAIN project, program developers stated that recruitment was difficult because some students could not afford to travel to the campus for courses and/or could not afford to quit their jobs in rural areas so that they could enroll (Reid & Bross, 1993).

Disadvantages of university-based training programs for rural practitioners are obvious. Although they are more convenient for university personnel and for practitioners living in nearby communities, students with family and job commitments often cannot take advantage of these opportunities. Tuition costs may also be a barrier for prospective students, requiring that universities provide some form of financial support for rural students.

Statewide Combined Training

A final approach for training of rural personnel is statewide collaborative efforts among local school districts, extension services, community colleges, higher education institutions, and medical and/or public health agencies or programs. Agencies may be able to offer diverse and specialized training programs to providers in sparsely populated rural areas by pooling resources.

In Utah, the university and local school districts have collaborated to offer off-campus in-service training to early childhood personnel within the state (Rule et al., 1993). In addition to the slow-scan televised courses and off-campus extension offerings, Utah State University collaborated with individual school districts to offer courses in larger districts having sufficient personnel in need of training. Instructors modified the content to address individual needs of districts and staff in a particular region. For example, cultural diversity issues could be targeted in districts with large Native American populations. In addition, staff from a variety of disciplines, including program supervisors, could participate in trainings, enhancing team functioning and implementing changes.

A second example of statewide combined training is in Illinois where training was planned and offered by the Illinois Technical Assistance Project and the Regional Technical Assistance System, coordinated through the State Department of Education (Crews, 1990). The state was divided into six regions for delivery of technical assistance and training for early intervention personnel in order for the training needs of rural as well as urban areas to be recognized. Needs assessment, in-service training, consultation, and dissemination of resource materials were among the activities offered. The system offered specialized training to early intervention teams within each region, tailored to meet the needs of particular regions and locales.

In Hawaii, the Healthy Start Training and Technical Assistance (HSTA) team (Eggbeer, Latzko, & Pratt, 1993), sponsored by the Departments of Health and Human Services with participation by early intervention agencies, provided in-service training throughout the state. In addition to providing training to professionals and other personnel working in the Healthy Start abuse and neglect prevention program, the HSTA team trained home visitors from the Kamehameha Early Education Center for Native Hawaiians and the military home visitor programs. The training curriculum was developed through a community-wide effort involving educators, human services providers, medical professionals, home visitors, and social services administrators. Although this model was used primarily for in-service training, such teams could be employed for preservice training in areas where a campus was not easily accessible.

An advantage of collaborative efforts is that the comprehensive and coordinated use of resources and the capability to meet needs can be better met. Often, if the CSPD in a state is involved, a needs assessment can serve as the foundation for joint efforts, ensuring that diverse areas of the state are served and that a transdisciplinary, interagency approach is used. Standardized features of such a system can ensure quality training and meeting of statewide competency objectives while provisions for individualization of training to programs and staff may be made (Eggbeer et al., 1993). With collaborative projects, duplication may be avoided, making better use of limited training dollars.

RECOMMENDATIONS

Training programs need to be tailored to the specific rural regions and service providers where they are offered because of the diversity in rural settings and service delivery systems. Climate, geography, specific needs of children and families, availability of service facilities, and location of students vary from region to region and present different challenges.

Multicomponent Training Programs

In order to tailor training programs to meet these diverse needs, the first recommendation is that rural training programs be composed of at least four distinct components: needs assessment, courses, practical experiences, and evaluation.

Needs Assessment

Before beginning instruction, a needs assessment should be completed by prospective students. Through this process, issues unique to an area (e.g., strategies for working with linguistically diverse families, assistance with service delivery in remote areas) can be identified. The training content can then be focused toward these identified student needs. Questions regarding knowledge and skills in early intervention competency areas, the accessibility of professional resources, service delivery issues, and needs related to providing culturally sensitive intervention can be included on the needs assessment.

Courses

In addition to a focus on specific needs, a core of courses aimed at providing general foundations and methods in early intervention should be provided. Telecommunications-based courses and condensed on-site courses are among options for delivery of course content. Courses should include the following:

1. Educational foundations (e.g., social and philosophical foundations, life-span human development, professional development)
2. Foundations in early intervention (e.g., child development, atypical development, survey of exceptionalities)
3. Methods of early intervention (e.g., families, assessment, curriculum, physical and medical management, environmental and behavioral management, transdisciplinary and interagency teaming) (McCollum, McLean, McCartan, & Kaiser, 1989)

Practical Experiences

In addition to didactic information about intervention approaches, practical field-based experiences should be included in early intervention personnel preparation programs. Recommended practice for adult learners includes the opportunity to transfer learning into daily practice (Knowles, 1980; Sprinthall & Thies-Sprinthall, 1983). Application of training principles may be encouraged and long-term behavior change may be enhanced through inclusion of a practical applications component (Bruder & Nikitas, 1992). Practical experiences with a variety of young children from birth to 5 years and their families are essential.

Equally important is that students are supervised while they are engaged in practical experiences. Supervision provides students with ongoing feedback on their newly acquired skills and an opportunity to modify and improve these skills (Klein & Campbell, 1990). In addition, the supervisor can assist students in integrating and applying theoretical information presented in the courses. Although on-site supervision of students may be impossible, additional options for supervising practical experiences in rural programs follow. These options are listed in Table 2.

Table 2. Options for practical applications components in early intervention rural training

Option	Description
1. On-site supervision (Squires & Ryan-Vincek, 1994)	Supervisor or instructor travels to rural locale once or twice a month for observation at practicum or jobsite.
2. Portfolio assignments (Watson & Bennett, 1993)	Students are given applied problems or assignments, which the instructor reviews and assists with as needed. These problems and assignments may be accompanied with follow-up visit by instructor.
3. Videotaped teaching sample (Rule et al., 1993)	Students videotape a specific lesson and mail it to the instructor for review.
4. Microteaching model (Widerstrom et al., 1986)	Instructor videotapes a lesson, which is viewed and practiced by students who in turn videotape an example for the instructor to review.

A first option includes on-site supervision in a practicum or work environment (Ludlow, 1994; Squires & Ryan-Vincek, 1994). By using this strategy, a supervisor or instructor can observe students in early intervention sites on a regular basis for a fixed time period (e.g., twice a month for one semester). Individually identified needs, training competencies, and state personnel standards can serve as a basis for targeting objectives and subsequent observations.

A second option involves the use of supervised portfolio assignments in which students are given applied problems or assignments that they must complete, with an instructor available for review and help (Bruder & Nikitas, 1992; Watson & Bennett, 1993). For example, an assignment could be given to design a group activity that would embed individualized family service plan objectives for five children of varying skill levels. The instructional plan, data collection system, and videotape of the lesson could be included in the student's portfolio. During a follow-up site visit, the instructor could collect and discuss the assignment with students either individually or in small groups.

A third option is to use videotaped teaching samples (Rule et al., 1993). Students videotape a specific lesson or application and mail it to the instructor for review. Feedback is given to students via mail or telephone. For this option, no on-site visits are made by the supervisor.

A fourth option is the microteaching strategy (Widerstrom et al., 1986) in which the instructor videotapes lessons or activities, which are then viewed and practiced by students who in turn videotape an example for instructor review. An advantage of this strategy is the modeling of positive examples by the instructor on the videotape.

A combination of strategies can be used, with on-site observation combined with distance techniques such as videotaped teaching samples and microteaching strategies. Additional recommended practices, such as ongoing systematic evaluation and adherence to effective adult learning strategies, are also recommended.

Evaluation

Program components should be evaluated to provide both formative and summative information (Snyder & Sheehan, 1993). Ongoing feedback will allow program modifications to better address student needs (Knowles, 1980) as well as increase overall program effectiveness. Students can be provided with forms each quarter to evaluate program components, such as courses, instructors, delivery approach (e.g., on-site, via satellite), supervisors, practical experiences, and general satisfaction with the program. A rating system such as a Likert-type scale can be used with additional space provided for comments and feedback. It is suggested that these evaluation forms be completed and returned to program administrators so that student anonymity is preserved. In this way, students can give feedback to the program without fear of reprisal. In addition, informal means of feedback (e.g., comments to instructors, reflections in student journals) can be gathered and used to make program modifications. Follow-up information can also be gathered from students after graduation regarding job placement, promotions, and retrospective ratings of program components and overall program quality.

Training in the Rural Setting

A second recommendation is to offer training, either on-site or through telecommunications-based distance education technologies, in the rural locale if possible. These training approaches allow less time away from work, less expensive travel for students, and the possibility of more effective training because it occurs in the environment where delivery of services will take place. Local supervisors and administrators will be more aware and more likely to support changes if training takes place locally than if students travel out of the area (Bennett, Watson, & Raab, 1991). In addition, clustering of students within an area for training encourages networking and exchange of information, which can continue after training. Networking may offset feelings of isolation and work stress reported by rural service providers (Carlson, 1992). In addition to professional networking, the clustering of rural practitioners may result in an increased awareness of services and available personnel in specific areas, leading to a more coordinated, interagency, transdisciplinary approach to service delivery.

On-Site Training

A third recommendation is to offer some on-site training at a designated location, if possible, rather than presenting training solely through telecommunications approaches. Face-to-face contact may be the most effective learning model because of increased interactions between the learner and instructor and among learners (Henri & Kaye, 1993) and enhanced ability for learners to make direct applications to current roles (Knowles, 1980). Instructors also may be able to make learning more effective through the use of pertinent examples from the community, allowing students to make a direct transfer and application of knowledge. At the same time, university–community partnerships may be formed through the use of community representatives in classes and the presence of university personnel at the rural site. As previously mentioned, the opportunity is present for students to form a network of fellow professionals that may facilitate professional collaboration and support as well as provide professional and personal resources. Although on-site instruction is not always possible because of financial and physical barriers, the combination of on-site approaches with distance education technologies similar to those used by the University of West Virginia and the University of Alaska captures the best of both worlds.

Locale-Specific Training Programs

A fourth recommendation is to adjust training programs to take heed of local social, political, and cultural values (Lynch & Hanson, 1992) and to target content to meet these needs (Marrs, 1984; Reid & Bross, 1993). There is an intrinsic social and cultural diversity in rural areas (Carlson, 1992), and one "rural" training program cannot be applied to every area within a state. Topics such as community networking, family access to services, and fulfilling multiple diverse roles should be individualized if they are to be effective (Watson & Bennett, 1993).

For example, in some rural areas, interventionists may need information about selecting language interpreters and translators and about including the interpreter on the intervention team. In other areas, interventionists may need information about certain religious and cultural practices before making home visits and suggesting home intervention activities with families. In addition, because values among families from the same cultural or ethnic background may differ, some discussion among service providers about how to identify values and tailor intervention strategies to value systems is suggested.

Collaboration

A fifth recommendation is that collaboration among institutes of higher education, state departments of education, and local agencies (e.g., school districts, health departments) will improve the quality of training. When resources are pooled, more ambitious and comprehensive efforts can be targeted. Because higher education is often driven by student tuition and numbers, many institutions may not be able to develop rural training programs without the support and encouragement of state departments of education and state CSPDs (Widerstrom et al., 1986). In addition, the likelihood that changes and improvements in early intervention practices will occur and that the accomplishments of students will be recognized is likely increased with the participation of a greater number of personnel and agencies (Rule et al., 1993; Squires & Ryan-Vincek, 1994). Involvement of state and local interagency councils, including early intervention coordinating councils, can help ensure that training is provided to those in need and that services are not duplicated.

Regionalized delivery of training under the auspices of the state lead agency and CSPD requires coordination. Figure 1 illustrates a regionalized organizational structure for the coordination of training and technical assistance (Bricker, 1989). In this example, the state is divided into six early intervention regions under one centralized training project providing technical assistance and evaluation. This training project assists sites in each region in developing their training and technical assistance expertise. In this example, each region has one selected training site, although the number may vary according to the population density and needs of the region. A variety of model community-based satellite programs is associated with each of the six training sites. Community colleges, regional education and health agencies, local education and health agencies, early childhood programs, and local early intervention interagency coordinating councils are involved with planning and coordinating training efforts within each region. In this model, specific training needs of personnel in rural areas can be addressed as well as the provision of coordinated, comprehensive personnel training throughout the state.

CONCLUDING REMARKS: FUTURE DIRECTIONS

Delivery of quality training to personnel living in rural areas poses great challenges due to barriers such as geographic terrain, conflicting work schedules, and lack of professional resources. Training approaches exist, however, that minimize these problems and allow for delivery of quality early intervention personnel preparation. On-site training in which intensive courses are taught in rural areas is one approach; telecommunications-based distance training in which

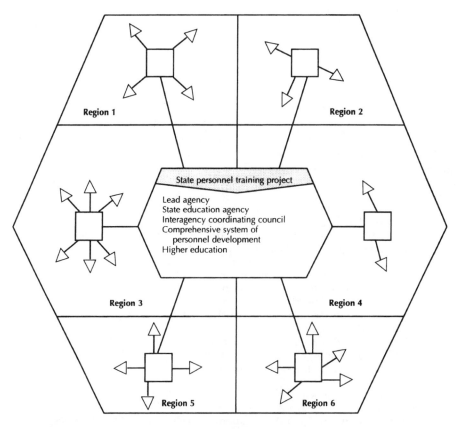

Figure 1. An example of a collaborative, statewide personnel training project. (□ = training site, △ = model community-based satellite programs.) (Adapted from Bricker [1989].)

technologies such as satellite broadcasts and computer networks are combined is a second approach. A third approach is for universities to offer training on campus, adjusting class schedules and content to meet the needs of personnel working in rural areas. Statewide combined trainings presented by local school districts, extension services, community colleges, higher education institutions, and medical and public health agencies are a fourth approach.

Personnel preparation programs in which local providers are clustered and trained at sites in a rural locale is the ideal approach for many reasons. While rural personnel are receiving training as a group, their sense of isolation may be lessened and sources of support may be increased. Collaborative programs with involvement by state, regional, and local early intervention agencies as well as higher education institutions are also recommended. Through statewide collaborative efforts, duplication may be avoided and a more coordinated and comprehensive training system may result.

Because there is an intrinsic diversity in rural areas, one rural training program will not address the needs of every area within a state. Therefore, programs will need to be designed to address the specific needs of a geographic locale, including the students who will receive training, the types of early intervention services provided, and the cultural and ethnic diversity of the area. Through careful planning and provision of training, children and families in rural areas will likely benefit by having personnel who are well trained in delivering a high quality of services.

REFERENCES

Barker, B., Frisbie, A., & Patrick, K. (1993). Broadening the definition of distance education in light of the new telecommunications technologies. In K. Harry, M. John, & D. Kugan (Eds.), *Distance education: New perspective* (pp. 39–47). New York: Routledge.

Bennett, T., Watson, A., & Raab, M. (1991). Ensuring competence in early intervention personnel through personnel standards and high-quality training. *Infants and Young Children, 3*(3), 49–58.

Bricker, D. (1989). *Early intervention for at-risk and handicapped infants, toddlers and preschool children.* Palo Alto, CA: VORT Corp.

Bricker, D., & Slentz, K. (1988). Personnel preparation: Handicapped infants. In M. Wang, H. Walberg, & M. Reynolds (Eds.), *The handbook of special education: Research and practice* (Vol. 3, pp. 319–345). Elmsford, NY: Pergammon.

Bruder, M., & Nikitas, T. (1992). Changing the professional practice of early interventionists: An inservice model to meet the service needs of Public Law 99-457. *Journal of Early Intervention, 16,* 173–180.

Carlson, R. (1992). What does it mean to work in a rural setting? A study of rural influences. *Journal of Rural and Small Schools, 5,* 43–47.

Crews, S. (1990, July). *Building a statewide technical assistance program.* Paper presented at the Early Childhood Intervention Conference, Lincoln City, OR.

Early Intervention Program. (1994, September). *Student handbook.* Eugene: University of Oregon.

Education for All Handicapped Children Act of 1975, PL 94-142. (August 23, 1977). Title 20, U.S.C. 1400 et seq: *U.S. Statutes at Large, 89,* 773–796.

Education of the Handicapped Act Amendments of 1986, PL 99-457. (October 8, 1986). Title 20, U.S.C. 1400 et seq: *U.S. Statutes at Large, 100,* 1145–1177.

Eggbeer, L., Latzko, T., & Pratt, B. (1993). Establishing statewide systems of inservice training for infant and family personnel. *Infants and Young Children, 5,* 49–56.

Gallagher, J.J., Trohanis, P.L., & Clifford, R.M. (Eds.). (1989). *Policy implementation and PL 99-457: Planning for young children with special needs.* Baltimore: Paul H. Brookes Publishing Co.

Hebbeler, K. (1994). *Shortages in professions working with young children with disabilities and their families.* Chapel Hill, NC: National Early Childhood Technical Assistance System.

Helge, D. (1981). Problems in implementing comprehensive special education programming in rural areas. *Exceptional Children, 47,* 514–520.

Helge, D. (1983). Increasing preservice curriculum accountability to rural handicapped populations. *Teacher Education and Special Education, 6,* 137–142.

Helge, D. (1984). The state of the art of rural special education. *Exceptional Children, 50,* 294–305.

Helge, D. (1990). At-risk students—A national view of problems and service delivery strategies. *Rural Special Education Quarterly, 10,* 42–52.

Henri, F., & Kaye, A. (1993). Problems of distance education. In K. Harry, M. John, & D. Kugan (Eds.), *Distance education: New perspective* (pp. 25–31). New York: Routledge.

Huntington, L. (1988). *Issues in personnel preparation in Utah.* Report submitted to the Utah State Office of Education. Salt Lake City: Utah State University, Early Intervention Research Institute.

Hutinger, P. (Ed.). (1981). *What's rural? An overview of successful strategies used by rural programs for young handicapped children.* Handicapped Children's Early Education Program Rural Network Monograph.

Individuals with Disabilities Education Act Amendments of 1991, PL 102-119. (October 7, 1991). Title 20, U.S.C. 1400 et seq: *U.S. Statutes at Large, 105,* 587–608.

Klein, N., & Campbell, P. (1990). Preparing personnel to serve at-risk infants, toddlers, and preschoolers. In S. Meisels & J. Shonkoff (Eds.), *Handbook of early childhood intervention* (pp. 679–699). New York: Cambridge University Press.

Knowles, M. (1980). *The modern practice of adult education: From pedagogy to androgyny.* Chicago: Association Press Follet Publishing Company.

Ludlow, B. (1994). Using distance education to prepare early intervention personnel. *Infants and Young Children, 7,* 51–59.

Lynch, E.W., & Hanson, M.J. (Eds.). (1992). *Developing cross-cultural competence: A guide for working with young children and their families.* Baltimore: Paul H. Brookes Publishing Co.

Marrs, L. (1984). A bandwagon without music: Preparing rural special educators. *Exceptional Children, 50,* 334–342.

McCollum, J., & Bailey, D. (1991). Developing comprehensive personnel systems: Issues and alternatives. *Journal of Early Intervention, 15,* 57–65.

McCollum, J., McLean, M., McCartan, K., & Kaiser, C. (1989). DEC White Paper: Recommendations for certification of early childhood special educators. *Journal of Early Intervention, 13*(3), 195–211.

Meisels, S., Harbin, G., Modigliani, I., & Olson, K. (1988). Formulating optimal state early intervention policies. *Exceptional Children, 55,* 159–165.

Mills, P., Vadasy, P., & Fewell, R. (1987). Preparing early childhood special educators for rural settings: An urban university approach. *Topics in Early Childhood Special Education, 7,* 59–74.

Need for early intervention professionals detailed. (1985, October). *Teaching Research Newsletter, I*(3), 1–2.

Parsons, A. (1990). A model for distance delivery in personnel preparation. *Journal of Visual Impairment and Blindness, 11,* 445–450.

Reid, B., & Bross, M. (1993). Project TRAIN: Training Rural Area Interventionists to Meet Needs. *Rural Special Education Quarterly, 12,* 3–8.

Royce, P., Cummings, R., & Cheney, C. (1990). Project NETWORC: A distance learning model in early childhood special education. *Rural Special Education Quarterly, 10,* 2–4.

Rule, S., Fiechtl, B., & Huntington, L. (1993). Preparation of early intervention personnel in a rural state. *Rural Special Education Quarterly, 12,* 9–14.

Shaeffer, M., & Shaeffer, B. (1993). Audio teleconferencing: Creating a bridge between rural areas and the university in early childhood/special education. *Rural Special Education Quarterly, 12,* 23–29.

Shaw, R., & Nye, J. (1993). An off-campus college program to prepare rehabilitation teachers of visually impaired students. *Journal of Visual Impairment and Blindness, 93,* 273–274.

Smith, B. (Ed.). (1988). *Mapping the future for children with special needs PL 99-457.* Iowa City: University of Iowa, Administration on Developmental Disabilities.

Smith, Q., Fasser, C., Wallace, S., Richards, L., & Potter, C. (1990). Children with disabilities in rural areas: The critical role of the special education teacher in promoting independence. *Rural Special Education Quarterly, 11,* 24–30.

Snyder, S., & Sheehan, R. (1993). Program evaluation in early intervention. In W. Brown, S. Thurman, & L. Pearl (Eds.), *Family-centered early intervention with infants and toddlers: Innovative cross-disciplinary approaches* (pp. 269–302). Baltimore: Paul H. Brookes Publishing Co.

Sontag, J., Schacht, R., Horn, R., & Lenz, D. (1993). Parental concerns for infants and toddlers with special needs in rural vs. urban counties of Arizona. *Rural Special Education Quarterly, 12*(1), 36–46.

Sprinthall, N., & Thies-Sprinthall, L. (1983). The teacher as an adult learner: A cognitive-developmental view. In G. Griffin (Ed.), *Staff development* (pp. 13–35). Chicago: University of Chicago Press.

Squires, J., & Ryan-Vincek, S. (1994). The rural early intervention training project. *Rural Special Education Quarterly, 13*(4), 17–27.

Starlings, C., Wheeler, J., Ryan-Vincek, S., Schnoor, J., & Barrett, H. (1993). *Alternative education: An integrated distance model for teacher training in Alaska.* Unpublished manuscript. Anchorage: University of Alaska–Anchorage, School of Education.

Watson, A., & Bennett, T. (1993). A model for training early childhood special educators in rural settings. *Rural Special Education Quarterly, 12,* 15–22.

Widerstrom, A., Domyslawski, D., & McNulty, B. (1986). Rural outreach training in early childhood special education: A cooperative model. *Journal of the Division for Early Childhood, 10,* 84–92.

III

TOWARD COLLABORATION AND EFFECTIVE PRACTICES

14

PREPARING PERSONNEL TO WORK WITH FAMILIES

Paula J. Beckman, Sandra Newcomb, Nancy Frank, Lynn Brown, Jennifer Stepanek, and Deirdre Barnwell

During an exchange between a service provider and a mother that occurred nearly 20 years ago, the mother shared a sentiment that the service provider still recalls. The mother had an 18-month-old son who had multiple disabilities. As part of a parent training program, the mother was given a form on which she was asked to select among a list of potential objectives for her son. These objectives were relatively broad and organized in the domains of language, cognition, motor, self-help, and social skills.

At the time, this approach was considered quite innovative. Programs for infants and toddlers were relatively new and the concept of "parent involvement" was beginning to grow in popularity. The mother took her time and thoughtfully considered each of the possible objectives based on her experience with her son. When she was finished, she handed the form back to the service provider, frowned, and said, "Well, I did the best I could . . . but frankly, it seems like he cries nearly 18 hours a day. I'm not sure I care about any of this; all I want him to do is stop crying."

In many ways this story illustrates the reasons that a growing number of professionals has sought new ways to work with families. It exemplifies how easy it can be for professionals to overlook fundamental concerns that families may have about their children, although they are making efforts to work in partnership with families. This example also reflects the extent to which conceptualizations of intervention based primarily on traditional developmental domains may not fully address the needs of children and families. In addition, it suggests that even service providers who are committed to working collaboratively with families may need special preparation to be effective in their efforts.

THE IMPORTANCE OF WORKING WITH families has become increasingly apparent to service providers in early intervention. Recognition of the family's role in early intervention is reflected in Part H of PL 101-476, the Individuals with Disabilities Education Act (IDEA) of 1990. This act requires service providers to include families in the process of planning and implementing intervention programs in ways that are unprecedented in most disciplines. Even service providers who provide excellent direct services to children may have concerns about working with families because they have had little specific training (Bailey, McWilliam,

& Winton, 1992; Mahoney, O'Sullivan, & Fors, 1989). Service providers need preparation to work effectively with families as partners on early intervention teams. This chapter is intended to provide a framework for preparing professionals to work with families. The chapter begins with a review of the theoretical basis for working with families, an overview of the philosophy of family-centered services, and a description of the roles of family members and service providers on early intervention teams. This is followed by a description of potential barriers to working effectively with families, a description of critical dimensions of preparing personnel to work with families, and an overview of the family specialization training area in the Department of Special Education at the University of Maryland. Finally, this chapter reviews the knowledge and competencies that are recommended when preparing personnel to work with families along with some specific strategies that can be used to teach those competencies.

THEORETICAL BASIS

Views of recommended practice in early intervention have been heavily influenced by theoretical perspectives that emphasize the family as a system (Bronfenbrenner, 1979; Minuchin, 1974; Turnbull, Summers, & Brotherson, 1986). From a family-systems perspective, factors that influence one part of the family system also exert an influence on other parts of the family. For families of children with disabilities, one implication is that factors that influence the parent (e.g., values and beliefs, economic circumstances, time demands) also influence the child and may influence the family's participation in intervention programs. Similarly, the needs of the child ultimately influence other members of the family as well as the interactions among family members.

A similar, though somewhat different, perspective is the *transactional model* of child development formulated by Sameroff and Chandler (1975). The transactional model emphasizes the dynamic interplay between environmental circumstances and biological influences in the development of children over time. When applied to work with families (Beckman, 1984; Beckman-Bell, 1981), this model emphasizes the reciprocal and changing impact of child and family factors. From this perspective, the family is seen as both influencing the child and being influenced by the child over time.

The emergence of the family-systems and transactional perspectives has been important because both perspectives create a broad and dynamic framework from which to view the child and family. They emphasize the importance of multiple influences on child development and family adaptation. As such, they provide an important basis for a shift in the way that professionals work with families in early intervention.

FAMILY-CENTERED SERVICES

These theoretical formulations, as well as a growing body of research concerned with families, have led to a major shift in the way that families are viewed by professionals. Initial efforts to involve parents in their children's programs were focused primarily on parent training efforts and on obtaining parental approval of professional recommendations (Beckman, Robinson, Rosenberg, & Filer, 1994; Dunst, Johanson, Trivette, & Hamby, 1991; Johnson, Jeppson, & Redburn, 1992; McGonigel & Garland, 1988). McGonigel and Garland (1988) have noted that early approaches toward families were often overly directive and intrusive. These authors argued that recent conceptualizations recognize the parent as the decision maker and emphasize family strengths. Family-systems theory provides the basis for a shift in emphasis to the entire family. As applied to early intervention, this shift is frequently described as a shift toward *family-centered* services.

Although the concept of family-centered services has been defined somewhat differently by various authors, it generally includes 1) a focus on the needs of the entire family rather than only on the needs of the child, 2) respect for family diversity, 3) an emphasis on flexible and responsive service delivery, and 4) an emphasis on parental choice and decision making (Dunst et al., 1991; Leviton, Mueller, & Kaufmann, 1992; McGonigel, Kaufmann, & Johnson, 1991; Minke & Scott, 1993). In describing the implications of a family-centered philosophy on team participation, McGonigel and Garland (1988) noted that families should be able to choose the level of team participation that is most comfortable for them. Some families will choose a leadership role, whereas others may not.

As professionals have struggled to define and implement family-centered services, family-centered approaches have often been contrasted with more *child-centered* approaches to intervention (Able-Boone, Sandall, & Loughry, 1989; Bailey, Buysse, Edmondson, & Smith, 1992; Bailey, McWilliam, & Winton, 1992; Dunst et al., 1991; McBride, Brotherson, Joanning, Whiddon, & Demmitt, 1993; Raver & Kilgo, 1991). Drawing this contrast has been important in that it highlights the need to consider the entire family system in planning interventions. However, it would be unfortunate if this contrast were interpreted to suggest that the interventionist must choose between focusing on the needs of the child and focusing on the needs of the family. It may be more useful to contrast services that are family centered with those that are *program centered.* Viewing the contrast in this way highlights the difficulties of creating programs and services that put the needs of the service system and the professionals who work in it before the needs of the children and families whom they are paid to serve. Although the interests of children may, from time to time, test the resources of the family system, it is rare that the needs and interests of families are completely at odds with those of the children who are a part of the family. Most families want their children to have an effective intervention program. Their search for appropriate programs, their advocacy efforts, and their confrontations with the system are typically on *behalf* of their children and are often expressions of frustration about the way the system has worked for them. Indeed, in a study involving focus groups of families of 40 children with special needs, one of the most commonly expressed service needs was for appropriate, high-quality intervention programs (Petr & Barney, 1993). Thus, even when families have pressing concerns that are not directly related to their children's disabilities, high-quality direct services for their children are likely to remain important to them and are an important component of a family-centered program.

The evolution of family-centered services has led to a shift away from more traditional views of teachers, therapists, and other professionals as the primary decision makers with respect to services for a child (Bailey, Buysse, et al., 1992). From a family-centered perspective, families are central players in making decisions about the type and amount of intervention their children receive as well as their own level and type of involvement in those services (Bailey, 1987; Bailey, Buysse, et al., 1992; Gill, 1993; McGonigel & Garland, 1988; Raver & Kilgo, 1991). Using a family-centered approach requires collaboration with parents as members of the assessment, planning, and service delivery team.

The Role of Families and Service Providers on Teams

An integral part of a family-centered philosophy involves a fundamental shift of the families' roles on intervention teams. A substantial body of literature suggests that, all too often, parents have been relegated to the role of receiving information from professionals and have not been viewed as equals in the decision-making process (Beckman, in press; Beckman, Boyes, & Herres, 1993; Leviton et al., 1992; McBride et al., 1993; McGonigel & Garland, 1988; Minke & Scott, 1993). The move toward family-centered services acknowledges parents' contributions and represents an effort to establish more equality in the parent–professional partnership.

Viewing family members as full and equal participants on decision-making teams does not lessen the role of service providers or diminish the value of their perspectives. Service providers bring their disciplinary expertise, their experience with a variety of different children and disabilities, and their knowledge of the service system to the intervention team.

In contrast, parents are often the ultimate, yet unrecognized, coordinators of their children's services (Lash & Wertlieb, 1993). They are central to communication with medical, educational, therapeutic, financial, and insurance personnel, as well as with other individuals who may be involved in some aspect of their children's lives. Parents know many things about their children from which professionals can benefit (e.g., what makes them happy or sad, excited or frightened, motivated or hesitant). Parents know how their children respond in different contexts and how they adapt to new situations. This knowledge makes parents a critical source of information when planning and implementing early intervention programs.

Open and honest sharing of ideas, knowledge, and skills can lead to a collaborative team process and result in better services for the child. In a study of parent and professional focus groups by Summers et al. (1990), communication and interactions between families and professionals were reported as the most critical elements in the process of collaboration. An example of the importance of such communication can be drawn from the initial process of placing and serving a child. Initial assessment data may be inadequate or insufficient to make appropriate decisions. Service providers benefit from information provided by people who are familiar with the child across a variety of contexts. Family perceptions, assessments, and contributions to the decision-making process are often critical to obtaining an accurate perspective of each child's needs (Leff, Chan, & Walizer, 1991).

A new balance is emerging between a professional's disciplinary expertise and the family's decision-making authority and responsibility. One way to achieve this balance is through the process of informed decision making. By using such a process, parents share their knowledge, expertise, and priorities for their children. Similarly, service providers share their observations, knowledge, and recommendations with parents. Parents can make an "informed decision" using all of the information available to them. The parents and service providers can work together to integrate the parents' unique knowledge of the children with the service providers' knowledge of their disciplines and service systems.

Personnel Preparation Barriers to Working with Families

Despite the increased recognition that children are part of a larger family system and the movement toward collaborative relationships with families, barriers to the implementation of such services have been identified. Bailey, Palsha, and Simeonsson (1991) studied the professional skills and concerns of professionals in moving toward a more family-centered approach to providing services in early intervention. They found that service providers were frequently concerned about whether their skills were adequate and about the potential impact these changes would have on children and families (e.g., concern about reduced quality of services available for children). There was also concern about collaboration (e.g., how roles are divided). Similarly, Mahoney et al. (1989) studied the family practices of early interventionists and identified several impediments to implementation of a systems-based, family-centered philosophy. One major difficulty was that even when they were working with families, the service providers believed that they did not have adequate preparation. These providers reported relying primarily on intuition rather than on specific training. A family-systems approach and a family-centered philosophy in early intervention require specific preparation to work with families.

The necessary preparation involves more than a simple orientation to a family-centered philosophy. Rather, such training must be focused on specific skills and strategies for working with families; such skills and strategies include how to interview families, how to conduct home visits, and how to conduct individualized education program (IEP) and individualized family service plan (IFSP) meetings. This view is supported by the work of Bailey et al. (1991), who found that although many participants in their study were already familiar with the general philosophy, these professionals expressed concern that they did not possess adequate skills to implement a family-centered approach. There is still a paucity of preservice and in-service training for both educational and medical professionals that provide specific strategies about ways to enhance communication, to increase awareness of and respect for family diversity, and to build working partnerships with families (Bailey, in press; Bailey, Simeonsson, Yoder, & Huntington, 1990; Lynch & Hanson, 1992; Stepanek, in press).

Bailey and his colleagues (Bailey, Palsha, et al., 1990; Bailey, Simeonsson, et al., 1991) surveyed more than 500 personnel preparation programs spanning more than 10 disciplines and found that most students received little specific training in working with families. Even when training in these areas does exist, it rarely involves family input and participation (Bailey, McWilliam, & Winton, 1992; Stepanek, in press; Widrick et al., 1991).

Dimensions of Preparing Personnel to Work with Families

Taken together, the acceptance of theoretical perspectives emphasizing the family as a system, the philosophical shift toward family-centered services, and

IDEA's Part H requirements concerning service coordination and the IFSP have converged to create a significant change in early intervention. These changes have resulted in a corresponding shift in the skills needed by individuals providing early intervention services.

A comprehensive program to prepare personnel to work with families should include at least three major dimensions. These dimensions are considered important in many aspects of personnel preparation and have either individually or collectively been described in the literature (Eggbeer, Fenichel, Pawl, Shanok, & Williamson, 1994; Fenichel, 1991; Moss & Wightman, 1993; Valli, 1992; Zeichner & Liston, 1987). The dimensions include knowledge acquisition, supervised practice, and reflection.

Acquisition of a Fundamental Knowledge Base

In early intervention, the acquisition of a fundamental knowledge base includes a familiarity with current literature and standards of recommended practice for young children and their families. As is typical in most programs, this knowledge base, as it relates to families, is primarily provided through courses and readings that include the theory, philosophy, and empirical basis for including families in early intervention as well as methods for working with families.

Opportunities for Supervised Practice

The second dimension, opportunities for supervised practice, may take a range of forms including interviews and role-playing experiences that are part of courses. In addition, supervised practice is a part of more intensive experiences, such as practicum experiences and student teaching. To be optimal, such practice should provide students with the opportunity to work with families from diverse backgrounds, families who have children with many different needs, and families who are involved with multiple agencies (e.g., social services and education). Practical experiences are vital because it is in such contexts that students can begin to integrate and apply didactically learned skills. Experiences should include opportunities to practice the skills students will need as they interact with families on early intervention teams, which include developing respectful and supportive relationships with families; providing service coordination; working with families to identify their resources, priorities, and concerns; and helping families gain access to needed services.

It is important to emphasize the value of *supervised* experiences. The dynamics of working with families can often be complex, both for the service provider and for the family. Early interventionists will encounter families who have a range of strengths and needs. Chan and Leff (1994) have argued that good supervision helps students integrate theory with the individual situations in which they find themselves as they work with children and families. It also helps them integrate their own personal reactions with what they experience and with what they have learned in coursework. Families also vary with respect to their degree of adaptation to the children's disabilities (Beckman, in press). For example, although some studies have reported increased stress, isolation, and/or depression in families of children with disabilities (Dyson & Fewell, 1986; Kazak & Marvin, 1984; Stagg & Catron, 1986), other studies have provided evidence that not all families experience such effects (Frey, Greenberg, & Fewell, 1989;

Gowen, Johnson-Martin, Goldman, & Appelbaum, 1989). For example, one family may be coming to terms with the long-term impact of their child's disability, while another is having difficulty adapting to a life-threatening medical condition. These circumstances demand that service providers be mature, sensitive, and flexible. Moreover, such circumstances often elicit personal reactions in the service provider that have been shaped by his or her own life experiences. Appropriate supervision is essential in order for students to learn healthy and effective strategies for working in a variety of circumstances (Chan & Leff, 1994). Fenichel (1991) has argued that, among other things, supervision and mentorship provide opportunities to deepen and broaden knowledge, model collaborative relationships, respond to the student's immediate needs, and support students as they deal with particularly stressful aspects of their work.

Reflection

The importance of supervision highlights the third dimension of the personnel preparation process, reflection. Once students have had the opportunity to practice their skills, it is important that they analyze and reflect on their actions. Many authors have emphasized the importance of reflection. Sokoly and Dokecki (1992) have argued that to provide ethical early intervention, the ability to use self-reflection is essential. Taylor and Valli (1992) have described reflection as the ability to critically examine one's actions and the context of those actions. They have argued that the importance of this self-examination helps create consciously driven means of engaging in professional intervention rather than basing intervention on habit, tradition, or impulse. Zeichner and Liston (1987) summarized the work of eight studies concerned with the effectiveness of a preparation program that emphasized reflection. These authors noted several positive outcomes. For example, supervisors were more consistent in asking their students to question their teaching practice and evaluate it based on ethical criteria. Students also began to engage in the critical analysis of their practicum situations.

During supervision and in courses, opportunities for students to use reflection can be emphasized. Students can be asked to reflect by doing such things as describing how a specific reaction from a parent made them feel, what they were thinking about when they took a particular action, or how they might have handled a given situation differently. Students can also be encouraged to think about their own temperaments and values and to reflect about ways in which these characteristics influence their work with families. Taylor and Valli (1992) have suggested that the quality of students' reflections can be assessed by their ability to relate knowledge to practice, their ability to view a situation from multiple perspectives, and their ability to see alternatives to their thinking and actions.

Coursework and Field Experiences

Because of the need to prepare personnel to work with families of young children with disabilities, a *family specialization* for students in early childhood special education has been developed at the University of Maryland. Students who participate in this specialization often have experience in the area of infancy and are specifically seeking additional training to work with families. The family specialization provides opportunities to develop expertise in working with families in three ways: 1) coursework, 2) practicum experiences, and 3) assistantships. All students in this specialization are required to take a course on working with families that covers the theoretical and empirical literature concerned with families and introduces students to basic strategies for developing and maintaining positive working relationships with families. Students are also required to take a course focused on service coordination. Finally, students select two electives from outside the department that apply to work with families (e.g., courses in adult learning, family crisis and intervention, family counseling, conflict resolution). Students apply information from courses during field experiences (through practicum placements and assistantships) that specifically focus on families (e.g., working with a service coordinator, facilitating parent groups). Practical experiences are supervised by university personnel with extensive experience in working with families (e.g., a special educator, a parent, a social worker). In addition to meeting individually with students, these supervisors conduct seminars that provide an opportunity for the students to apply knowledge gained in courses, reflect on experiences, discuss issues that arise during practica, and receive additional information and support.

Knowledge, Competencies, and Strategies for Working with Families

The ability to work with parents on early intervention teams involves a number of specific skills that have often been absent in personnel preparation programs that focus only on direct intervention skills with children. In this section, knowledge and competencies are identified that are important for preparing service providers to work effectively with families. Strategies that have been found useful in helping students develop these competencies are also described. The knowledge, competencies, and strategies described in this section are derived from the literature (Able-Boone et al., 1989; Bailey, 1987; McGonigel et al., 1991; Minke & Scott, 1993) as well as from the experiences of the authors of this chapter. These areas, described below, are summarized in Table 1.

Familiarity with the Theoretical and Empirical Literature Concerned with Families

The theoretical and empirical literature provides a critical basis for understanding the importance of collaboration with families. Such a basis includes an understanding of family systems, family life cycles, the ways in which a disability affects the family, family stress, and family coping and adaptation.

Many traditional strategies (e.g., lectures, classroom discussions, readings) remain important mechanisms for providing students with a theoretical and empirical foundation. However, principles of adult learning suggest that for such information to be meaningful for students, it should be tied to direct practice (Knowles, 1984). One particularly effective strategy is to have a family member(s) share his or her perspective and describe the impact the child with a disability has on the family system. When discussing such issues as family-systems theory, it is especially helpful if more than one member of the family (e.g., a mother and a father and/or an older sibling) is willing to share individual perspectives. Such real-life examples not only illustrate important concepts for students but provide a common basis for discussion and application. Some authors

Table 1.　Knowledge and competency areas to work effectively with families

  1.　Familiarity with the theoretical and empirical literature concerned with families
  2.　Ability to work with families from diverse backgrounds
  3.　Ability to build relationships with families
  4.　Familiarity with local, state, and federal policies
  5.　Ability to function as a service coordinator
  6.　Ability to provide support
  7.　Ability to provide information and training to families
  8.　Understanding the role and contributions of other team members
  9.　Ability to resolve conflicts
 10.　Self-reflection
 11.　Understanding barriers to effective communication with families

have suggested that reading personal accounts or reading literature from a parent perspective enhances sensitivity to such issues as well (Seligman & Darling, 1989).

Another useful strategy for acquiring a knowledge base involves the presentation of case studies. The value of case studies as a personnel preparation strategy has gained considerable attention over the years (McWilliam & Bailey, 1993). Case studies can illustrate many points. For example, they can be used to have students practice identifying family priorities, resources, and concerns; identify the family's coping strategies; and discuss the most appropriate use of formal supports.

Ability to Work with Families from Diverse Backgrounds

Early interventionists have increasingly recognized the growing diversity within and across families (Beckman & Bristol, 1991; Harry, 1992; Lynch & Hanson, 1992; Shapiro & Simonsen, 1994). Diversity can be reflected in many ways, including values, culture, ethnicity, education, spirituality, geographic location, economic circumstances, and family composition. Such differences are the source of considerable variation in how families perceive and react to disability, communicate, cope with problems, and manage their day-to-day lives. These differences can, in turn, influence other variables that are closely associated with early intervention, such as child-rearing styles, parent–child interaction patterns, and when and how families seek help.

To be effective, early intervention personnel need to understand and respect family diversity. Bailey (in press) has argued that service providers must ultimately accept that, except for cases of child abuse and neglect, families have a right to the values they hold. Providing materials and suggestions that take into consideration the family's beliefs and values can contribute to positive relationships between families and service providers.

These goals are not easy to accomplish. They can be infused across a variety of courses and practical experiences and can become an ongoing subject of reflection and self-appraisal for students. In-class activities can include values-clarification experiences in which students explore their own system of beliefs and values and reflect on ways their values may differ from those of others. As part of this process, it is important to ask students to analyze how their values and beliefs influence their exchanges with families. Another strategy is to have students in field placements analyze their lesson plans in terms of their relevance for children and families from diverse backgrounds. Students can then reflect upon ways they could adapt their lesson plans to include a range of cultural practices. Finally, case studies are powerful ways to illustrate how an interventionist's personal values and beliefs may conflict with those of a family. By confronting these issues during relatively neutral, in-class discussions, it is often possible to sensitize students to issues they may encounter while working in the field.

Ability to Build Relationships with Families

A critical element in working effectively with families involves the ability to establish and maintain positive relationships (Beckman, Frank, Newcomb, & Brown, in press; Eggbeer et al., 1994; Kalmanson & Seligman, 1992; McGonigel et al., 1991). Kalmanson and Seligman (1992) have argued that the success of virtually all interventions depends on the quality of the service provider's relationship with the family, even when the relationship is not, in and of itself, the focus of the intervention. The ability to establish relationships is essential to all aspects of working with families, including the development and implementation of an IEP or IFSP. Several critical factors are important in the ability to establish positive working relationships with families. For example, Shulman (1978, 1992, 1993) has demonstrated that the capacity for empathy is one of the most important factors associated with effective relationships. Seligman and Darling (1989) have emphasized the importance of being both nonjudgmental and trustworthy. In a qualitative study, Greig (1993) found that honesty and trust were highly salient determinants of whether a family member found his or her relationship with service providers to be helpful. McGonigel et al. (1991) defined quality interpersonal relationships as ones in which active listening takes place; individuals are treated with respect and dignity; individual family values, customs, and beliefs are respected; communication is open and honest; complete and unbiased information is shared with families; strengths as well as needs are recognized; and family choices and decision-making processes are honored. To achieve this type of relationship, service providers need to engage in active and focused listening, elaborate and expand on the family's ideas, and provide appropriate feedback for the family's concerns.

Strategies for teaching these competencies can include role playing and specific practica. For example, students can be asked to engage in mini-interviews in which they practice the use of open and closed questions or practice active listening (Hutchins & Cole, 1992). Case studies can be used to discover how professionals communicate and build trust. Another strategy is to ask students to identify a family and to develop a relationship over an extended period of time for the purpose of providing support. The value of such experiences has been stressed elsewhere in the literature (Seligman & Darling, 1989). Such one-to-one experiences can help sensitize students to the needs of families as well as to the interpersonal issues that can arise as they offer support to the family. However, while students are engaged in this relationship, it is important that they have intensive supervision by an experienced professional.

Familiarity with Local, State, and Federal Policies

Familiarity with local, state, and federal guidelines governing early intervention services is important for several reasons. This knowledge is critical to ensure that students 1) comply with requirements pertaining to parental participation, 2) provide appropriate services, 3) adhere to designated timelines, and 4) are prepared in the event of due process challenges. In addition, knowledge of current regulations may help professionals provide accurate information to families concerning their rights. Several strategies can be used to prepare personnel who understand local, state, and federal policy. During a course, students can analyze local implementation of particular policies. Representatives from local and state agencies can offer class presentations concerning legal requirements and the issues involved in implementing policies at their levels. Contacts with state and local providers also offer students opportunities to ask questions in areas they find confusing.

Student placements in federal, state, and local agencies and advocacy organizations may be helpful in providing real-world experience concerned with policy issues. Opportunities to attend meetings of state and local interagency coordinating councils provide useful ways to learn how policies are established as well as the issues with which state and local agencies must contend as they implement Part H. Students can frequently observe and participate in IEP and IFSP meetings. It may also be useful to have students attend these meetings with a family and to analyze the meetings from a family perspective. Such experiences can provide the basis for a reaction paper or class discussion regarding the extent to which the family's rights and perspectives were respected, as well as what parts of the meeting might have presented difficulties. The extent to which it is possible to involve students in IEP and IFSP meetings is likely to vary. Some programs may limit the accessibility of these meetings for reasons of confidentiality. To ensure the availability of such experiences, it is helpful to establish and maintain ongoing relationships with direct services programs.

Ability to Function as a Service Coordinator

General responsibilities of service coordinators include coordinating assessments and evaluations, facilitating the development and evaluation of IEPs and IFSPs, informing families about the availability of advocacy services, coordinating the services provided to the child, and facilitating transitions (Zipper, Weil, & Rounds, 1993).

Unfortunately, early interventionists are often not adequately prepared to coordinate services. For example, Coulter, Wallace, and Laude (1993) interviewed service providers in five counties to obtain their perspectives on the early intervention system. They found a significant lack of information among agencies about the services provided by other agencies.

In addition to basic information about community services, service coordinators need strategies for facilitating interagency communication and cooperation. These include the ability to work with a variety of disciplines; conduct family interviews; and identify family concerns, priorities, and resources. Because service coordinators often negotiate with a range of individuals who have differing agendas, they need to understand team dynamics and the roles of specific disciplines, and they need skills in conflict resolution (Zipper et al., 1993).

Many of these skills can be taught as part of course activities. For example, role-playing activities can be designed so that students can practice such skills as conducting interviews with families. It is also useful to have students conduct and audiotape an interview with a family. The audiotape can then be reviewed and analyzed with respect to the dynamics of the interview, the information obtained, the interview skills used, and the alternative strategies that may have better facilitated the interview process. Students can also observe videotaped examples of IEP and IFSP meetings and analyze the dynamics of the meeting, identify exchanges that were supportive to family members, and discuss incidents that might have proven stressful. As a group, students can brainstorm alternative approaches and reflect upon the impact of each one.

Another activity that can be used to improve service coordination skills is to have students prepare a resource file for a specific family. When conducting this activity, it helps to require students to do more than prepare a list of potential resources. Rather, the students can be required to actually contact each potential resource and determine eligibility requirements, restrictions on the service, how to apply, and other issues relevant to obtaining the service. By requiring students to take this additional step, they not only become more familiar with the service system but also come face to face with the limitations of those services. For example, although the students may initially report that respite services are available for families, actually pursuing this resource often reveals limitations due to lack of income, limits on the number of hours available, or restrictions based on the child's medical status.

Ability to Provide Support

As service providers become more involved with families, they often find themselves providing many types of support (e.g., emotional support, concrete help). To do this effectively, students need to demonstrate the skills necessary to develop supportive relationships with families. This includes the ability to conduct home visits and to facilitate the development of support groups and support networks. In a qualitative study using focus groups, Petr and Barney (1993) found that parents emphasized the importance of receiving emotional support. The parents in this study reported that although informal sources of support (e.g., family, church, friends) were important, they could not always depend on these systems. Parents indicated that the most reliable source of emotional support was other parents of children with disabilities. Thus, it is also helpful if service providers can go beyond direct services and understand how to address the networking, informational, and emotional needs of families.

Again, a variety of strategies can be used to prepare personnel to provide such support. Videotapes can be used as a way of sensitizing students to family needs and analyzing positive and negative examples of support to families (Edelman, 1991; Edelman, Greenland, & Mills, 1992). Students can also be asked to identify and describe various models available in the literature for providing social support (Beckman, Newcomb, Frank, Brown, & Filer, 1993; Zeitlen & Williamson, 1988). Once such models have been identified, students can discuss ways to integrate all or part of these models into local intervention programs. Students can be asked to attend support groups and reflect upon the dynamics they encounter as well as the issues that are presented by families.

Part of learning to provide support in this way means learning to understand one's own personal boundaries and limitations. Thus, an important part of preparation efforts should involve helping students recognize circumstances in which they need help from other professionals (e.g., therapist, counselor). One way of addressing this issue is through weekly meetings in which students discuss issues with which they are confronted and identify the appropriate responses.

Ability to Provide Information and Training to Families

Interventionists need to provide information to families in ways that are understandable and applicable and that demonstrate a respect for the family's unique knowledge of their child. The literature has suggested that honest information about the child is a need that is consistently expressed by parents (Bailey, Blasco, & Simeonsson, 1992; Beckman, in press; Greig, 1993; Leff et al., 1991; Petr & Barney, 1993). In fact, in 1993, Greig found that the perceived quality and availability of information received from service providers is a major criterion by which parents judge the support they receive from professionals. Similarly, in a focus group study, Petr and Barney (1993) reported that an important source of frustration for families in IEP meetings was a lack of information provided by school staff.

Again, several approaches can be used to teach students strategies for providing information. Students might develop informational or training materials for a family of a specific child. The students might also develop a resource file of information geared specifically for parents and family members that can be used when they enter the field. Such materials might include specific curriculum materials designed for parents (e.g., Hanson, 1987; Hanson & Harris, 1986), information about specific disabilities, or books designed to provide information to families about the early intervention system (e.g., Beckman & Boyes, 1993). It is especially helpful to organize a cooperative project among class members in which materials are shared so as to maximize the resources available to all members.

Understanding the Role and Contributions of Other Team Members

For a team to work effectively, it is essential that both family members and service providers see themselves as respected partners and that team members understand and value the expertise of other members. Unfortunately, this is not always the case. The literature has suggested that parents are frequently not viewed as equal participants in the IEP and IFSP processes (Beckman, Boyes, & Herres, 1993; Brinkerhoff & Vincent, 1986; Gilliam & Coleman, 1981; Souffer, 1982). For example, there is evidence that a relatively large percentage of IEPs are developed prior to the actual team meeting (Souffer, 1982).

Students can be taught to create more family-friendly team meetings. For example, making sure that the family has been introduced to everyone on the team may seem obvious, but such small insensitivities are frequent complaints of families (Beckman, in press; Beckman, Boyes, & Herres, 1993). Other strategies, such as *beginning* the meeting by asking the parents how they feel about the progress that has been made and discussing *their* priorities before starting a discussion of the goals of service providers, send a message of respect and concern for the family. Brinkerhoff and Vincent (1986) studied the effects of an experimental program designed to increase the participation of parents in the IEP process. They found that an intervention package that included providing more information to parents prior to the meeting as well as training staff in strategies for including parent input was effective at increasing parent participation.

One strategy for teaching students about the role of various team members is to have students interview professionals from other disciplines regarding 1) their role on the team, 2) ways that they work with other team members and families, and 3) the benefits and difficulties that they have experienced. Another strategy is to have students observe team members from other disciplines who are working with the same child. Students can then be asked to integrate the goals of multiple team members within the context of their own intervention activities and to reflect upon the ways in which the goals and activities of team members are consistent or in conflict. They might also be asked to put themselves in the role of the family and think about the impact of trying to implement the combined set of proposed activities. Such an exercise can provide an important "reality check" for service providers by helping them appreciate the impact of their recommendations on families.

Ability to Resolve Conflicts

Given the range of individuals who are on the early intervention teams, it is not unusual for disagreements to arise. Bailey (1987) has argued that nonresolution of such differences among team members can undermine the relationship with the family. Conflict resolution strategies are helpful so that disagreements can be resolved quickly.

Ways to familiarize students with the importance of conflict resolution strategies include observing a due process hearing, interviewing a parent who has been through due process, or having a parent describe his or her experience with due process. Such activities provide the basis for discussions about the impact of such an adversarial proceeding. Students can then be introduced to alternatives to due process, such as mediation. Students can also be taught specific strategies to use in the conflict resolution process. Students can then practice those strategies during in-class simulations. For example, Turnbull and Turnbull (1990) suggested that when a family becomes angry it may be helpful to engage in such strategies as writing down the parents' complaints, showing parents the list and asking if there are additional complaints, soliciting suggestions, writing down suggestions, and so forth. After such a simulation, participants can reflect upon their reactions to the process. Case studies that illustrate examples of conflicts also provide valuable opportunities for students to analyze the conditions that led to the conflict and identify points at which conflicts can be resolved. Another helpful exercise is to have students play the role of advocate for the family in a dispute and then play the role of advocate for the program or agency. They can then reflect on what they learned as a result of experiencing each perspective.

Self-Reflection

The ability to develop and maintain strong, positive relationships with families requires an adequate understanding of one's own personal style and the factors that influence personal behavior (Seligman & Darling, 1989). The development of such insights requires students to become familiar with their own system of beliefs, their unique working styles, and their own temperaments. Such characteristics will influence their reactions to individual family circumstances as well as their recommendations for intervention.

It is important for students to examine how their own styles and personal strengths interact with those of the family. Self-reflection requires constant examination of individual interactions with families and the effect of personal style on these exchanges. For example, does the student enjoy being with people from diverse groups? Does the student prefer exchanges with families to be organized neatly around distinct tasks or is the student more comfortable with an open-ended approach? How does this intervention style affect the way the student works with families? There is no one intervention style that is "right." However, professionals need to be aware of their own styles and how they affect different families.

Understanding Barriers to Effective Communication with Families

Whether a parent believes he or she is encouraged to participate in a team process and delivery of his or her child's services depends on a number of factors. Considerable evidence has suggested that parents frequently experience frustration and concern about their interactions with professionals (Beckman, Boyes, & Herres, 1993; Brinkerhoff & Vincent, 1986; Johnson et al., 1992; Seligman & Darling, 1989; Shelton & Stepanek, 1994). Therefore, personnel who provide early intervention must recognize potential barriers to communication between parents and service providers. Programs that prepare personnel to work with parents must help students understand and overcome these barriers. Some barriers that have been identified in the literature include differing service priorities; differing values, beliefs, and language; failing to listen; negative attitudes; and the use of professional jargon. These are described in more detail below.

Differing Service Priorities   Of particular concern for family participation on early intervention teams are problems that arise when parents and service providers differ with respect to their priorities for goals and services. Even when parents and service providers have common goals (e.g., appropriate care, intervention for a child), each may have different approaches to reaching those goals (Thomas, 1990). The success of intervention may be limited if the interventionist attempts to impose goals and activities that are not acceptable or important to the family. Focusing on outcomes that are important to the family helps ensure that the family's perspective has been respected and accepted by the service providers on the team.

Differing Values, Beliefs, and Language   As indicated previously, interventionists are serving an increasingly diverse group of young children and families. There are many sources of this diversity, which may include such factors as culture, ethnicity, religious affiliation, education, and income. Whatever the source, it is helpful for service providers to be aware of differences so they can maximize the potential for helping the family.

Such differences may pose barriers to communication for several reasons. Cultural groups often have different expectations about the roles of families in the education of children. Lynch and Stein (1987) reported differences between ethnic groups in the level of involvement parents had in their children's programs. A major barrier to participation for Latino families was language and communication difficulties. Communication difficulties influenced families' understanding of the services provided. Other authors have reported that the lack of language-appropriate information and materials for non–English-speaking families was a barrier to involvement as was a shortage of bilingual personnel (Chan, 1990; Lynch & Stein, 1987).

Differences in values and beliefs can present significant barriers to interaction with families. Although not always stated openly, these values may be evident in subtle ways (e.g., how a parent phrases a concern, describes the family's needs, organizes family life). Differences in beliefs are often unrecognized or unstated until they are challenged by exposure to different values. Thus, interventionists and families both may experience a range of reactions. When interventionists are unaware of a discrepancy in values, conflicts may arise that adversely affect families. For example, a common goal of intervention programs is to facilitate the child's independence. When working with a family for whom interdependence is valued, stressing the child's future independence may create a sense that the family's values and goals for their child are not appreciated.

Shapiro and Simonsen (1994) have noted that it may be difficult to get Latino families to participate in support groups because groups are often organized in ways that ignore fundamental values common to many Latino families. For example, these authors noted that for many Latino families of Mexican origin, the concept of *simpatico* is a significant factor mediating behavior. For these individuals, there is an emphasis on politeness and respect in their desire to promote harmony and avoid conflict. These tendencies may make families reluctant to challenge authorities in IEP and IFSP meetings. In a group, simpatico might cause a family to refrain from making comments that would be difficult for other members.

Failing to Listen   Families have frequently reported that a major barrier to communication with service providers occurs when service providers do not listen to them (Segal, 1985; Seligman & Darling, 1989). Communication breakdown can occur when service providers do not acknowledge or consider information provided by parents. It can also occur when professionals fail to respond when families express a concern, ask for information, or express an objection to a professional recommendation.

Negative Attitudes   Another potential barrier to communication between parents and professionals may be the attitude of service providers (Gill, 1993). Parents may have difficulty voicing an opinion that is not consistent with that of the professional for fear of being judged "noncompliant," "angry," "hostile," "demanding," or "hard to work with." Several authors (e.g., Lipsky, 1985; Seligman & Darling, 1989) have argued that such labels are often overgeneralized, and therefore, no matter what role the family assumes, there is the potential for negative interpretation. Parents may also be concerned that a negative judgment may adversely affect the quality and/or quantity of services their children receive.

Use of Professional Jargon   Another barrier to communication with families is the use of professional jargon. Acronyms or technical terminology used without explanation can lead to misunderstandings and even to unnecessary feelings of inferiority. Explaining or eliminating such jargon can help avoid potential communication barriers. Students should understand that, in some instances, parents who appear passive may simply be unfamiliar with terminology, eligibility requirements, or other aspects of service delivery.

Many of the strategies identified previously will help students overcome the barriers to effective communication. An awareness of these barriers may help students be more sensitive to circumstances in which they might arise. Case studies, videotaped examples, role playing, and simulation activities are all important techniques that can be used to sensitize students to the potential barriers that can occur in working with families as part of an early intervention team.

CONCLUDING REMARKS: FUTURE DIRECTIONS

The increased emphasis on such concepts as family-systems and family-centered services has resulted in many challenges for individuals involved in personnel preparation. Preparation must now go beyond the provision of discipline-specific skills related to the development of young children. Equally important are the philosophy, personal qualities, and skills of the people working with families. The basic philosophical approach to preparing effective service providers should be one of working with families on the basis of their strengths and capabilities. Personnel must truly believe that families are raising their children to the best of their abilities. When working with a family on an early intervention team, the role of the early interventionist is to enhance the family's sense of their own competence and capabilities. Increasingly, the emphasis on working with families leads to an emphasis on the importance of developing positive relationships, collaborating, and respecting diversity. There must be permission within personnel preparation programs to set standards for students and to direct into other endeavors students who are unable to achieve sensitivity and respect for families.

Preservice programs must creatively provide opportunities for students to learn skills for working with families in a safe and supervised setting. The focus of these opportunities must be on simulating experiences so that students can expand their knowledge, broaden their frame of reference, sensitize their reactions, reflect on their interactions, and deepen their empathy for the families with whom they work.

REFERENCES

Able-Boone, H., Sandall, S., & Loughry, A. (1989). Preparing family specialists in early childhood special education. *Teacher Education and Special Education, 12*(3), 96–102.

Bailey, D. (1987). Collaborative goal setting with families: Resolving differences in values and priorities for services. *Topics in Early Childhood Special Education, 7*(2), 59–71.

Bailey, D. (in press). Preparing early intervention professionals for the 21st century. In M. Brambring, H. Rauh, & A. Beelman (Eds.), *Early childhood intervention: Theory, evaluation and practice.* Berlin: de Gruyter.

Bailey, D.B., Blasco, P.M., & Simeonsson, R.J. (1992). Needs expressed by mothers and fathers of young children with disabilities. *American Journal on Mental Retardation, 97*(1), 1–10.

Bailey, D.B., Buysse, V., Edmondson, R., & Smith, T. (1992). Creating family-centered services in early intervention: Perceptions of professionals in four states. *Exceptional Children, 58,* 298–309.

Bailey, D.B., McWilliam, P.J., & Winton, P. (1992). Building family-centered practices in early intervention: A team-based model for change. *Infants and Young Children, 5*(1), 73–82.

Bailey, D.B., Palsha, S.A., & Simeonsson, R.J. (1991). Professional skills, concerns, and perceived importance of work with families in early intervention. *Exceptional Children, 58,* 156–165.

Bailey, D.B., Simeonsson, R.J., Yoder, D.E., & Huntington, G.S. (1990). Preparing professionals to serve infants and toddlers with handicaps and their families: An integrative analysis across eight disciplines. *Exceptional Children, 57*, 26–35.

Beckman, P.J. (1984). A transactional view of stress in families of handicapped children. In M. Lewis (Ed.), *Social connections beyond the dyad* (pp. 281–298). New York: Plenum.

Beckman, P.J. (in press). The service system and its effects on families: An ecological perspective. In M. Brambring, H. Rauh, & A. Beelman (Eds.), *Early childhood intervention: Theory, evaluation and practice.* Berlin: de Gruyter.

Beckman, P.J., & Boyes, G.B. (1993). *Deciphering the system: A guide for families of young children with disabilities.* Cambridge, MA: Brookline Books.

Beckman, P.J., Boyes, G.B., & Herres, A. (1993). The IEP and IFSP meetings. In P.J. Beckman & G.B. Boyes (Eds.), *Deciphering the system: A guide for families of young children with disabilities* (pp. 81–100). Cambridge, MA: Brookline Books.

Beckman, P.J., & Bristol, M.M. (1991). Issues in developing the IFSP: A framework for establishing family outcomes. *Topics in Early Childhood Special Education, 11*(3), 19–31.

Beckman, P.J., Frank, N., Newcomb, S., & Brown, L. (in press). Developing relationships with families. In P.J. Beckman (Ed.), *Strategies for working with families of young children with disabilities.* Baltimore: Paul H. Brookes Publishing Co.

Beckman, P.J., Newcomb, S., Frank, N., Brown, L., & Filer, J. (1993). Providing support to families of infants with disabilities. *Journal of Early Intervention, 17*(4), 445–454.

Beckman, P.J., Robinson, C.C., Rosenberg, S., & Filer, J. (1994). Family involvement in early intervention: The evolution of family-centered services. In L.J. Johnson, R.J. Gallagher, M.J. La Montagne, J.B. Jordan, J.J. Gallagher, P.L. Hutinger, & M.B. Karnes (Eds.), *Meeting early intervention challenges for children and their families: Providing services from birth to three* (pp. 13–31). Baltimore: Paul H. Brookes Publishing Co.

Beckman-Bell, P. (1981). Child-related stress in families with handicapped children. *Topics in Early Childhood Special Education, 1*(3), 45–54.

Brinkerhoff, J.L., & Vincent, L. (1986). Increasing parental decision-making at the individualized education program meeting. *Journal of the Division for Early Childhood, 11*(1), 46–58.

Bronfenbrenner, U. (1979). *The ecology of human development: Experiments by nature and design.* Cambridge, MA: Harvard University Press.

Chan, J.M., & Leff, P.T. (1994). Educating students in providing humanistic care: The significant contribution of the health care professional. *The ACCH Advocate, 1*(2), 37–45.

Chan, S. (1990). Early intervention with culturally diverse families of infants and toddlers with disabilities. *Infants and Young Children, 3*(2), 78–87.

Coulter, M.L., Wallace, T., & Laude, M. (1993). Early intervention services in selected Florida counties: The provider perspective. *Children's Health Care, 22*(2), 125–141.

Dunst, C.J., Johanson, C., Trivette, C.M., & Hamby, D. (1991). Family oriented early intervention policies and practices: Family-centered or not? *Exceptional Children, 58*(2), 115–126.

Dyson, L., & Fewell, R.F. (1986). Stress and adaptation in parents of young handicapped and nonhandicapped children: A corporative study. *Journal of the Division for Early Childhood, 10*, 28–35.

Edelman, L. (1991). *Delivering family-centered home-based services.* [Videotape and Facilitator's Guide]. Baltimore: Project Copernicus.

Edelman, L., Greenland, B., & Mills, B.C. (1992). *Building parent/professional collaboration.* [Videotape and Facilitator's Guide]. St. Paul, MN: Pathfinder Resources.

Eggbeer, L., Fenichel, E., Pawl, J.H., Shanok, R.S., & Williamson, G.G. (1994). Training the trainers: Innovative strategies for teaching relationship concepts and skills to infant/family professionals. *Infants and Young Children, 7*(2), 53–61.

Fenichel, E. (1991). Learning through supervision and mentorship to support the development of infants, toddlers, and their families. *Zero to Three, 12*(2), 1–26.

Frey, K.S., Greenberg, M.T., & Fewell, R.F. (1989). Stress and coping among parents of handicapped children: A multidimensional approach. *American Journal of Mental Retardation, 94*(3), 240–249.

Gill, K.M. (1993). Health professionals' attitudes toward parent participation in hospitalized children's care. *Children's Health Care, 22*(4), 257–271.

Gilliam, J.E., & Coleman, M.C. (1981). Who influences IEP committee decisions. *Exceptional Children, 47,* 642–644.

Gowen, J.W., Johnson-Martin, N., Goldman, B.D., & Appelbaum, M. (1989). Feelings of depression and parenting competence of mothers of handicapped and nonhandicapped infants: A longitudinal study. *American Journal of Mental Retardation, 94*(3), 259–271.

Greig, D.L. (1993). *Extremely low birthweight infants (800 grams or less): Medical and developmental outcome at one to five years and social support needs of their mothers.* Unpublished doctoral dissertation, University of Maryland, College Park.

Hanson, M.J. (1987). *Teaching the infant with Down syndrome: A guide for parents and professionals.* Austin, TX: PRO-ED.

Hanson, M.J., & Harris, S.L. (1986). *Teaching the young child with motor delays.* Austin, TX: PRO-ED.

Harry, B. (1992). Developing cultural self-awareness: The first step in values clarification for early interventionists. *Topics in Early Intervention, 12*(3), 333–350.

Hutchins, D.E., & Cole, C.G. (1992). *Helping relationships and strategies.* Pacific Grove, CA: Brooks/Cole Publishing Company.

Individuals with Disabilities Education Act (IDEA) of 1990, PL 101-476. (October 30, 1990). Title 20, U.S.C. 1400 et seq: *U.S. Statutes at Large, 104*(Part 2), 1103–1151.

Johnson, B.H., Jeppson, E.S., & Redburn, L. (1992). *Caring for children and families: Guidelines for hospitals.* Bethesda, MD: Association for the Care of Children's Health.

Kalmanson, B., & Seligman, S. (1992). Family–provider relationships: The basis of all interventions. *Infants and Young Children, 4*(4), 46–52.

Kazak, A.E., & Marvin, R.S. (1984). Differences, difficulties, and adaptation: Stress and social networks in families with a handicapped child. *Family Relations, 33,* 67–77.

Knowles, M.S. (1984). *The adult learner.* Houston, TX: Gulf.

Lash, M., & Wertlieb, D. (1993). A model for family-centered service coordination for children who are disabled by traumatic injuries. *The ACCH Advocate, 1*(1), 19–41.

Leff, P.T., Chan, J.M., & Walizer, E.M. (1991). Self-understanding and reaching out to sick children and their families: An ongoing professional challenge. *Children's Health Care, 20*(4), 230–239.

Leviton, A., Mueller, M., & Kaufmann, C. (1992). The family-centered consultation model: Practical implications for professionals. *Infants and Young Children, 4*(3), 1–8.

Lipsky, D.K. (1985). A parental perspective on stress and coping. *American Journal of Orthopsychiatry, 55*(4), 614–617.

Lynch, E.W., & Hanson, M.J. (Eds.). (1992). *Developing cross-cultural competence: A guide for working with young children and their families.* Baltimore: Paul H. Brookes Publishing Co.

Lynch, E.W., & Stein, R.C. (1987). Parent participation by ethnicity: A comparison of hispanic, black, and anglo families. *Exceptional Children, 54*(2), 105–111.

Mahoney, G., O'Sullivan, P.S., & Fors, S. (1989). The family practices of service providers for young handicapped children. *Infant Mental Health Journal, 10*(2), 75–83.

McBride, S.L., Brotherson, M.J., Joanning, H., Whiddon, D., & Demmitt, H. (1993). Implementation of family-centered services: Perceptions of families and professionals. *Journal of Early Intervention, 17*(4), 414–430.

McGonigel, M.J., & Garland, C.W. (1988). The individualized family service plan and the early intervention team: Team and family issues and recommended practices. *Infants and Young Children, 1*(1), 10–21.

McGonigel, M.J., Kaufmann, R.K., & Johnson, B.H. (1991). *Guidelines and recommendations for the individualized service plan.* Bethesda, MD: Association for the Care of Children's Health.

McWilliam, P.J., & Bailey, D.B. (Eds.). (1993). *Working together with children and families: Case studies in early intervention.* Baltimore: Paul H. Brookes Publishing Co.

Minke, K.M., & Scott, M.M. (1993). The development of individualized family service plans: Roles for parents and staff. *The Journal of Special Education, 27*(1), 82–106.

Minuchin, S. (1974). *Families and family therapy.* Cambridge, MA: Harvard University Press.

Moss, B., & Wightman, B. (1993). From the use of skills to use of self: Professional development through training to enhance relationships. *Zero to Three, 14*(1), 1–8.

Petr, C.G., & Barney, C.G. (1993). Reasonable efforts for children with disabilities: The parents' perspective. *Social Work, 38*(3), 247–254.

Raver, S.A., & Kilgo, J. (1991). Effective family-centered services: Supporting family choices and rights. *Infant Toddler Intervention, 1*(3), 169–176.

Sameroff, A., & Chandler, M.J. (1975). Reproductive risk and the continuum of caretaking casuality. In F.D. Horowitz (Ed.), *Review of child development research* (Vol. 4, pp. 189–244). Chicago: University of Chicago Press.

Segal, M.M. (1985). *An interview study with mothers of handicapped children to identify both positive and negative experiences that influence their ability to cope.* Paper presented at the Fourth Annual Conference of the National Center for Clinical Infant Programs, Washington, DC.

Seligman, M., & Darling, R.B. (1989). Professional–family interaction: Working toward partnership. *Ordinary families, special children* (pp. 214–244). New York: Guilford Press.

Shapiro, J., & Simonsen, D. (1994). Educational/support group for Latino families of children with Down syndrome. *Mental Retardation, 32*(6), 403–415.

Shelton, T.L., & Stepanek, J.S. (1994). *Family-centered care for children needing specialized health and developmental services* (3rd ed.). Bethesda, MD: Association for the Care of Children's Health.

Shulman, L. (1978). A study of practice skill. *Social Work, 23,* 274–281.

Shulman, L. (1992). *The skills of helping: Individuals, families and groups.* Itasca, IL: F.E. Peacock.

Shulman, L. (1993). Developing and testing a practice theory: An interactional perspective. *Social Work, 38*(1), 91–97.

Sokoly, M.M., & Dokecki, P.R. (1992). Ethical perspectives on family-centered early intervention. *Infants and Young Children, 4*(4), 23–32.

Souffer, R.M. (1982). IEP decisions in which parents desire greater participation. *Education and Training of the Mentally Retarded, 17*(2), 67–70.

Stagg, V., & Catron, T. (1986). Networks of social supports for parents of handicapped children. In R.R. Fewell & P.F. Vadasy (Eds.), *Families of handicapped children: Needs and supports across the life span* (pp. 279–296). Austin, TX: PRO-ED.

Stepanek, J.S. (in press). *Moving beyond the medical/technical: Analysis and discussion of psychosocial practices in pediatric hospitals.* Bethesda, MD: Association for the Care of Children's Health.

Summers, J.A., Dell'Oliver, C., Turnbull, A.P., Benson, H.A., Santelli, M.C., Campbell, M., & Siegel-Causey, E. (1990). Examining the individualized family service plan process: What are family and practitioner preferences? *Topics in Early Childhood Special Education, 10*(1), 78–99.

Taylor, N.E., & Valli, L. (1992). Refining the meaning of reflection in education through program evaluation. *Teacher Education Quarterly, 19*(2), 33–47.

Thomas, R. (1990). A foundation for clinical family assessment. *Children's Health Care, 19,* 244–250.

Turnbull, A., Summers, J., & Brotherson, M. (1986). Family life cycle. In A. Turnbull & H.R. Turnbull (Eds.), *Families, professionals and exceptionality: A special partnership* (pp. 85–112). Columbus, OH: Charles E. Merrill.

Turnbull, A.P., & Turnbull, H.R. (1990). *Families, professionals, and exceptionality: A special partnership* (2nd ed.). New York: Macmillan.

Valli, L. (1992). *Reflective teacher education: Cases and critiques.* New York: SUNY Press.

Widrick, G., Whaley, C., DiVenire, N., Vecchione, E., Swartz, D., & Stiffler, D. (1991). The medical education project: An example of collaboration between parents and professionals. *Children's Health Care, 20*(2), 93–100.

Zeichner, K.M., & Liston, D.P. (1987). Teaching student teachers to reflect. *Harvard Educational Review, 57*(1), 23–48.

Zeitlin, S., & Williamson, G.G. (1988). Developing family resources for adaptive coping. *Journal of the Division for Early Childhood, 12*(2), 137–146.

Zipper, I.N., Weil, M., & Rounds, K. (1993). *Service coordination for early intervention: Parents and professionals.* Cambridge, MA: Brookline Books.

15

A SYSTEMS APPROACH

Pamela J. Winton, Camille Catlett, and Alison Houck

Ann, a speech-language pathologist, received a telephone call from Pat, a parent of a 4-year-old boy with disabilities. Pat called to express her dissatisfaction with a report Ann wrote that summarized a lengthy language assessment that Ann conducted with Andrew, Pat's son. Pat complained that the report could not be understood and did not provide any helpful information about what could be done to help Andrew. Ann responded by offering to try to explain the report. Pat was uninterested, stating that she knew there were better ways to conduct an assessment, and she hoped that Ann could find some ways to improve her practices with children and families.

Ann, who is very hardworking, was upset by the angry telephone call. On one hand, she was upset because of the anger and hostility she felt from Pat, which she felt was not justified. On the other hand, she had been reading and hearing about new approaches to child assessment that sounded similar to what Pat was requesting. Ann had just received a flyer from the state Part H early intervention agency about an upcoming workshop entitled "A Family-Centered Approach to Child Assessment." She decided to call the Part H coordinator and ask for more information. She had some doubts about the value of the workshop, based on past experiences in which workshops on early intervention topics that sounded interesting on paper turned out to be abstract, theoretical presentations that provided absolutely no practical information she could use. But she needed to update her credentials, and if the workshop offered continuing education units (CEUs) from her professional organization, then it was worth exploring.

Hal, the Part H coordinator, responded as best as he could to Ann's telephone call and her questions about the workshop. Hal tried to assure Ann that the information would be practical, but when he said that the presenter would likely be a faculty member from the state university, Ann had her doubts. Hal said he was "working on" the CEUs and hoped to have the paperwork in place. The telephone call did not convince Ann that the workshop would help her implement the kind of assessment that Pat wanted for her child.

Meanwhile, Hal called Fay, the university faculty member who was supposed to plan and implement the workshop. Unfortunately, the state contract to support the workshop had been delayed for political reasons, which meant that Hal was having to play "catch up" to get arrangements made. When Hal and Fay had first talked about the workshop, they had identified a number of dates that had come and gone while they waited for the contract. Now that a

The authors wish to thank Janet Bagby, who assisted with qualitative data analysis, and Ann Vaughn, who assisted with manuscript preparation.

date had been set, Fay was trying to back out because of other commitments and pressures. Her tenure and promotion review process was in full swing, and the pressures to publish articles and conduct research were strong. The telephone conversation between Fay and Hal was tense, as Hal tried to convince Fay that she was the best person in the state to conduct the workshop. Fay felt that the timing was bad in terms of her priorities, and she honestly expressed her concern that she would not be able to answer questions that the providers who attended the workshop might have about state regulations and reimbursement procedures that affected the way that they conducted assessments. She felt that the last workshop she gave for Hal had not met the expectations of the participants, simply because she was not able to deal with many of the practical questions; Fay felt she needed someone to co-present with her who was in touch with both state and community perspectives. She also had talked with Hal on previous occasions about her interest in trying to conduct a small evaluation study within the context of some of the state training efforts. On both fronts, Fay found Hal sympathetic and interested at a personal level; however, the demands of his job and the resources he had at his disposal made the research and additional support for the workshops difficult, if not impossible, to obtain. Fay and Hal had been colleagues for a long time and had respect for each other's opinions and good intentions; however, the pressures on both were great as they tried to resolve how to proceed with the workshop.

In the end, Fay agreed to conduct the workshop, and Hal agreed to send one of his support staff to assist with questions. Ann decided to attend the workshop and received her CEUs. From a certain point of view, the workshop was a success. Hal provided statewide training to a large number of providers on an important topic. The providers received credits that meant they were more "competent" to serve children and families. Fay fulfilled an obligation to a colleague and provided a more practical workshop while learning more about the state system as a result of support from Hal's office. However, what about Pat and her son Andrew? What are the chances that Pat will see changes in Ann's assessment procedures and report writing as a result of the energy, money, and effort expended on everyone's part? That is a question that lingers.

ONE OF THE GREATEST CHALLENGES facing states as they work to implement Part H of PL 101-476, the Individuals with Disabilities Education Act (IDEA) of 1990, is ensuring that there is an adequately trained cadre of professionals able to provide quality services to young children from birth to age 3 and their families (Harbin, Gallagher, & Batista, 1992). Because of the Part H emphasis on new content areas and service delivery approaches not typically covered in professional training programs (Bailey, Simeonsson, Yoder, & Huntington, 1990), states are under tremendous pressure to develop strategies for delivering up-to-date and relevant training to large numbers of people across a number of disciplines at both the inservice and preservice levels. An analysis of the states' progress toward implementing Part H suggests that personnel development is one of the areas in which the least amount of progress has been made (Harbin, Gallagher, & Lillie, 1991). One logical explanation for the slow progress is the lack of skilled trainers organized and ready to respond to the training challenges inherent in the early intervention legislation. The new roles being defined for professionals require rethinking traditional disciplinary boundaries, re-creating service delivery systems, and reconceptualizing family–professional partnerships (Shonkoff & Meisels, 1990). Likewise, training must be reconceptualized to reflect the changing relationships among disciplines, agencies, and families. This suggests that trainers should not only have expertise in newly identified content areas and training strategies, but also have expertise in facilitating change. University programs and various state agencies (e.g., physical and mental health, social services, human resources, education) need help in making these transitions.

Higher education faculty are a potential resource for addressing the early intervention personnel shortages and training needs (Bruder, Klosowski, & Daguio, 1989; Gallagher, 1989). Case study research conducted by the Carolina Policy Studies Program indicated that one of the keys to the states' successes in meeting the personnel preparation challenges is the existence of linkages between university and state agency efforts (Rooney, Gallagher, Fullagar, Eckland, & Huntington, 1992). However, linking faculty and state agency personnel is only a piece of the picture. A key to successful personnel preparation is bridging the traditional "tower–trench" gap; that is, ensuring that those in the "trenches" (families and providers who are caring for and educating young children with disabilities) are provided with the support, education, and information they need by those in the "towers" (university faculty and state agency officials who are entrusted with training dollars and responsibilities). Likewise, those in the "towers" need help from the "trenches" to ensure that the training and information they provide is grounded in real-world problems and solutions. Both of these groups have their own unique set of challenges and perspectives that must be taken into account in order to ensure progress in preparing quality personnel to implement early intervention legislation in the states. Attempts to address personnel preparation without taking a holistic approach are likely to result in ineffective and partial solutions.

The existing literature has yet to identify the barriers and facilitators of "tower–trench" linkages. What factors facilitate and strengthen those linkages and what factors create barriers? Specifically, what kinds of supports and resources do interdisciplinary groups of faculty identify as being important in terms of their effective participation in providing quality early intervention training? And furthermore, what is most likely to maintain their participation?

The purpose of this chapter is threefold: 1) to describe the components of a model for supporting university faculty in their personnel development roles through a holistic, systems-change approach designed to bridge the "tower–trench" gap; 2) to describe what has been learned from this model regarding the progress of states and individuals in implementing effective personnel preparation; and 3) to make recommendations for future directions based on findings from implementing this model.

THE SOUTHEASTERN INSTITUTE FOR FACULTY TRAINING MODEL

The Southeastern Institute for Faculty Training (SIFT) is one of four regional faculty training institutes funded by the U.S. Department of Education, Early Education Program for Children with Disabilities, from 1992 to 1995. These four regional institutes were funded for the purpose of providing support and training to university faculty in order to facilitate faculty involvement in providing early intervention in-service training within their states. SIFT worked with 15 southeastern states and jurisdictions in three cohorts of 5 states at a time. *Cohort 1* states were Arkansas, Louisiana, North Carolina, South Carolina, and Tennessee. *Cohort 2* states were Florida, Kentucky, Mississippi, the jurisdiction of

Puerto Rico, and West Virginia. *Cohort 3* states were Alabama, the District of Columbia, Georgia, Virginia, and the jurisdiction of the Virgin Islands. SIFT approached this mission from a systems-change perspective, based on the knowledge that making a meaningful and long-lasting impact on personnel preparation efforts would require attention to all aspects of the complex early intervention system. The goals of the project were to 1) facilitate personnel preparation linkages among families, professionals from different disciplines, state agencies, and institutions of higher education; 2) increase higher education faculty members' knowledge and skills related to early intervention content and instructional strategies; and 3) assist faculty in applying what they learned through their participation in the SIFT project to the training they provide others. The SIFT implementation plan is outlined in Figure 1.

Data from 300 university faculty, families, providers, and state early intervention leaders representing nine southeastern states and the jurisdiction gathered through multimethod strategies (needs assessment measures, follow-up surveys, and interviews) provide the basis for the information presented in this chapter. These 300 individuals participated in the SIFT project as either members of state leadership groups or state faculty teams from the nine states and the jurisdiction that comprised Cohorts 1 and 2. In some instances, data reported are from only Cohort 1 participants, rather than combined Cohorts 1 and 2 because Cohort 1 is the only cohort for which 6-month follow-up data have been analyzed. This qualification is noted in the text.

CRITICAL COMPONENTS OF THE SYSTEMS-CHANGE MODEL

In implementing the SIFT model, certain components of the implementation plan were critical to promote change. Figure 2 shows these critical components.

Support and Vision of State Leaders

A major goal of the SIFT project was to support and extend existing state efforts, which was in keeping with the assumption that creating long-lasting change requires maximizing the fit among new information, existing priorities, and available resources. One of the first SIFT activities was to secure support for the SIFT project from the Part H agency and the director of the university affiliated program (UAP) in each of the SIFT states. Part H and UAP representatives were asked to identify a group of important early intervention leaders in their states with power, resources, and expertise related to early intervention personnel preparation who would serve as a state leadership training team (SLTT) to assist with the SIFT effort in each of their states. They were also asked to ensure family representation and cultural diversity in this group.

The Identified State Leaders in Early Intervention Personnel Preparation

Table 1 provides summary data on the characteristics of the people invited by the Part H and UAP representatives to serve as SLTT members. The number of people identified as state leaders ranged by state from 7 to 41 with a mean number of 17 per state. Among these participants, the number of years experience in personnel preparation ranged from none to 47 with a mean of 12 years.

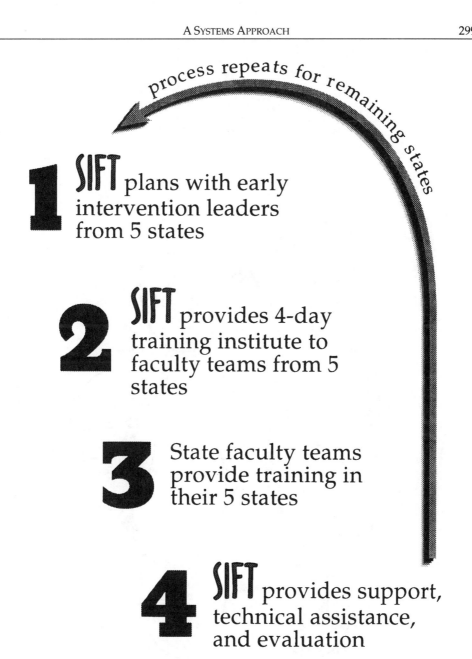

process repeats for remaining states

1 **SIFT** plans with early intervention leaders from 5 states

2 **SIFT** provides 4-day training institute to faculty teams from 5 states

3 State faculty teams provide training in their 5 states

4 **SIFT** provides support, technical assistance, and evaluation

Figure 1. An outline of the Southeastern Institute for Faculty Training (SIFT) implementation plan.

Status and Future Directions

The SLTT group in each state was convened for a 1- to 2-day meeting held in a central location in the state. The purpose of this meeting was to share information about personnel preparation and develop a vision or plan for where their state could focus future state efforts. To prepare the leaders for their participation in this meeting, a questionnaire entitled *Surveying the Personnel Preparation Landscape* was developed by the SIFT project and mailed to each participant in advance. The questions concerned personnel preparation issues of coordina-

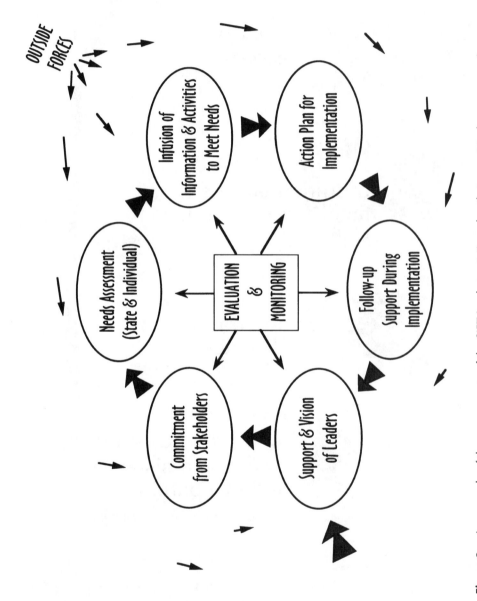

Figure 2. An example of the components of the SIFT implementation plan that are critical to promote change.

Table 1. State leadership training team characteristics

Characteristic	Percent
Ethnicity	
European American	90.5
African American	4.2
Latino/Hispanic	4.2
Native American	1.2
Parent of a child with a disability	17.0
Responsible for disbursement of training dollars	46.0
Primary work setting	
University	33.9
State agency	31.5
Community agency	14.3
University affiliated program	8.9
Community college	1.8
Other	9.5

Note: N = 169.

tion, collaboration, preservice and in-service linkages, family involvement, certification, and planning. These questions were based on the literature on recommended in-service practices and research on effective early intervention personnel preparation conducted through two previous research institutes (Winton, 1994).

Certain themes and priorities across states emerged from data collected and perspectives shared in the SLTT meetings. One theme was the need for more collaboration. Evidence for this statement comes from two sources: data from the *Surveying the Personnel Preparation Landscape* questionnaire and leaders' comments and priorities for future direction. One question asked on the measure was, "Does your state have a comprehensive system of personnel development (CSPD)?" A CSPD is a required component of each state's application for Part H dollars; therefore, each state participating in Part H presumably has a written plan. The federal intent in requiring the CSPD plan is to encourage a comprehensive, coordinated approach to training. One would expect that if the plan were indeed a blueprint for planning early intervention training, most early intervention leaders in personnel preparation would know of its existence. Figure 3 is a bar graph of the responses of the nine different states and the jurisdiction in Cohorts 1 and 2 to the above-mentioned question. Figure 3 shows that 1) there is considerable variation across the nine states and the jurisdiction in terms of the leaders' familiarity with CSPD, and 2) there were leaders in every state who had never heard of the CSPD. Anecdotal evidence supported the questionnaire data; collaboration across agencies and institutions regarding comprehensive planning for personnel preparation was rare.

Table 2 provides a summary of the leaders' responses (medians and quartiles) to the other questions on the measure. The responses to these questions suggest that every state has room for improvement in all areas addressed through the survey. Anecdotal information provides more detail about the leaders' concerns related to quality and collaboration in personnel preparation. What leaders describe as happening in many states is "parallel play"; each agency funds and im-

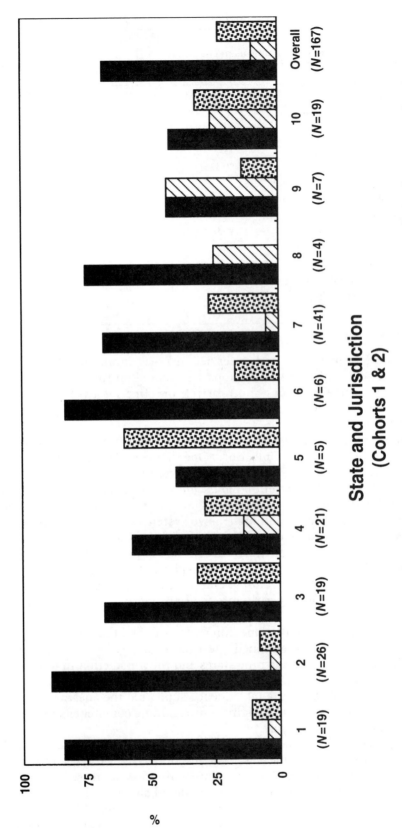

Figure 3. Responses of early intervention leaders in personnel preparation to the question, "Does your state (jurisdiction) have a comprehensive system of personnel development (CSPD)?" (■ = yes; ▨ = no; ▨ = don't know)

Table 2. Median responses of state leaders to *Surveying the Personnel Preparation Landscape* questionnaire

Question	Cohort 1 Pre-Institute[a]	Cohort 1 Postinstitute[a]	p value
Extent comprehensive system of personnel development used to plan and implement early intervention in state	3 (2, 4)	3 (2, 4)	
Extent in-service training efforts coordinated	3 (3, 3)	3 (3, 4)	
Extent in-service training efforts planned and implemented collaboratively	3 (3, 3)	3 (2, 4)	
Extent representatives of higher education involved in planning and implementing early intervention in-service training	3 (2, 3)	3 (2, 4)	
Extent higher education does adequate job providing preservice training in early intervention	2 (2, 3)	3 (2, 3)	.001[b]
Extent professional organizations involved in planning, implementing, and participating in personnel preparation efforts	3 (2, 3)	3 (2, 3)	
Extent families involved in planning, implementing, and evaluating personnel preparation activities	3 (2, 3)	3 (3, 4)	
Extent in-service and preservice training efforts linked	2 (2, 3)	3 (2, 4)	.005[b]
Extent preservice training opportunities tied to infant, toddler, and preschool certification and credentialing	3 (1, 4)	3 (2, 4)	
Extent in-service training opportunities tied to infant, toddler, and preschool certification and credentialing	3 (1, 4)	3 (2, 4)	
Extent family-centered philosophy infused into preservice training efforts	3 (2.5, 4)	3 (2, 4)	
Extent family-centered philosophy infused into in-service training efforts	3 (3, 4)	4 (3, 4)	
Extent preservice training activities planned by representatives from across disciplines and implemented with interdisciplinary audiences	3 (2, 3)	3 (2, 4)	
Extent in-service training activities planned by representatives from across disciplines and implemented with interdisciplinary audiences	3 (3, 4)	3 (3, 4)	

Note: Scale 0–5 (0 = no idea; 1 = never; 2 = seldom; 3 = sometimes; 4 = usually; 5 = always).
[a]Median (25th, 75th); $n = 61$.
[b]Wilcoxen test for paired data.

plements its own separate training initiatives. Comments made by leaders suggest that separate training initiatives are the result of many factors. For example, leaders commented, "There are too many players. The quantity of trainings and training providers makes it difficult to coordinate and collaborate," "Agencies are not seeing eye to eye," and "There is no central point or place from where you can obtain information [about early intervention personnel preparation]." The end result is that teachers are being trained through one initiative, allied health professionals through another, nurses through still another, and so forth.

This approach is unlikely to create the interdisciplinary, interagency systems of services intended by PL 99-457, the Education of the Handicapped Act Amendments of 1986 (which has been reauthorized as PL 102-119, the Individuals with Disabilities Education Act Amendments of 1991). Collaboration through the sharing of money and resources was rare. Agencies felt obligated and responsible to serve their constituent groups; relinquishing that responsibility and the money to support efforts of another agency was described as being difficult and risky. Leaders referred to this lack of collaboration between agencies as "guarding," "territoriality," and "turfism." Leaders indicated that quality was often sacrificed because of the demands for training large numbers of individuals through statewide or regional workshops.

As part of the SLTT meeting, participants were asked to prioritize a direction in which they believed personnel preparation activities in their states needed to go. Although the specifics varied from state to state, the need for collaboration and the need for the development and implementation of effective training models were themes that emerged across states in terms of future efforts. In one state, there was a strong desire to implement collaborative training efforts across three state agencies—the Part H lead agency, the department of education, and the department of health—in an attempt to build teamwork among teachers, home-based providers, and allied health personnel. In another state, the desire was to replicate a successful training model that involved families, direct services providers, and university faculty as community-based training teams whose purpose was to assist local programs in becoming more family centered. In yet another state, there was a desire to coordinate personnel preparation planning and implementation activities by engaging faculty from different disciplines and regions in the state to participate in the inactive CSPD subcommittee of the interagency coordinating council (ICC). In another state, the desire was to coordinate in-service and preservice efforts between the two major universities.

Data from the *Surveying the Personnel Preparation Landscape* questionnaire and from the priorities identified through the SLTT meeting have indicated that collaboration and effective training practices are important issues that need attention. In every state this priority was reflected in the process used to select faculty team members. State leaders believed it was imperative to have interdisciplinary and interagency representation. The issues of effective training practices and collaboration were addressed through subsequent activities that were part of the SIFT model; the evaluation data, from the authors of this chapter, as described in a later section of this chapter, suggest that more work needs to be done.

Commitment from and Support to Stakeholders

It has been the observation of the authors of this chapter that early intervention personnel preparation has not been a priority issue in many states; there have been too many other pressing concerns related to Part H planning and implementation. However, in almost every state there has been one individual or a small group of individuals who have been committed on a statewide basis to personnel preparation, including state agency staff and higher education faculty, who have been actively involved on a personnel preparation or CSPD subcommittee of the ICC or through a higher education consortium. The enthusiasm and commitment of these individuals have played a critical role in each state's ability to take advantage of the opportunity that a project like SIFT might bring to a state. These people were often selected to be on the state faculty team, and they often played a critical role in keeping the momentum going in terms of accomplishing plans made at the faculty training institute.

An integral part of SIFT was a 4-day, intensive training institute provided for each cohort in which faculty teams from each of the five states in a cohort would have the opportunity to plan and learn about innovative strategies for teaching early intervention content. The SIFT project asked the SLTT in each state to select 12–15 individuals from their state to make up the state faculty team that would participate in the 4 days of training. In making their selections, they were asked to choose faculty who were the "cream of the crop," that is, those faculty in whom they entrusted the important job of providing in-service training to providers. In addition, SIFT required that the faculty teams represent multiple disciplines, cultural diversity, family members, Part H agencies, and the UAP. States identified additional criteria to match their visions and plans for future personnel preparation efforts, such as geographic representation or links with existing initiatives. SIFT defined "faculty" in an inclusive fashion. Practica supervisors and adjunct instructors were included on teams to ensure inclusion of the perspectives of direct services providers. In addition, SIFT encouraged states to include important state agency personnel or any other individual viewed as critical to a statewide training effort by the SLTT. In all states there are some individuals who were members of both the SLTT and the state faculty team.

Table 3 provides summary data on the characteristics of the state faculty teams in Cohorts 1 and 2. The 128 participants in Cohorts 1 and 2 represented 16 different disciplines with a mean of 12.8 years of service delivery experience and 9.9 years of personnel preparation experience. Although the majority of the participants came from academic settings, significant numbers were drawn from state and community agencies. Approximately 20% of the participants were family members with children with disabilities, and 24.6% of the participants were from ethnic groups other than European American.

Once faculty were identified in states in Cohort 1, two questions surfaced for SIFT staff: 1) Would it be possible to entice faculty to participate? and 2) Would support for their participation and travel be forthcoming from their higher education institutions? Involvement in in-service training is not usually a priority for faculty; research, publication, and preservice teaching are their primary responsibilities. As it happened, faculty were eager to participate. Competition for places on the state faculty teams was so great in some states that in the second cohort, additional team slots (three) were provided to states who were willing to underwrite the total cost for the extra faculty members' participation. In some states, the leadership groups would select only faculty team members who were willing to commit a certain number of days to in-service training. As part of the SIFT evaluation process, state faculty team members were asked how many days they would be willing to commit to in-service training. On average, faculty team members were willing to commit to 15.8 days a year. This represented a commitment to be involved in in-service training that surpassed expectations. There was also strong support of administrators for faculty participation. Only 8 of the 128 participants did not receive institutional support from within their states for their travel to the 4-day faculty training institute.

Table 3. Characteristics of state faculty teams

Characteristic	Percent
Ethnicity	
European American	75.4
African American	11.9
Latino/Hispanic	11.1
Native American	1.6
Parent of a child with a disability	20.0
Primary work setting	
University	49.6
State agency	22.8
University affiliated program	8.9
Community agency	7.3
Community college	2.4
Other	8.9
If university affiliated program,	
type of faculty appointment	
Tenure track	36.1
Tenured	21.7
Clinical or adjunct	15.7
Practicum supervisor	3.6
Other	22.9

Note: N = 128.

Responsiveness of SIFT Project to State and Individual Needs

A major goal for the SIFT staff was to ensure that the 4-day, intensive faculty training included what states and individual state team members believed would enhance their ability to deliver quality personnel preparation. As mentioned previously, state priorities were identified through data gathered in conjunction with the SLTT meeting in each state. Individual needs assessment data were collected from each faculty team member before the training.

How SIFT Could Help

The needs assessment measure focused on how the faculty training institute could enhance faculty members' effectiveness as trainers. Faculty were asked to indicate their priorities in terms of which of the 10 early intervention content areas (those that are emphasized in Part H) they wanted covered in the 4-day faculty training institute. These 10 content areas are as follows: family-centered practice, individualized family service plan (IFSP), IDEA, inclusion and/or integration, service coordination, cultural diversity, interdisciplinary training, interagency collaboration, assessment and/or evaluation, and transitions. The three content areas chosen most frequently were 1) IFSP development with families, 2) inclusion, and 3) IDEA (laws and regulations). These choices may not represent a one-to-one correlation with the content areas in which faculty perceived themselves to be least competent, but likely are a reflection of current or future areas in which faculty are expected to train others. Faculty also were asked to prioritize which of seven training strategies they wanted to be covered in the

4-day faculty training. The training strategies from which they chose are as follows: principles of adult learning, self-assessment procedures, families as co-teachers, cross-disciplinary co-teaching, case method of instruction, team training, and interactive techniques. The following areas received the highest ratings: 1) team training (strategies for training entire teams), 2) families as co-teachers, and 3) cross-disciplinary co-teaching. These choices seem to indicate that faculty share the interest and desire for collaboration expressed by the leaders in their state.

Participants were asked to rank, using a 1–5 scale with 5 being "high priority," a list of resources that would assist them in conducting in-service training in early intervention in their states. Table 4 contains the response choices and mean ratings. The three highest priority items were 1) having access to training resources (e.g., curricula, videotapes), 2) having access to other faculty doing early intervention training, and 3) interest from the Part H agency. It is interesting to note that reimbursement for time and travel received the lowest priority, evidence of the commitment participants had made to in-service training as part of their involvement in the SIFT project.

Another question asked participants to rank training materials according to their potential usefulness. Table 5 provides a list of the response choices and the mean rating for each on a 1–5 scale, with 5 being "extremely helpful." The resources that were perceived as being the most useful were 1) a packaged curriculum including all of the elements in the list, 2) videotapes, and 3) interactive and experiential training activities.

The 4-day faculty training institutes for Cohorts 1 and 2 were planned on the basis of the needs assessment. The focus of the individual sessions was on demonstrating and modeling a variety of training strategies and innovative materials rather than simply providing content in a didactic, traditional style. Providing faculty with time to preview innovative, interdisciplinary, family-centered training materials through an on-site collection was another strategy used to meet the need for access to materials. Time was devoted to state planning to encourage interdisciplinary and interagency collaboration and networking related to state-specific personnel issues.

Table 4. Mean rating of resource priority in conducting in-service training

Resource	Mean	SD
Access to training resources	4.59	.67
Access to other faculty and programs doing early intervention training	4.24	.87
A show of interest from Part H system	4.22	1.11
Faculty members with whom to co-teach	4.13	.89
Family members with whom to co-teach	4.13	.98
Commitment from institution to support in-service training activities	4.07	1.30
Further training in a variety of training processes and models	4.01	1.09
Reimbursement for travel	3.86	1.30
Reimbursement for time	3.34	1.43

Note: Scale 1–5 (1 = not helpful; 5 = extremely helpful);   N = 125.

Table 5. Mean rating of resources to assist faculty in training efforts

Resource	Mean	SD
Packaged curriculum containing items listed	4.62	.71
Videotapes	4.48	.75
Interactive and experiential training activities	4.36	.82
Overhead transparencies	4.30	.79
Case studies	4.22	.99
Discussion questions	4.16	.86
Evaluation measures	4.13	.90
Lecture outlines	3.87	1.11

Note: Scale 1–5 (1 = not helpful; 5 = extremely helpful); *N* = 125.

Development and Implementation of Action Plans

One of the assumptions underlying the SIFT project was that for change to occur attention must be paid during the faculty training institute to the application of new ideas to the workplace. To that end, each state faculty team and each individual participant was asked to develop a "back home" plan that would clearly delineate how they would embed what they had learned through SIFT into personnel preparation activities in their state. As part of the SIFT evaluation process, follow-up data were collected 6 months after the 4-day faculty training institute to assess progress and satisfaction related to the goals. An analysis of the types of goals and the extent to which they were accomplished provides some interesting and provocative information about the change process.

Developing State Plans

In Cohort 1, the SIFT staff made the assumption that each state team would arrive at the 4-day faculty training institute with some knowledge of how and why members had been selected. Familiarity with the vision for personnel preparation that had been developed by the SLTT who selected the team members was also expected. One of the lessons learned from Cohort 1 was that clear communication between the SLTT and the state faculty teams prior to the 4-day institute did not necessarily occur. Therefore, in Cohorts 2 and 3 it was strongly suggested to the SLTT that faculty be convened prior to the training institute to discuss these issues. This communication was deemed critically important for teams to be able to develop during the training institute state plans that were consistent with the leaders' priorities and that could be supported by state resources. When the process worked well, the state vision, the faculty selection process, and the state and individual plans developed during the training were consistent and reflected a shared knowledge and values base related to early intervention personnel preparation. As expected, the state plans varied considerably from state to state in focus and specificity.

Implementing State Plans

Follow-up visits with the combined faculty and SLTT groups in each state were conducted 6 months after the training institute. Using a Likert-type scale, participants were asked to rate the extent to which progress had been made on each objective identified as part of the state plan. Results indicated that progress was made on all objectives; however, no state achieved all of its objectives.

Barriers and Facilitators

A variety of roadblocks interrupted state plans. Roadblocks included changes in key leadership positions and unexpected administrative red tape at the state agency level. For example, in three of the five Cohort 1 states, there was turnover in the Part H coordinator position during the states' involvement with SIFT. Another barrier identified across all states related to the amount of time and effort required to implement the state plans. Because most members of the state faculty teams were serving as volunteers without pay when they agreed to commit to a state plan, often no one was available to serve as the catalyst for maintaining the momentum when setbacks occurred. Having someone with the ultimate responsibility for implementation is critical. Ironically, one of the central features of interagency and interinstitution efforts—shared responsibility and leadership—can serve as an inherent barrier if no one is assigned ultimate responsibility to implement interagency plans.

Facilitators of progress toward shared goals were also identified during the follow-up visits. State team members most commonly identified each other as the strongest facilitator, noting that "person-to-person links make the difference and account for systems change."

Another observation that continues to be validated is that 6 months is a short time period in which to implement a state plan. It has been more than a year since the Cohort 1 faculty training institute was held. Most state teams in that cohort continue to meet and report back to SIFT on progress that continues to be made related to their plans.

Developing Individual Plans

As expected, there was considerable variability in the focus and number of selected objectives in individual plans that faculty developed (with a range of 2–8). Some individual objectives were directly linked to the broader state plan; therefore, completion was dependent more or less on the state team's success at implementing plans. Other objectives could be completed by the individual, such as trying out an activity demonstrated by SIFT in a university course. Many of the objectives involved collaboration with other faculty members, such as co-teaching a course or working in collaboration on a grant.

The individual objectives were analyzed according to whether the focus was preservice or in-service training or whether they had a dual focus (i.e., addressed both preservice and in-service training). The largest percentage of the objectives had a dual focus (43.7%). Examples might be inviting a university colleague to join the state CSPD subcommittee of the ICC or using some of the interactive activities demonstrated at SIFT in both preservice and in-service training. The focus of 34.4% of the objectives was in-service training (e.g., collaborating with a colleague to plan and offer a workshop). The focus of 21.9% of the objectives was on preservice training (e.g., inviting a family member to present to students in a course, writing a preservice grant with a colleague).

Implementing Individual Goals

As part of the SIFT evaluation plan, follow-up telephone interviews were conducted with each participant 6 months after the faculty training institute to determine the amount of progress and the extent to which they were satisfied with the progress made in reaching their individual goals. To collect the data, the objectives the participants had developed at the faculty training institute were read to them over the telephone by a research assistant, and the participants were asked to rate progress and satisfaction for each objective on a 1–5 Likert-type scale.

Participants reported moderate progress and satisfaction with their accomplishments. Participants indicated higher mean levels of progress (3.62 versus 3.37) and satisfaction (3.68 versus 3.45) on preservice training as opposed to in-service training goals. This difference was statistically significant ($p < .01$). A possible explanation for these differences could be that the in-service training goals were more likely to be linked with the overall state plan, which had an in-service focus because of the nature of the grant that funded the SIFT project. This meant that the in-service training objectives were more likely to be dependent on the accomplishment of a larger, more complicated plan.

Barriers and Facilitators

One of the questions asked of participants during the 6-month follow-up interview was to describe the barriers and facilitators to accomplishing their objectives. A content analysis of this information was conducted using techniques described by Miles and Huberman (1994). Four broad categories related to the barriers and facilitators were identified: 1) individual related, 2) trainee related, 3) organization and/or institution related, and 4) SIFT related. Within those broad categories, subcategories were identified. All comments were coded into the subcategories by three coders. Consistent patterns of barriers and facilitators were noted by all three coders.

The barriers and facilitators related to in-service training goals and dual (in-service and preservice training) focus goals were similar. The most frequently mentioned barrier was time. Individuals reported that when they got back into their job settings they simply did not have the time to pursue some of the goals that they had set for themselves; frequently other job-related priorities interfered. The following three major facilitators were mentioned: 1) support and interest of colleagues; 2) existing grants, structures, or initiatives that supported their goals; and 3) the follow-up support and technical assistance from SIFT. SIFT provided technical assistance to states for 6 months following the 4-day faculty training institute, which included two on-site state meetings and long-distance support that took a variety of forms. Technical assistance most often provided included 1) support for grant-writing efforts, 2) brainstorming with faculty teams or individuals related to training events or state planning, 3) sharing new materials, and 4) linking states and individuals for problem solving. This information provides further evidence of the importance of colleagues in keeping the momentum going, of linking projects like SIFT with existing initiatives, and of follow-up support in a training project.

The most frequently mentioned barrier to attaining preservice training goals was the resistance to change encountered in the higher education institutions. Problems mentioned in this regard included crammed curricula, which makes it hard to insert new materials or coursework, and lack of control over how money is spent and allocated. For instance, faculty who wanted to hire parent consultants were frustrated by the lack of money to pay parents. Although institutional resistance to change was mentioned to some degree as an in-service barrier, it was not mentioned with as much frequency. An interesting preservice and in-service training difference was related to trainee interest and receptivity. This was described as a facilitator in regard to preservice goals being accomplished, with comments such as, "Students are so eager for this information. It is motivating to continue to try these ideas." Trainee interest and receptivity were more likely to be mentioned as a barrier than a facilitator to accomplishing in-service goals with comments such as, "Professionals are resistant to making changes; new ideas are threatening."

EVALUATION

As indicated in Figure 2, evaluation and monitoring occurred during each component of the SIFT project. The data reported address the following three questions related to the goals of the SIFT project:

1. Did the SIFT model facilitate linkages between institutions of higher education and their state agencies?
2. Did the SIFT model increase faculty self-efficacy related to early intervention content and training strategies?
3. Did the SIFT model assist faculty in applying knowledge and skills in the training they conduct in their states?

Did the SIFT Model Facilitate Linkages?

Approximately 450 qualified and competent individuals representing a diversity of disciplines, agencies, roles, and backgrounds were brought together through SIFT in structured activities related to personnel preparation. Measures of satisfaction indicated that these activities were perceived to be useful for the participants in Cohorts 1, 2, and 3. The continued involvement of individuals with SIFT over time has suggested that participants perceived value in these activities.

During the follow-up telephone interview, 78% of the Cohort 1 participants indicated that SIFT had provided them with access to new faculty. Another question asked during this interview was, "What has been the major impact that SIFT has had on you?" The open-ended responses to this question were analyzed using techniques suggested by Johnson and LaMontagne (1993) and Miles and Huberman (1994). Table 6 provides a description of the categories and subcategories that were identified and the percentages of statements assigned to each category. The greatest number of responses (51.8%) was in the category of networking. As Table 6 indicates, the largest number of new relationships are with other faculty. Given that this was a priority on the needs assessment, it appears that the SIFT model met this need and that linkages were made on the individual level.

A question of importance is whether the SIFT model improved linkages at the systems level. The questionnaire *Surveying the Personnel Preparation Land-*

Table 6. The major impact of SIFT

Category	Percentage
Networking total	51.8
With faculty	[23.5]
With state agencies, institutions, organizations	[12.9]
With SIFT	[8.2]
With other states	[4.7]
With families	[2.3]
Training strategies	20.0
Training materials	14.1
Training content	8.2
Addressed "big picture"	8.2
Felt supported and validated	4.7
Motivation	2.3
No impact	2.3
No response	2.3

Note: Number of statements coded = 85; percentage of relevant statements coded into each category and subcategory.

scape, which was administered to SLTT members at the beginning of their states' involvement in the project (pre-institute), was administered again by mail 6 months after the state faculty team participated in the 4-day faculty training institute (postinstitute). A comparison of pre- and postresponses (medians, quartiles, and significance levels) on this measure for the Cohort 1 leaders who responded at both data collection points is shown in Table 2. These data suggest that positive change occurred in two areas; leaders were more likely to perceive that institutions of higher education are doing an adequate job of providing preservice training in their state ($p < .001$), and leaders were more likely to perceive that preservice and in-service efforts are linked in their state ($p < .005$). Providing higher education faculty and agency personnel with the opportunity to share, learn, and problem-solve together seemed to create *at least* the perception of positive change. The fact that there were no other significant differences on this measure validates the idea that changing systems is difficult.

Did the SIFT Model Increase Participants' Self-Efficacy?

One of the variables identified in the literature as being associated with the implementation of innovative practices is self-efficacy (Stein & Wang, 1988). Self-efficacy, as defined by Bandura (1977), is a broad concept related to a sense of overall mastery of behavior and coping skills. Bandura maintained that people make judgments about their ability to perform a behavior or task and that people select tasks or activities that they believe they are capable of handling. According to Bandura (1993), those who have a strong belief in their self-efficacy will find ways of exercising control to accomplish goals even in the face of obstacles and constraints.

Self-efficacy was measured in two ways: self-ratings of knowledge and skill related to early intervention content and training strategies and a willingness to provide early intervention training. Faculty were asked to rate their current levels of knowledge and skill in two areas: 1) early intervention content, and 2) training strategies for conveying the content at two points in time—prior to participation in the faculty training (pre-institute) and 6 months after participation (postinstitute). As shown in Tables 7 and 8, a statistical analysis of the comparison indicates that faculty self-ratings improved in all areas.

A statistical analysis also was conducted to compare self-ratings of competence in the 10 knowledge and skill content areas (see Table 7) with self-ratings of competence in the seven training strategies (see Table 8). The results indicated that faculty were more confident of their content knowledge and skill than they were of their training strategies. This difference was statistically significant pre-institute ($p < .0001$) and postinstitute ($p < .01$). These findings supported the importance of focusing on training strategies in faculty training institutes.

The other way that changes in self-efficacy were measured was by asking participants to rate on a 1–5 scale their willingness to provide training at three levels (preservice, in-service, and technical assistance). At the end of the 4-day faculty training institute they were asked to rate their willingness before the training institute and their willingness after the training institute. There were significant differences in their ratings at all three levels ($p < .0001$), and their willingness to conduct early intervention training increased as a result of participation. These findings indicated that the SIFT model was successful at increasing the self-efficacy of participants.

Did the SIFT Model Have Application to the Workplace?

No matter how satisfied, confident, and enthusiastic participants may be, the true test of effectiveness depends on how much existing programs and structures are changed. This evaluation question addressed three areas: faculty participa-

Table 7. Cohort 1 faculty self-ratings of knowledge and skill in 10 content areas—Pre- and postinstitute

Content area	Cohort 1 pre-institute[a]	Cohort 1 postinstitute[b]	p value
Family-centered practice	4 (3, 4.5)	5 (4, 5)	.0001[c]
Individualized family service plan	3 (3, 4)	4 (4, 5)	.0001[c]
IDEA	3 (2, 4)	4 (4, 5)	.0001[c]
Inclusion and integration	4 (3, 4)	4 (4, 5)	.0001[c]
Service coordination	4 (3, 4)	4 (4, 5)	.0001[c]
Cultural diversity	3.5 (3, 4)	4 (3, 5)	.0001[c]
Interdisciplinary teaming	4 (4, 5)	5 (4, 5)	.0045[c]
Interagency collaboration	4 (3, 4)	4 (3.5, 5)	.0097[c]
Assessment and evaluation	4 (4, 5)	5 (4, 5)	.0019[c]
Transitions	3 (3, 4)	4 (3, 5)	.0001[c]

Note: Scale 1–5 (1 = low; 5 = high).
[a]Median (25th, 75th); $N = 57$.
[b]Median (25th, 75th); $N = 44$.
[c]Wilcoxen test for paired data.

Table 8. Cohort 1 faculty self-ratings of knowledge and skill in seven training strategies—Pre- and postinstitute

Training approach	Cohort 1 pre-institute[a]	Cohort 1 postinstitute[b]	p value
Principles of adult learning	3 (2, 4)	4 (3, 5)	.0001[c]
Self-assessment procedures	3 (2, 3.5)	4 (3, 4)	.0001[c]
Families as co-teachers	3 (3, 4)	4 (3.5, 5)	.0001[c]
Cross-disciplinary co-teaching	3 (2.5, 4)	4 (3, 5)	.0001[c]
Case method of instruction	3 (2, 4)	4 (3.5, 5)	.0001[c]
Team training	3 (2, 4)	4 (3, 5)	.0001[c]
Interactive techniques	3 (2, 4)	4 (3.5, 4)	.0001[c]

Note: Scale 1–5 (1 = low; 5 = high).
[a]Median (25th, 75th); N = 57.
[b]Median (25th, 75th); N = 44.

tion in conducting in-service training, faculty success at embedding effective practices into in-service training, and the overall impact of the program.

Did SIFT Participants Increase Their Involvement in Local and State Early Intervention In-Service Training?

Although there is anecdotal evidence that participants who had not been previously involved in in-service training became involved as a result of SIFT, these differences in involvement were not supported by statistical evidence. At the 6-month follow-up data collection point, participants were asked to estimate the number of days they had provided in-service training in their state during the last 6 months using a 1–5 scale with 1 = none, 2 = 1 day, 3 = 2–5 days, 4 = 6–10 days, and 5 = 11 days or more. The median response was 3 on the scale, signifying 2–5 days of training. They had been asked this same question prior to their participation in SIFT, using the same response format. There were no significant differences. In other words, despite their increased self-confidence and willingness, more involvement in providing in-service training did not occur at a level that was statistically significant. It should be noted that participants may have been involved in planning and other related activities; the question focused on actual delivery of training. Follow-up interview data suggested that some participants were waiting to be asked to conduct in-service training activities but the invitation never came from state or community agencies. Other participants were still involved in the planning process, which was taking longer than they anticipated. One explanation for this delay is the bureaucratic red tape encountered in some states related to trying to finance some of the state plans and the time it took to get some of the training efforts organized. State agency personnel sometimes encountered difficulties in engaging faculty because of their busy schedules. The phrase "use it or lose it" might be applicable here. If too much time expired before participants were provided an opportunity to use their in-service plans and ideas, momentum seemed to be lost. This outcome reinforces the importance of setting manageable and achievable goals, experiencing success, and building relationships for further activities. It might also mean that the availability of faculty willing to conduct in-service training needs to be widely advertised to state and community agencies and those with training money.

Did SIFT Participants Improve the Quality of In-Service Training They Provided to Others?

Another strategy for examining the application of ideas received in training was a pre- and postinstitute assessment of questions related to the "quality indicators." The quality indicators are listed as a checklist in Figure 4; they are based on the literature related to recommended in-service practices and effective early intervention personnel preparation (Winton, 1994) and represent a summary of the policies and practices that SIFT hoped to promote. Participants were asked at the end of the 4-day faculty training institute (after they had some exposure to how these quality indicators were being defined) to estimate on a 1–5 scale the extent to which the training they had conducted during the last 6 months reflected each quality indicator with 1 being never and 5 being always. They were asked the same question 6 months later.

Table 9 provides a summary of Cohort 1 pre- and postinstitute responses (medians, quartiles, and significance levels). Significant differences were found on only two items: item 11 (extent experiential activities and modeling and/or demonstration opportunities were provided as part of the training) and item 15 (extent of impact the training had on practices). An examination of the items on the quality indicator checklist reveals that they can be placed into two groups: those over which participants had some degree of control (items 11–16) and those over which they had little control (items 1–10). The Cronbach alpha statistic, which describes the internal consistency of the responses to these items, was .75 for both groups indicating good consistency. Interviews with participants revealed the difficulty they had in creating the kinds of changes suggested by items

---

Is the training you are planning coordinated with your state's CSPD [comprehensive system of personnel development] plan?

Will you ensure that certification or licensure credits are available to all trainees who participate?

In planning and conducting this training, will you work as part of an interdisciplinary instructor team?

Will family members of children with disabilities (consumers of services) participate as part of the instructor's team?

In terms of the target audience, will efforts be made to conduct team-based training [including as many of the key professionals who work together on a team as possible]?

Will efforts be made to attract an interdisciplinary audience [at least three or more disciplines are well represented]?

Will family members be involved as participants?

Will the training be actively endorsed and/or attended by administrators?

Will experiential activities and modeling/demonstration opportunities be provided as part of the training?

Will handouts be provided [for review of content by trainees at a later time]?

Will training strategies be varied and sequenced in such a way as to meet the needs of different learning styles?

Will training strategies be used for embedding/applying the training ideas to the workplace?

Will trainees identify specific ideas/practices that they desire to try in the workplace [an action plan]?

Will ongoing support, monitoring, or technical assistance be provided to trainees?

Will the actual impact of training on practices be measured or evaluated?

Figure 4. Checklist of quality indicators related to early intervention in-service training. (Reprinted with permission from Early Childhood Report (ECR). Copyright 1994 by LRP Publications, 747 Dresher Road, P.O. Office Box 980, Horsham, PA 19044-0980. All rights reserved. For more information on other products published by LRP Publications, please call 1-800-341-7874, ext. 281.)

Table 9. Extent to which training conducted by Cohort 1 participants reflected quality indicators

Items	Pre-institute[c]	6-month follow-up[d]	p value
"No control" items[a, b]			
1. Extent training coordinated with state comprehensive system of personnel development	1.5 (0, 2.5)	2 (1, 3)	
2. Extent certification or licensure credits available to trainees	2 (0, 4)	2 (0, 3)	
3. Extent worked as an interdisciplinary instructor team	2 (0, 3)	2 (1, 3)	
4. Extent family members of children with disabilities participated in training	2 (0, 3)	1.5 (0, 2)	
5. Extent training was team based	2 (1, 3)	2 (1, 3)	
6. Extent the audience was interdisciplinary	3 (2, 3)	3 (2, 4)	
7. Extent family members involved as participants	2 (1, 3)	3 (1, 3)	
8. Extent the training was actively endorsed by administrators	4 (3, 4)	4 (3, 4)	
9. Extent the training was attended by administrators	2 (1, 2)	2 (2, 3)	
10. Extent ongoing support or technical assistance was provided to trainees	2 (1, 3)	2 (1, 3)	
"Control" items[e]			
11. Extent experiential activities and modeling and/or demonstration opportunities provided as part of training	2 (2, 3)	3 (2, 4)	.007[f]
12. Extent training strategies used for embedding or applying the training ideas to the workplace	3 (2, 3.5)	3 (2.5, 4)	
13. Extent training strategies varied and sequenced to meet different learning styles	3 (2, 3)	3 (3, 4)	
14. Extent trainees identified specific ideas and practices to try in the workplace	2 (1, 3)	2 (2, 3)	
15. Extent actual impact of training on practices was measured or evaluated	2 (1, 3)	2.5 (1, 4)	.01[f]
16. Extent handouts and written materials provided to participants	4 (4, 4)	4 (4, 4)	

Note: Scale 0–4 (0 = never; 4 = always); N = 34; Cronbach's alpha = .75.
[a]Items over which participants had little control or power to change.
[b]Performed at 6-month follow-up.
[c]Median (25th, 75th); N = 57.
[d]Median (25th, 75th); N = 44.
[e]Items over which participants were more likely to have control.
[f]Wilcoxen text for paired data.

1–10 on the checklist. Participants stated that they were often not "in charge" of in-service training and could not determine who came, how it was planned, and how it was linked with CSPD, certification, and follow-up technical assistance. The fact that participants were more likely to include experiential activities and evaluation in training they conducted postinstitute as compared to pre-institute suggests that the faculty training institute, with its emphasis on interactive training strategies and evaluation strategies, was successful in changing practices in these two areas.

Did SIFT Participants Actively Use the Resources of SIFT Beyond the 4-Day Faculty Training Institute, and Did They Perceive SIFT as Having a Lasting Impact?

In the follow-up interviews with Cohort 1, 83% of the participants said they had used materials discovered at SIFT, and 74% had used SIFT as a resource. At the 6-month state follow-up meetings, 96.7% of those in attendance indicated that SIFT had made a difference in their state, and 96.7% thought their participation with the SIFT project contributed to their knowledge of personnel preparation activities in their states. This quote from one participant illustrates the kinds of changes described by some faculty:

> Since my participation in the SIFT training, I have truly re-created my training approach. In addition, I am systematically reworking the courses I teach at the preservice level to more readily represent what I have learned through SIFT. My course evaluations have always been strong, but this semester's were "off the chart." The techniques and activities modeled by the SIFT faculty, the ready-to-use materials, the annotations and exposure to training resources saved me countless hours of preparation time.

CONCLUDING REMARKS: FUTURE DIRECTIONS

SIFT clearly made an impact at the individual level. The members of the state faculty teams experienced significant increases in their knowledge and skill related to early intervention content and training strategies. They developed new collaborative relationships, used new materials and resources that they found through SIFT, and accomplished individual and collective goals related to embedding new ideas into the training they conducted. They made some progress toward improving the quality of the in-service training they provided to others.

The impact SIFT made related to changing early intervention systems is not as clear or evident at this point. Data have indicated that changes at these levels are difficult and take longer than the 6-month follow-up evaluation period. The difficulties in making changes in systems described by SIFT participants are similar to research reported in the business literature. Making changes at an organizational level has been described as extraordinarily difficult and taking at least 3–5 years to accomplish (Kanter, Stein, & Jick, 1992). The fact that collaborative relationships across agencies and institutions were being promoted, thus changing several organizations, contributed to the complexity and difficulty of the task.

In spite of these difficulties, it is evident that in some states there are positive changes in the way some personnel preparation activities are now being funded, planned, and implemented that are the result of the states' participation in the SIFT project. The following examples are representative of some of these changes:

- One state, in which the SIFT team included Part H representatives, a Part B representative, and the ICC chair, has worked with the other team members to design statewide training on transitions. Part H and Part B have provided funding for the training. SIFT team members have identified key stakeholders within communities, provided training and resources to them, and supported their development of local transition policies and plans that are also consistent with state policies. SIFT team members will also provide follow-up technical assistance.
- Three members of one SIFT team (a physical therapist, a psychologist, and a speech-language pathologist) coordinated a statewide project to provide training about assistive technology for very young children with disabilities that featured strong parent–professional collaboration. They invited family members to participate and asked them to invite professionals who they thought could also benefit from the training. The result was a diverse audience learning together to design and implement collaborative goals. This approach to statewide training is continuing to be pursued at the state level.
- In one state, a community college faculty member and a 4-year university faculty member have crafted articulation agreements that will foster the transition of students from community college programs (2 year) into Part H discipline-specific training programs (4 year). This state is working to promote similar articulation agreements as a strategy for addressing personnel shortages.

What is apparent is that every state has a great deal of work left to be done. What follows are recommendations based on observations and findings from the SIFT project.

- Faculty are willing to commit time to in-service training and are eager for support that will improve their effectiveness as trainers. Higher education administrators are supportive of opportunities for faculty to develop skills. Investing in faculty training is a critical component to states' progress in personnel preparation.
- Making changes that move state systems toward effective practices and collaboration among agencies, disciplines, and levels of service delivery related to personnel preparation is a slow and time-consuming process. Ongoing support, monitoring, and evaluation are necessary components to projects whose goals are related to systems change.
- The financial resources that have been directed at personnel preparation have been limited; a larger contribution from agencies and institutions is needed if quality is to be improved.
- In many states there is a core group of individuals who are committed to improving the quality of personnel preparation, often as volunteers on ICC subcommittees. These individuals are often faculty at institutions of higher education. Supporting and sustaining these human resources and ensuring that state agency leaders are part of these efforts are critical to future progress.
- Personal relationships are an important element in these changes being made. Relationships among personnel at all levels (state, community, universities, consumers) seem to sustain "bottom-up" and "top-down" efforts. Structuring opportunities for these individuals to develop the solutions to the personnel preparation challenges that will work in their states should be part of the state and federal early intervention agenda.

• Developing new relationships between higher education faculty and state agencies takes time and trust. Outside initiatives, like SIFT, can help with initial contacts but cannot guarantee that linkages will be sustained.

Each state has its story. The SIFT project has had the privilege of being invited to become a minor character in the story for a very short time for the purpose of supporting the other characters and contributing positively to change. These stories will continue, and staff of projects similar to SIFT that follow should remember that the solutions to personnel preparation challenges lie within, not outside, state systems. The challenge is identifying, supporting, and enhancing the resources and strengths; providing additional resources; and serving as a catalyst for helping states move toward future goals.

REFERENCES

Bailey, D.B., Simeonsson, R.J., Yoder, D.E., & Huntington, G.S. (1990). Preparing professionals to serve infants and toddlers with handicaps and their families: An integrative analysis across eight disciplines. *Exceptional Children, 57*(1), 26–35.

Bandura, A. (1977). Self-efficacy: Toward a unifying theory of behavioral change. *Psychological Review, 84*(2), 191–215.

Bandura, A. (1993). Perceived self-efficacy in cognitive development and functioning. *Educational Psychologist, 28*(2), 117–148.

Bruder, M., Klosowski, S., & Daguio, C. (1989). *Personnel standards for ten disciplines servicing children under P.L. 99-457: Results from a national survey.* Farmington: Division of Early Childhood and Family Studies, Department of Pediatrics, University of Connecticut Health Center.

Education of the Handicapped Act Amendments of 1986, PL 99-457. (October 8, 1986). Title 20, U.S.C. 1400 et seq: *U.S. Statutes at Large, 100,* 1145–1177.

Gallagher, J. (1989). *Planning for personnel preparation: Policy alert (P.L. 99-457, Part H).* Chapel Hill: Carolina Policy Studies Program, Frank Porter Graham Child Development Center, University of North Carolina at Chapel Hill.

Harbin, G.L., Gallagher, J., & Batista, L. (1992). *Status of states' progress in implementing Part H of IDEA: Report #4.* Chapel Hill: Carolina Policy Studies Program, Frank Porter Graham Child Development Center, University of North Carolina at Chapel Hill

Harbin, G.L., Gallagher, J., & Lillie, T. (1991). *Status of states' progress in implementing Part H of IDEA: Report #3.* Chapel Hill: Carolina Policy Studies Program, Frank Porter Graham Child Development Center, University of North Carolina at Chapel Hill.

Individuals with Disabilities Education Act (IDEA) of 1990, PL 101-476. (October 30, 1990). Title 20, U.S.C. 1400 et seq: *U.S. Statutes at Large, 104*(Part 2), 1103–1151.

Individuals with Disabilities Education Act Amendments of 1991, PL 102-119. (October 7, 1991). Title 20, U.S.C. 1400 et seq: *U.S. Statutes at Large, 105,* 587–608.

Johnson, L., & LaMontagne, M. (1993). Using content analysis to examine the verbal or written communication of stakeholders within early intervention. *Journal of Early Intervention, 17*(1), 73–79.

Kanter, R.M., Stein, B.A., & Jick, T.D. (1992). *The challenge of organizational change: How companies experience it and leaders guide it.* New York: Free Press.

Miles, M., & Huberman, A. (1994). *Qualitative data analysis* (2nd ed.). Beverly Hills: Sage Publications.

Rooney, R., Gallagher, J., Fullagar, P., Eckland, J., & Huntington, G. (1992). *Higher education and state agency cooperation for Part H personnel preparation.* Chapel Hill: Carolina Policy Studies Program, Frank Porter Graham Child Development Center, University of North Carolina at Chapel Hill.

Shonkoff, J.P., & Meisels, S.J. (1990). Early childhood intervention: The evolution of a concept. In S.J. Meisels & J.P. Shonkoff (Eds.), *Handbook of early childhood intervention* (pp. 3–31). Cambridge, MA: Cambridge University Press.

Stein, M.K., & Wang, M.C. (1988). Teacher development and school improvement: The process of teacher change. *Teaching and Teacher Education, 4*(2), 171–187.

Winton, P. (1994). Early intervention personnel preparation: The past guides the future. *Early Childhood Report, 5*(5), 4–6.

16

BUILDING A COLLABORATIVE TEAM

Elizabeth Straka
and Diane Bricker

Guided by the literature and professional experiences, I began to assist teams in developing a transdisciplinary approach to assessment and intervention for young children with disabilities and their families. I recall the excitement of having the opportunity to assist teams who were committed to the concept of transdisciplinary teamwork. Although I approached the transdisciplinary training with enthusiasm, I found myself experiencing uneasiness as I prepared training agendas. My agendas reflected a straightforward step-by-step process, yet I knew that the training process needed to be more interactive than linear.

It was important that my training assist teams in developing transdisciplinary assessment and intervention efforts. However, it was equally important to teach teams that the ongoing process (rather than the final product) was the key to successful transdisciplinary efforts. I recall a team telling me that it attempted a transdisciplinary arena assessment and was frustrated because it was unsuccessful. After this same team participated in team-building and communication activities, explored its service delivery system, and participated in ongoing training to expand its knowledge and expertise across disciplinary boundaries, it began to experience success with the transdisciplinary approach. The training helped team members realize that their initial failure with transdisciplinary efforts was a result of not participating in an ongoing process to prepare for and support teaming efforts. The ongoing process that the team participated in allowed team members to 1) develop an equal and open relationship through trust and communication, 2) incorporate a problem-solving attitude, and 3) develop team competencies that lead to successful teaming efforts.

The transdisciplinary approach to assessment and intervention services for young children with disabilities and their families involves a cooperative venture among early intervention professionals. Research has shared the complex challenges of transdisciplinary practices. Ongoing training and staff development have been cited as integral factors in addressing the challenges of transdisciplinary team efforts. My commitment and enthusiasm regarding transdisciplinary services persists as team members and families who engage in the ongoing process of transdisciplinary teaming share how they are able to work closely with each other and recognize that obtaining multiple perspectives is critical in fully understanding and meeting the diverse needs of children with disabilities.

Support for writing this chapter came in part from Grant #H029D40067 from the U.S. Office of Special Education Programs to the Center on Human Development and from Grant #HQ29Q3007 from the U.S. Office of Special Education Programs to the University Affiliated Program of Georgia, University of Georgia.

The authors would like to thank Kristie Frontczak for her critical reading and constructive feedback on an earlier draft of this chapter.

The author of this case scenario is Elizabeth Straka.

THE PRECEDING CHAPTERS HAVE PRESENTED a variety of information considered essential in the training and preparation of personnel who provide services to young children who are at risk and/or have disabilities and their families. A review of these chapters reveals attitudes, shared principles, and competencies that, although articulated differently across disciplines, are essential to the development of effective and efficient team collaboration. The information presented in this chapter is designed to help professionals begin the process of exploring beliefs, principles, and competencies that will lead to effective collaborative team practices.

Before moving forward in the discussion of how to build collaborative teams, it may be useful to define what is meant by *collaboration*. In a general sense, collaboration means people working together to achieve a greater efficiency; however, in this chapter, and throughout this book, collaboration has added meaning when applied to early intervention teams. In this chapter, collaboration has three essential elements: 1) a commitment to developing and using a common goal that guides and directs the team's activities, 2) an agreed-upon process that is respectful of each member's contribution, and 3) an outcome that is coordinated and integrated in order to produce more effective and satisfactory outcomes.

Because collaborative teams are different from traditional multidisciplinary teams, they require different procedures. Effective collaboration among team members requires professionals to understand their specific areas of expertise as well as integrate their knowledge and skills with those of other professionals and caregivers. Employing and coordinating an array of strategies that are thought to lead to effective team collaboration is a significant challenge. As more professionals acknowledge the value of collaborative team efforts, the need for guiding principles, specific competencies, effective strategies, and useful examples becomes evident.

This chapter offers suggestions and practical strategies to assist professionals and teams in moving toward effective team collaboration. Specifically, the goal is to synthesize the information addressing effective team practice presented in previous chapters and to offer guidelines for the application of this information. To address this goal, the authors discuss 1) an environment that fosters collaborative practices, 2) a set of principles that underlies effective team collaboration, 3) global team competencies, 4) two case studies that compare a traditional and a collaborative team approach, and 5) one case study emphasizing a collaborative team approach for assessment and intervention purposes. The first two case studies are presented and analyzed to examine collaborative team practices or team competencies that were or were not used. The first case study describes traditional assessment procedures used to determine the eligibility of a child for early intervention services and a multidisciplinary team process to develop an individualized family service plan (IFSP) or an individualized education program (IEP). The second case study describes an intervention program developed for a young child with disabilities. The final case study presents collaborative team efforts while assessing and intervening with a child with disabilities and his family.

AN ENVIRONMENT THAT FOSTERS COLLABORATION

Changing to a collaborative team model requires both the development of specific competencies and the commitment to building an environment that supports collaborative interactions among team members. An essential element of a supportive "environment" is the beliefs or attitudes that team members bring to the table (Kovarsky, 1992). Successful collaboration requires that team members believe that collaborative practices will yield more effective and satisfactory outcomes for them and the families and children they serve than employing noncollaborative practices (Fullan & Stiegelbauer, 1991; Lester & Onore, 1990). Moving from traditional to collaborative team practices will likely not endure unless the professionals involved have or develop attitudes and beliefs that support and sustain the necessary change.

PRINCIPLES THAT FOSTER COLLABORATION

Bringing positive beliefs and attitudes to the team about the need for collaboration does a great deal in setting the stage for collaborative team practices to occur; however, successful team collaboration efforts are also dependent on employing a set of principles that will ensure that collaborative team practices occur. The authors of this chapter have identified five principles that they believe are essential for effective team collaboration:

1. Having a common goal or purpose
2. Involving caregivers
3. Developing joint outcomes from assessment
4. Coordinating intervention and evaluation activities
5. Evaluating team functioning

These principles are discussed in the following sections.

Having a Common Goal or Purpose

The formal definition of teamwork is "joint action by a group of people, in which each person subordinates his individual interests and opinions to the unity and efficiency of the group" (*Webster's New Universal Unabridged Dictionary*, 1983, p. 1871). In order to fulfill this definition, it seems that agreement upon a common goal or purpose is essential. For collaborative practices to occur consistently, the group or team needs a clarifying and unifying direction that can be provided, in part, by developing a common goal or purpose. Teams that are able to agree upon and articulate their common purpose are teams that are likely to be successful in their collaborative efforts. Team collaboration is more than an integrated team effort; it is "a way of being" that is maintained by professionals who trust and respect each other and who are guided by a common purpose and philosophy (Pugach & Johnson, 1995, xii).

Involving Caregivers

Underlying the notion of collaborative teams is the principle that caregivers are active participants on the team. If given proper support and preparation (e.g., providing background information on how the team functions, conducting preassessments in the home, offering individual preparatory sessions), most caregivers want to be involved in service delivery efforts for their children. Professionals should approach parents and other caregivers with the attitude that these individuals wish to be involved with the assessment, intervention, and evaluation efforts directed to their children and families. A positive attitude toward caregivers in conjunction with offering families support and a variety of options for participation will likely result in significant success with involving caregivers as active members of the team.

Developing Joint Outcomes from Assessment

The goal of collaborative teams should be the gathering of information and the creation of written assessment reports (e.g., diagnoses, IFSPs, IEPs, evaluation) that involve joint efforts. The assessment information should be gathered and presented in an integrated fashion rather than as a series of individual observations and reports that are sequenced together. Reaching this goal will likely require the team to perform the assessment in a coordinated and integrated manner (e.g., an arena assessment). Following the assessments, the team should develop a group "sense" of the content of the report and how that content should be presented. The caregiver should, of course, participate in selecting goals and outcomes and setting priorities. Developing coordinated joint assessment outcomes will assist significantly in conducting intervention and evaluation activities that are also thoughtfully integrated.

Coordinating Intervention and Evaluation Activities

Most children who are eligible for early intervention programs have multiple service needs and many reside with families that face challenges in their day-to-day existence. It is therefore effective and efficient for teams, including family members, to develop intervention and evaluation activities designed to target a number of goals and objectives and to do so across a variety of settings. The development of documents, particularly IFSPs or IEPs with carefully chosen goals and objectives to target multiple skills or problem areas, is of great assistance in planning and executing coordinated and integrated intervention and evaluation activities. An essential principle for the functioning of collaborative teams is the need to design a set of cohesive and coordinated intervention and evaluation activities that are meaningful to children and families and that bring maximal efficiency to the professionals' efforts.

Evaluating Team Functioning

The final principle critical to the success of collaborative team efforts is the team's willingness to evaluate its performance on an ongoing basis. Without careful and ongoing evaluation of the team's progress toward its common purpose and objectives, team members cannot be sure their time and energy are being used in the most profitable manner for themselves and for the children and families with whom they work. The nature of the evaluation efforts undertaken must be tailored to the team's unique characteristics, structure, and goals; however, each team will likely want to determine how well it functions as a team (e.g., effectiveness of its communication, ability to resolve differences), how successfully it meets its stated purpose, how effectively it involves caregivers, and how efficiently it uses allocated resources. Answers to these and other challenges will be instrumental in assisting teams in using genuine collaborative practices.

TEAM COMPETENCIES THAT FOSTER COLLABORATION

After a team has created a supportive environment (e.g., members share positive attitudes about the need for collaborative efforts) and has agreed to employ the principles described above to build collaborative practices, the next step is for team members to target the development of competencies that will lead to effective collaborative practice. The development of team-building competencies is essential because discipline-specific training often addresses team-building competencies either only briefly or not at all. As many chapters in this book point out, preservice training is largely focused on assisting students to develop the knowledge and skill base that is specific to their discipline, and little information or practice is offered on how to coordinate assessment, intervention, and evaluation efforts with professionals from other disciplines. The need for developing team-building competencies is critical to instituting effective collaboration among team members.

In reviewing literature addressing team collaboration, including the chapters in this book, the authors of this chapter have identified five global team competencies that appear essential to the development of genuine collaborative practice. Figure 1 shows these five global competencies and their associated objectives. The five global competencies address the areas of communication, assessment, IFSP or IEP development, intervention, and evaluation.

Although the parent, caregiver, or other designated family member should be considered a participating member of the team, an important distinction concerning family member involvement is made in Figure 1. For the communication competency area, the caregiver is considered to be no different from other team members, and therefore the four associated objectives apply equally to caregivers and professional staff. For the remainder of the competency areas (2–5), the objectives listed are appropriate primarily for professional staff; for example, it is inappropriate to expect that caregivers will be able to match assessment purposes to measurement strategies. There may be parents who are interested in doing this and these parents should be encouraged to do so; however, it seems unwise to expect that all caregivers will have the interest or the information base to perform many of the specific competencies listed in Figure 1.

Communication

The authors believe that all competencies listed in Figure 1 are important; however, for most teams, competency 1, effective communication skills, should be

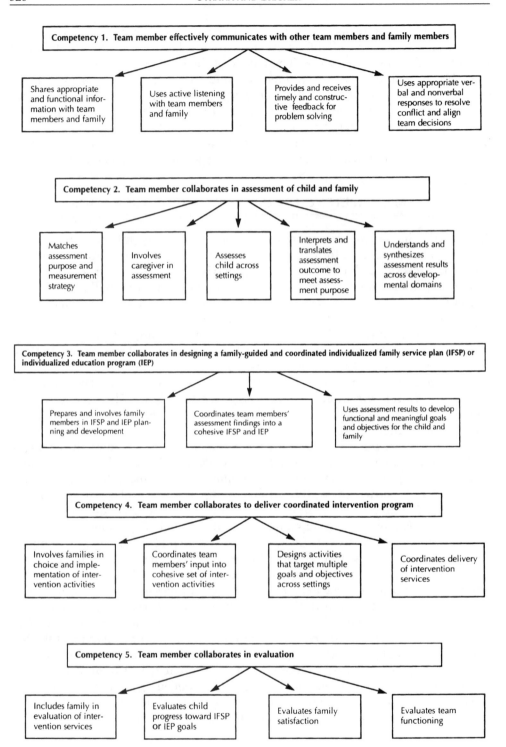

Figure 1. Five global competencies and their associated objectives that appear essential to the development of genuine collaborative practice.

addressed first and should continue to receive attention while the remaining team competencies are targeted. Effective communication skills are critical because communication is the foundation of all interactions. Effective communication allows individuals to exchange experiences and knowledge, develop trust and respect, and establish a sense of group unity and direction (Pugach & Johnson, 1995). In addition, competency 1 is pivotal because effective communication skills are needed by all team members in order to conduct collaborative discussions regarding team environment, team structure, and professional roles and responsibilities. Successfully meeting the competencies listed in the other four areas is contingent upon the development and use of effective communication skills.

Listed under the global communication competency are four specific objectives thought to enhance effective communication. These specific objectives include sharing appropriate and functional information, using active listening, providing timely and constructive feedback, and resolving conflict and aligning decisions. Clearly other skills may assist in developing and maintaining effective communication among team members, but the listed objectives are likely critical to satisfying and effective communicative exchanges.

Assessment

Competency 2, collaborating in the assessment of the child and family, addresses the initial stages and potential subsequent contact with the child and family. Group discussion regarding the purpose of the assessment and choice of an instrument will help ensure that the assessment process will yield useful and meaningful information. Specific objectives include matching the assessment purpose and measurement strategy, involving caregivers in the assessment process, assessing the child and family if appropriate across domains and across settings, translating assessment findings into functional outcomes, and synthesizing assessment findings across domains. Acquiring and using these objectives should result in collaborative efforts to administer a single or group of assessments, which reduces redundant testing and may yield information that can be more easily synthesized, interpreted, and translated into functional and coordinated outcomes.

Individualized Family Service Plan and
Individualized Education Program Development

Competency 3, collaborating to design a family-guided and coordinated IFSP or IEP, addresses the need for a collaborative plan that will guide intervention efforts. Collaborative discussion and joint decision making in developing and writing functional goals and objectives can result in a useful IFSP or IEP that guides the intervention efforts of all team members. The content of a quality IFSP or IEP provides the road map for the team to collaboratively move children from their present level of functioning to the acquisition of skills specified and prioritized by the family and other team members. Specific objectives include involving caregivers in the planning and development of the IFSP or IEP, developing functional and meaningful goals, and writing a cohesive and useful IFSP or IEP.

Intervention

Competency 4, collaborating to deliver a coordinated intervention program, involves the transfer of the functional goals and objectives into intervention activities that are appropriate and meaningful to children and families. Specific objectives again include involving family members in any way they deem appropriate, integrating service delivery elements, designing activities to target multiple goals and objectives across settings, and designing intervention activities to address targeted goals and objectives. Team members discuss the child and the child's environments and collaboratively determine when and how to embed child goals and objectives into routine, child-initiated, and planned activities. Success is dependent on the team members' abilities to discuss and coordinate their specific roles and responsibilities in the intervention process.

Evaluation

The last competency, competency 5, collaborating in the evaluation of child and family progress, focuses on determining the effect collaborative intervention efforts have on the child's IFSP or IEP goals, objectives, and family outcomes. Joint evaluations (e.g., family and professionals) should be conducted to determine the progress of the individual children and families and the generic impact of the program. At a minimum, evaluations should address family satisfaction and team functioning. The development and implementation of collaborative practices often require continual refinement as professionals practice new skills, employ principles that foster collaboration, and build an environment to support team efforts. Specific objectives include involving the caregiver in the evaluation process, coordinating evaluation efforts for children and families, and determining how effectively the team is functioning.

The competency areas and specific objectives associated with each area shown in Figure 1 represent the authors' opinions about the skills needed for successful collaboration to occur. Although available literature reinforces the choices (e.g., Pugach & Johnson, 1995), it does not provide empirical support for the selection of these or other competencies. No studies have been found that compare a team's use of collaborative skills with teams that do not have these skills, nor have any studies been found in which the skills or competencies of "collaborative" teams have been critically examined. It appears likely that for some time to come the professionals in the field will have to rely on clinical judgment to pinpoint competencies that appear to promote collaborative team practices; however, the authors of this chapter believe that individuals who acquire the competencies listed in Figure 1 will be able to successfully collaborate with parents and other professionals in designing and implementing assessment, intervention, and evaluation activities.

COLLABORATIVE PRACTICE

The remainder of this chapter is devoted to presenting three case studies of children with disabilities and their families. The first two case studies are designed to illustrate a traditional approach to assessment, IFSP development, and intervention. In the first and second case studies, an approach that does not include families as members of the team and that has professionals who collect individual assessment data and generate individual IFSPs, intervention and evaluation recommendations, and activities is described and then compared with an approach that employs collaborative practices listed in Tables 1 and 2. The last case study is designed to illustrate a team that has developed a supportive environment, applied collaborative principles, and developed the competencies described in this chapter to help the team members deliver quality assessment, intervention, and evaluation services to children with disabilities and their families.

Case Study 1: Assessment for Eligibility and Individualized Family Service Plan Development

Mr. and Mrs. Holt and their 24-month-old daughter, Jenny, have recently relocated to a new community. Jenny had been previously diagnosed with a developmental delay and was enrolled in a home-based infant program. Mr. and Mrs. Holt benefited from the home-based intervention program, as did Jenny; however, they are still concerned about Jenny's motor and communication development and they are having increasing difficulty managing Jenny's emotional outbursts.

Staff from the home-based program referred the Holts to a community-based diagnostic clinic located in their new community. The purpose for the referral was to determine if Jenny was eligible for local services and if eligible, to develop an IFSP. The clinic has an assessment team whose members include a psychologist, physical therapist, social worker, physician, and communication specialist. In general, these professionals assess and intervene independent of one another. After completing their individual assessment procedures, the team members convene to discuss their assessment results and to develop potential goals and objectives for the IFSP. Recommendations based on assessment results are written by each individual team member, combined into a report, and forwarded to families.

The Assessment Procedure

Jenny was brought to the clinic by her parents on a Monday morning and informed upon arrival of the following schedule:

8:30 A.M.–9 A.M.	*Intake with social worker.*
9 A.M.–10 A.M.	*Psychologist assesses Jenny with the Bayley Scales of Infant Development–Revised (Bayley, 1993) as the Holts watch.*
10 A.M.–10:30 A.M.	*Developmental pediatrician administers the Denver Developmental Screening Test (Frankenburg, Dodds, Fandel, Kazuk, & Cohrs, 1975) and also completes a pediatric evaluation.*
10:30 A.M.–11 A.M.	*Physical therapist conducts an informal motor evaluation.*
11 A.M.–12 P.M.	*Communication specialist administers the Sequenced Inventory of Communication Development (SICD) (Hedrick, Prather, & Tobin, 1975).*

The day began with the Holts being interviewed by the social worker. They were asked to complete a variety of paperwork prior to the 9 A.M. psychological evaluation. After the paperwork was completed, the social worker escorted the Holts to the small testing room and introduced them to Dr. Bender, the psychologist. Dr. Bender explained to the Holts that he was going to administer a standardized test to determine if Jenny was eligible for local early inter-

vention services. Before proceeding with the test, Dr. Bender obtained background informa-tion for 15 minutes. The Holts were uncomfortable because they could see that Jenny was al-ready antsy and Dr. Bender was asking them many of the same questions asked by the social worker. After interviewing the Holts, Dr. Bender picked up Jenny and placed her in a small chair in order to administer the standardized test. Jenny wiggled in the chair and tried re-peatedly to slip down to the floor. She also preferred to play with the test items according to her own interest rather than complete the tasks outlined by Dr. Bender. The Holts became anxious because they observed that Jenny was not engaging in behavior she often produced at home while playing on the floor with her familiar toys.

Dr. Bender finished his assessment at 10 A.M. and escorted the Holts to the reception area. The Holts were disappointed that Dr. Bender offered no comments on Jenny's perfor-mance. After a 10-minute wait, the secretary escorted the Holts and Jenny to the developmen-tal pediatrician's office. After answering a series of questions, many of them duplicating the social worker's and psychologist's queries, the pediatrician administered the Denver Develop-mental Screening Test to Jenny as she played on the floor. The Holts noticed that this test required Jenny to perform some of the same tasks the psychologist asked her to do earlier; however, this time Jenny was more cooperative and completed some of the tasks that she did not perform when given the Bayley Scales. The Holts mentioned this to the pediatrician and he commented that it was typical for that to occur with young children. Again, at the close of this session, the pediatrician offered the Holts no feedback on Jenny's performance.

The next meeting began about 10:30 A.M. and was with the physical therapist, Ms. Degas. Although Ms. Degas did not administer a formal test, she did ask Jenny to participate in a variety of activities. While Jenny engaged in these activities, Ms. Degas wrote a number of notes but she never asked the Holts if Jenny's responses were typical for her nor did she ask the Holts what their specific concerns were about their daughter's motor development. The Holts left this meeting again feeling unsatisfied.

The morning ended with the communication evaluation conducted from 11 A.M. to 12 P.M. By the time the Holts were introduced to the communication specialist, they wondered who was more exhausted, themselves or Jenny. Jenny would not use the few words she had and she fell asleep halfway through the session. Most of the information obtained by the com-munication specialist was through parent report. This was upsetting to the Holts because some of their major concerns with Jenny were in the area of communication. The Holts felt it was unfortunate that Jenny had fallen asleep during what they considered to be a critical assessment.

The Holts left the clinic with their sleeping daughter and the team convened that after-noon to discuss their findings. Team members reported Jenny's standard scores and dis-cussed her "weaknesses." The team agreed that Jenny was eligible for early intervention services and a referral report was developed. Given this decision, a preliminary IFSP was also developed. The social worker telephoned the Holts and conveyed the assessment findings and the team's decisions. An IFSP meeting was then scheduled at the Holts' convenience.

The Individualized Family Service Plan Meeting

The team was assembled around a table with its assessment findings and written reports when the Holts were escorted into the room by the social worker and were asked to be seated at the end of the table. The social worker opened the meeting explaining to the Holts that each professional would share his or her assessment results on Jenny and make recommendations. Each team member began by explaining his or her findings, often using technical jargon, and further discussing Jenny's problems from his or her perspective. For example, the physical therapist reported that Jenny had a moderate gross motor delay involving hypotonicity and weaknesses in her upper and lower extremities. The physical therapist recommended the following goals and objectives:

1. *Jenny will work on increasing tone.*
2. *Jenny will work on improving trunk control.*
3. *Jenny will work on pull-to-stand.*

The communication specialist's findings indicated that Jenny had a limited receptive and expressive vocabulary. Specifically, she noted that information obtained by parent report indicated that Jenny did not participate in interactive games, imitate basic motor actions or consonant–vowel combination sounds, or follow simple commands. The communication specialist recommended the following goals:

1. *Jenny will increase her spoken vocabulary by adding five nouns and five verbs.*
2. *Jenny will increase her understanding of the concepts in and on.*
3. *Jenny will use appropriate social greetings to other children and adults.*

In addition, other team members offered goals and objectives to be included on the IFSP. After the team members shared their findings and made their recommendations, the Holts were asked if they had anything to add. The Holts mentioned their concern about Jenny's tantrums; the professionals had not observed this behavior, and therefore indicated to the Holts that including this as a goal should wait until the professionals could obtain further information. In closing, the Holts were asked to sign the IFSP so Jenny could receive appropriate services as quickly as possible. The social worker gave the Holts the name and telephone number of the agency to which Jenny had been referred. The Holts were not given names of alternative placements or the opportunity to visit programs prior to placement determination.

The Analysis

An analysis of this case study is undertaken as a method for comparing a team whose members function using what is called a traditional approach with a team approach that uses collaborative practices. The traditional team is composed of a group of professionals who conduct independent assessments, arrive at disciplinary recommendations, develop separate goals and objectives for the IFSP, and create a series of unrelated intervention plans and activities. In this approach, parents tend not to be included as participating members of the team nor are the interventionists from the receiving program included. However, collaborative teams have developed an environment that supports collaboration, have adopted a set of principles that fosters cooperative efforts, and have worked to develop competencies that permit effective interactions that may result in the creation of coherent and cohesive assessment, IFSP or IEP, and intervention outcomes while making the parents feel included as partners in the process.

Table 1 presents a comparative analysis between the traditional and collaborative approaches specifically focused on team activities of assessment, caregiver participation, and IFSP or IEP development.

Table 1. Comparative analysis between traditional and collaborative approaches focused on competency areas 1, 2, and 3

Traditional team	Collaborative team
Team Activity: **ASSESSMENT** Competency 1 and Competency 2	
• The membership on the team is fixed. • The team assesses the child without consideration of individual or family characteristics or needs.	• The team composition is flexible and the individual needs of both the child and caregiver are the first priority for team members.
• The team does not collect information from the caregiver prior to the assessment and does not ask if a home visit could be made.	• The team collects pertinent information prior to the assessment and that information is shared among team members. • Assessment information can be collected in the home setting. Collecting the intake information during an initial home visit allows the caregiver and professionals to prepare for the assessment procedures. • The social worker explains the process and the caregiver is told what to expect during the assessment. • The social worker emphasizes the caregiver's role in the assessment process. • The caregiver is given an opportunity to ask questions and receive clarification prior to the assessment.
• Assessment measures used by the psychologist and pediatrician have numerous tasks that overlap.	• The social worker obtains extensive background information from the caregiver prior to the assessment. • Team members collaborate prior to the assessment to discuss and review intake information and decide which assessment measures are most appropriate to establish eligibility and intervention direction. • Team members discuss individual and team roles and responsibilities to eliminate overlap in assessment procedures. • Team members decide who will administer specific assessment items and if the assessment process will elicit the information they need and the family desires. • Team members coordinate schedules to ensure they are available to obtain relevant and useful information as another team member administers an assessment tool. For example, the communication specialist coordinates his or her schedule to obtain information at the same time the psychologist administers his or her assessment.

(continued)

Table 1. (*continued*)

Traditional team	Collaborative team
• Measurement tools (e.g., norm-referenced tools), although appropriate for determining eligibility for service, are not appropriate for developing intervention goals and objectives.	• Team members meet prior to administration of assessment to determine the purpose of the assessment process and then identify the tests that will be administered for eligibility purposes and the assessments that will be administered for programmatic purposes. Often team members can obtain assessment data by watching interactions between the child and another team member.
• Team members conduct the evaluation in isolation. No integration or coordination of the assessment process nor discussion of what each team member plans will occur.	• The team discusses and coordinates assessment tools and strategies for the child. • An arena assessment is used whenever possible because it permits the coordination of assessments across disciplines and is child and family friendly.

Team Activity:
CAREGIVER PARTICIPATION
Competency 1 and Competency 2

• The caregiver's input in terms of assessment information on the child in general and in the child's performance at home in particular is not obtained.	• The caregiver is asked for input at all stages of the assessment. • The caregiver is asked to assist in child's assessment and is expected to take an active role unless the caregiver specifically indicates that he or she does not want to participate. • Procedures and tools take into account the caregiver's values, background, and culture.
• The process is exhausting for children and parents. Thus, the validity of the results is highly questionable.	• The team coordinates schedules and consolidates assessment times to obtain quality information regarding the child's strengths and needs in the quickest and most efficient manner.
• No immediate feedback is given to the caregiver.	• Immediate feedback is given to the caregiver and he or she is given time to ask questions.

Team Activity:
IFSP DEVELOPMENT
Competency 1 and Competency 3

• The goals and objectives are developed from the results of standardized assessment tools.	• Appropriate tools (e.g., curriculum-based assessment and evaluation tools) and procedures are used to generate functional and appropriate goals and objectives.
• The caregivers are unprepared for the IFSP meeting. • The caregivers are not told what to expect or what will transpire during the meeting nor are they told what their role will be.	• The caregivers are adequately prepared before the IFSP meeting in terms of their role and their contributions.

(*continued*)

Table 1.   (*continued*)

Traditional team	Collaborative team
• Team members use jargon when presenting their reports to caregivers.	• Team members use terms that are family and interdisciplinary friendly.
• Team members present predeveloped goals and objectives that are not coordinated nor integrated into a functional plan.	• Goals and objectives are functional and include multiple developmental targets whenever possible.
• Input from caregivers regarding the selection of IFSP goals and objectives does not occur.	• Caregivers are the primary decision makers in choosing goals and objectives to be targeted and the priority of goals and objectives for their child.
• The caregivers are asked to sign the IFSP without being allowed time to consider the information presented.	• Caregivers are allowed time to process the information presented at the IFSP meeting prior to signing the IFSP.
• Critical players (e.g., early intervention teacher, parents) are not included in the development of the IFSP.	• Critical players (e.g., both sending and receiving teachers and therapists) attend and participate in the development of the IFSP.

Case Study 2: Early Intervention Services

Ben is a 4-year-old with developmental delays and a diagnosis of pervasive developmental disorder. Ben lives with his mother, Mrs. Conner, and his maternal grandmother. Ben attends a preschool program 2 days a week for 3 hours each day. The IEP developed for Ben contains 8 long-range goals and 13 associated objectives that are to be targeted throughout the day and include the following:

Social Goal and Objectives

Goal 1.   *Ben will initiate and maintain communicative exchange with familiar adults.*

   Objective 1.   *Ben will respond to communication from familiar adults.*

   Objective 2.   *Ben will initiate communication with familiar adults.*

Cognitive Goal and Objective

Goal 1.   *Ben will use functionally appropriate actions on objects.*

   Objective 1.   *Ben will use simple motor actions on different objects.*

Communication Goals and Objectives

Goal 1.   *Ben will use consistent word approximations.*

   Objective 1.   *Ben will imitate consonant–vowel combinations.*

   Objective 2.   *Ben will use consistent consonant–vowel combinations for five words.*

Goal 2.   *Ben will follow one-step directions without cues.*

   Objective 1.   *Ben will follow one-step directions.*

Fine Motor Goals and Objectives

Goal 1.   *Ben will assemble toys that require putting pieces together.*

   Objective 1.   *Ben will fit shapes into corresponding space.*

   Objective 2.   *Ben will fit objects into defined spaces.*

Goal 2.   *Ben will use his index finger to activate objects.*

   Objective 1.   *Ben will show interest in a toy's function.*

   Objective 2.   *Ben will use his hand to activate objects.*

Adaptive Goal and Objective
Goal 1. *Ben will indicate toileting need.*
　　　　Objective 1. Ben will demonstrate bowel and bladder control.
Gross Motor Goal and Objectives
Goal 1. *Ben will jump forward.*
　　　　Objective 1. Ben will jump from a low structure.
　　　　Objective 2. Ben will jump up and down.

In this preschool, each professional assesses the children on his or her caseload and independently determines goals and objectives for the IEP. When Ben entered the program, the professionals convened as a team to discuss the members' individual assessment findings and to discuss their IEP recommendations. Ben's mother and grandmother attended the IEP meeting. They listened to the professionals' recommendations and signed the IEP.

Ben's preschool program is located in a public school and employs Ms. Goldberg, an early interventionist, and Ms. Tatum, an instructional aide. A communication specialist visits the program 2 days per week and provides intervention services to children in the program who have communication goals on their IEPs. The physical therapist visits the program 2 half-days per month to work with the children who have motor disabilities. The communication specialist and physical therapist attend weekly team meetings infrequently because of scheduling problems.

Mrs. Conner takes Ben to his preschool program because this gives her a potential opportunity for observation and for talking to Ms. Goldberg. When Mrs. Conner and Ben enter the preschool, Ben breaks loose from his mother's hand and races across the room where he begins to play with a toy in the corner. Mrs. Conner follows Ben and attempts to get him to take his coat off and is unsuccessful. Ms. Goldberg is busy, which offers Mrs. Conner no opportunity to talk to her before she leaves.

Ben spends 30 minutes in free play, at which time he is allowed to choose from an array of toys that are placed on the shelf. Typically, Ben will choose one toy that he enjoys spinning and/or banging. Ben gets little supervision during free play and an IEP goal or objective is rarely targeted during this time. Today, as usual, Ben does not interact with the other children during free play but instead spends most of his time spinning wheels on a truck as he sits in the corner.

Ben does not independently follow directions; therefore, when circle time begins, Ms. Tatum takes Ben's hand and directs him to the appropriate classroom area. Ms. Goldberg uses songs and finger plays to help Ben work on imitating common actions, which is one of his communication goals. Following circle time the children move to the table for snack time. Ben does not follow the other children and requires Ms. Tatum's assistance to make it to the snack table. Ben appears to enjoy snack time and Ms. Tatum has noted that he demonstrates increased eye contact with her during snack time. In addition, he will attempt a variety of vocal imitations to obtain a desired snack item.

Two times each week, after snack time, the communication specialist escorts Ben from the classroom for 30 minutes of individual therapy. Ben receives his communication therapy in isolation and when Ben returns to the room today, the communication specialist confers briefly with Ms. Goldberg about Ben's progress.

During outside time Ben wanders about and eventually indicates by gesturing that he wants to be on the swing. Ben is placed on the swing where he is observed to laugh and babble. Ms. Tatum is delighted with Ben's behavior but disappointed because the communication specialist does not see the communication Ben is displaying.

Once a month, the physical therapist removes Ben from outside time to work on his gross and fine motor skills. The therapy consists of a series of unrelated activities designed to address Ben's IEP goals for motor development. After today's session in which Ben was uncooperative, the physical therapist returns Ben to the room and leaves a note for Ms. Goldberg indicating her concerns about his uncooperativeness; however, she does not suggest a meeting with Ms. Goldberg or Ben's mother.

During the next 30 minutes, a structured activity is introduced. Each child, including Ben, is directed to select a puzzle, take it to a table, and put it together. After finishing one puzzle, children are permitted to exchange it for another. During this time, Ben drops his puzzle pieces on the floor one by one. Both Ms. Goldberg and Ms. Tatum attempt to get Ben to complete his puzzle, but he is unwilling or perhaps unable to do so. Ms. Goldberg collects data during the structured activity time.

During the last 30 minutes of the day, the class has closing circle time. Ben is once again led to the circle area for songs and finger plays. He tries to run away, but Ms. Tatum sits him on her lap.

Ben's mother returns to the classroom and tries to help Ben put on his coat. Ben squirms and resists. Ms. Goldberg comes over and assists Mrs. Conner as she briefly tells her about Ben's day at school. After the children leave, Ms. Tatum and Ms. Goldberg discuss the morning and prepare for the afternoon group of children.

The Analysis

As with the first case study, the description provided reflects a traditional approach that does not emphasize collaborative practices. Table 2 presents a comparative analysis between the traditional approach and a collaborative approach to intervention and evaluation.

Learning to collaborate goes far beyond the exchange of technical knowledge and the ability to understand the jargon of other disciplines. If professionals are expected to understand and share roles and responsibilities, they must have a variety of competencies that enhance communication and cooperation across assessment, intervention, and evaluation activities. The final case study illustrates a collaborative team approach to assessment, intervention, and evaluation of young children with disabilities.

Case Study 3: Collaborative Assessment and Intervention

Marcus was born by emergency cesarean when Mrs. Johnson went into labor unexpectedly at 29 weeks' gestation. Her pregnancy was uneventful except for a severe flu 4 weeks prior to Marcus's birth. Marcus weighed 3 pounds, 3 ounces. He remained in the neonatal intensive care unit (NICU) for 8 weeks. During his stay at the hospital, he required a respirator twice and he spent his first month under an oxygen hood. The physician reported that Marcus had some lung damage but within an 8-week period he gained weight and was discharged.

The first 14 months of Marcus's life were difficult for Mr. and Mrs. Johnson because of Marcus's frequent respiratory infections and middle ear infections. On two occasions he was hospitalized with bronchitis. The infections appeared to slow Marcus's weight gain and overall development.

By the time Marcus was 16 months old, Mr. and Mrs. Johnson believed Marcus's health was improving. Once his health was not their major concern, they became worried about his development. During Marcus's 20-month physical evaluation, Mrs. Johnson expressed her concern regarding Marcus's development to his pediatrician, Dr. Loggin. She was particu-

Table 2. Comparative analysis between traditional and collaborative approaches focused on team activities of intervention and progress evaluation

Traditional team	Collaborative team

Team Activity:
INTERVENTION
Competency 4

Traditional team	Collaborative team
• Each team member independently writes goals and objectives, which results in the IFSP containing 6 goals and 14 objectives. • Efforts to collaborate in developing the goals and objectives do not occur. • The caregiver is not involved in developing the goals and objectives on the IFSP.	• The team, which includes the caregiver, collaborates to develop the IFSP goals and objectives. • The team ensures that the IFSP is a useful working document by limiting the number of goals and objectives and assuming they are functional for the child. • The team explains to the caregiver that many opportunities naturally occur throughout the preschool day for all of the child's objectives to be targeted and that the IFSP can be changed as often as needed.
• The team does not coordinate intervention planning. • The teacher independently decides when and how to target objectives throughout the preschool day.	• The classroom interventionist shares the classroom activity schedule with all service providers and the caregiver. • The team establishes an ongoing meeting time to discuss the classroom activities and how and when to embed goals across activities.

Team Activity:
INTERVENTION PLAN
Competency 4

Traditional team	Collaborative team
• The team does not involve the caregiver in the intervention process. For example, the caregiver may be available when he or she transports the child to and from school. He or she is not involved in embedding objectives during school drop-off and pick-up times.	• The interventionist uses opportunities to establish an ongoing routine with the caregiver for working on goals and objectives in a functional manner. For example, the interventionist and caregiver could work on greeting and departure social skills when the child arrives at and departs from school.
• The team environment and structure support the philosophy of related services occurring outside of the preschool classroom setting.	• The team creates an environment that allows related professionals to be "part" of the classroom routine. Most intervention services are delivered in the classroom. For example, the child is reported to demonstrate more eye contact during snack and more babbling when he or she is on the swing; therefore, this information would be shared with the communication specialist and the specialist might choose to work with the child during those activities or provide input to other service providers on how to elicit specific behaviors from the child during those activities.

(continued)

Table 2.   (continued)

Traditional team	Collaborative team
• Team members focus on individual domains and do not target multiple goals within activities.	• Team members focus on functional and appropriate goals. • Team members share knowledge and skills that assist interventionists and family members in targeting multiple goals during functional and routine activities.
• The interventionist targets goals during specific activities. • Related services providers target goals from individual domains.	• Team members collaborate to determine the most appropriate time to target specific goals and objectives. • Team members embed training of skills across contexts, which will provide greater opportunities for acquisition.
• Team members work independently of each other. • Team members do not share information on targeted skills.	• Team members work together and share knowledge and skills regarding how to deliver services.

Team Activity:
PROGRESS EVALUATION
Competency 5

• Data collection occurs during planned activities.	• Data collection occurs across professionals and across child-initiated, routine, and planned activities.
• Data collection is not shared across professionals.	• Professionals collaborate to determine data collection process and how to share information on an ongoing basis.

larly worried about the difficulty she was still having with feeding Marcus and his slow motor and communication development. Dr. Loggin completed a developmental screening and the results indicated the need for further testing to determine if intervention services were warranted.

Referral and Assessment

A referral was made by Dr. Loggin to Start Early, a program that provides comprehensive assessment and intervention services to young children with developmental delays. Ms. Clark, a social worker from Start Early, received the referral information and telephoned Mr. and Mrs. Johnson. Ms. Clark explained that their service system provided a variety of services and that an assessment would determine whether Marcus was eligible for services and, if so, what type of intervention services were needed. Ms. Clark made an appointment for a home visit to further explain the Start Early program and discuss options for assessment services.

During the home visit Ms. Clark collected pertinent intake information to share with other team members. Mr. and Mrs. Johnson expressed their concern with Marcus's slow development. After the background information was collected and Mr. and Mrs. Johnson were given an opportunity to ask questions, Ms. Clark explained the general team assessment procedures that would be used.

Ms. Clark inquired about what type of involvement they wanted in the assessment process and encouraged both parents to take an active role. Mr. and Mrs. Johnson were willing to participate in the assessment if it would help the professionals better understand Mar-

cus. Mr. Johnson asked that the assessment be conducted at the Start Early building, rather than in their home, because he wanted to see the facility. Before leaving, Ms. Clark said she would share the intake information with team members and coordinate schedules for Marcus's assessment.

Ms. Clark presented the intake information during the next team meeting. The team discussed schedules and determined that Dr. George (the psychologist), Ms. Heather (the communication specialist), and Ms. Rodman (the occupational therapist) would coordinate schedules for Marcus's assessment. After being informed that Mr. and Mrs. Johnson wanted to come to the facility for the assessment, the team suggested that the Johnsons bring some of Marcus's favorite toys. Understanding that feeding was of concern, they suggested the appointment be scheduled around a snack time to assess Marcus's eating skills. Although the team always functions in a flexible manner during assessments, in order to follow the child's lead the team members developed a tentative schedule and discussed roles and responsibilities. The tentative schedule was mailed to Mr. and Mrs. Johnson. The assessment schedule included the following activities:

8:50 A.M.	Meet with social worker
9:00 A.M.	Arena assessment with psychologist, occupational therapist, and communication specialist
10:00 A.M.	Feeding assessment
10:20 A.M.	Postteam–family assessment debriefing
10:40 A.M.	Postteam assessment debriefing

Mr. and Mrs. Johnson arrived on Monday morning and were greeted by Ms. Clark. They were escorted to a playroom and asked to make themselves comfortable. They sat on the floor and Marcus began to explore the playroom. Ms. Clark explained that this was a time for Marcus to adjust to the new surroundings and that she would answer any questions the parents might have before the other team members arrived.

At the same time Ms. Clark was answering questions, the assessment team was meeting to review its prior decisions regarding the assessment purpose and process to ensure it was organized to collect necessary and accurate assessment data. The occupational therapist indicated that she had arrived at 8:30 A.M. and prepared the playroom environment for the assessment. Team members reviewed roles and responsibilities. The psychologist planned to administer the Bayley Scales of Infant Development (Bayley, 1993) for eligibility purposes and to address cognitive development. The communication specialist and occupational therapist were planning to assess the other developmental domains by using a criterion-referenced curriculum-based assessment, which would collect functional and programmatic information. The team agreed to follow the child's lead whenever possible; however, Dr. George would take the lead when he needed to administer standardized test items.

Dr. George, Ms. Heather, and Ms. Rodman entered the playroom, sat on the floor, and introduced themselves. Marcus was busy playing with a pop-up toy as the professionals briefly chatted with Mr. and Mrs. Johnson. Dr. George asked how Marcus was feeling. Ms. Rodman noticed that Marcus was having a difficult time manipulating a button on the pop-up toy and attempted to assist him. Ms. Heather noted that he was vocalizing in response to his frustration with the pop-up toy and that he exhibited joint attention when Ms. Rodman started to interact with him. The team continued to gather pertinent and functional information to complete the assessment as Marcus played.

While Ms. Rodman was interacting with Marcus, she noted that he preferred to crawl around the room rather than walk. She continued to interact with Marcus in order to obtain her assessment information, while Dr. George observed and was able to score several standardized test items. When Ms. Rodman completed her assessment, Dr. George continued by introducing the remaining test items on the Bayley Scales. While Dr. George was interacting with Marcus, both Ms. Heather and Ms. Rodman asked Dr. George to try different strategies to elicit behaviors of interest. After completing the Bayley Scales, Marcus was offered a snack. As requested, Marcus's typical snack food had been brought and the team asked Mrs. Johnson to interact with Marcus as she usually did during snack. Ms. Heather and Ms. Rodman observed and answered questions posed by Mr. and Mrs. Johnson.

Following his snack, Marcus was taken from the high chair and placed on the floor near his favorite toys. At this time, Ms. Clark returned and the team obtained the final information it needed through a parent report. The team asked the parents about their impression of Marcus's performance during the assessment and shared its impressions by commenting on Marcus's strengths and areas where he showed significant developmental delays.

Ms. Clark informed Mr. and Mrs. Johnson that the team would write a comprehensive report regarding its assessment of Marcus and asked if there was anything they wanted included in the report. She explained that a meeting would be scheduled to discuss the report and to suggest possible referrals for services. She provided Mr. and Mrs. Johnson with a list of area programs. The team recommended two centers that might best meet Marcus's needs. They encouraged the parents to visit these centers and determine which one they might choose for Marcus in order to have an opportunity to invite the receiving agency staff to the IFSP meeting. In closing, the IFSP meeting was scheduled and a home visit was arranged to help prepare the family for the IFSP meeting.

The team convened for the postteam assessment debriefing. Dr. George asked how team members felt about the assessment process. Ms. Heather appreciated Ms. Rodman's verbal and nonverbal interactions with Marcus because they helped her quickly obtain a sample of his gestures and vocalizations. Ms. Rodman was pleased with the family interaction that occurred during the assessment because it allowed her to obtain essential data in a short time period. Dr. George believed the assessment went well and he had been able to administer all relevant items from the standardized test. Ms. Clark believed the family was involved in the assessment and reported that they left feeling satisfied and comfortable with the information they received.

Ms. Rodman agreed to write the interdisciplinary evaluation report. Team members were asked to give their assessment results to Ms. Rodman by a specific date to allow her to integrate the information into one report. Ms. Clark reminded the team that she was going to make a home visit to prepare Mr. and Mrs. Johnson for the IFSP meeting.

Individualized Family Service Plan

Mr. and Mrs. Johnson arrived at the IFSP meeting feeling apprehensive but prepared because Ms. Clark had told them what to expect and how they could contribute to the process. They were happy to know that Ms. Clark asked Ms. Lexington, the teacher from the Teeter Totter Toddler Program, to the IFSP meeting. Mr. and Mrs. Johnson observed various toddler programs and told Ms. Clark that their first choice was Ms. Lexington's program. It was agreed that the IFSP meeting would be held in two phases. Phase 1 would be a preliminary meeting to address eligibility and placement and to structure a preliminary IFSP. Phase 2 would be used to write the selected goals, objectives, and outcomes and would occur following the administration of program-relevant assessment measures.

The preliminary IFSP meeting began with Ms. Clark asking Mr. and Mrs. Johnson to share their impressions regarding Marcus's development and to talk about the goals that were important for them and Marcus. The Johnsons referred to a developmental child form, which had been provided by Ms. Clark. They found this form helpful because it was designed for parents and helped them better understand Marcus's development, contribute developmental information to the IFSP process, and suggest and prioritize goals for Marcus.

The professionals shared their assessment results and overall impressions, while using family-friendly terminology. Dr. George indicated the scores from the standardized test revealed Marcus was eligible for intervention services. He explained that the Bayley Scales of Infant Development was administered for eligibility purposes only and the intervention team would now need to administer a program-relevant, curriculum-based assessment tool. Ms. Rodman reported on Marcus's performance in the fine motor, gross motor, and adaptive areas. She recommended that Marcus be examined by a physical therapist. Ms. Heather discussed Marcus's emerging communication and social skills. Dr. George summarized the assessment outcome and recommended that Marcus receive intervention services. The team, including the Johnsons, discussed service possibilities and family desires. Mr. and Mrs. Johnson told the team that they had visited a number of sites and, as mentioned at the beginning of the meeting, they liked Ms. Lexington's program the best. The team agreed to reconvene in 3 weeks after Ms. Lexington had the opportunity to observe Marcus and administer a curriculum-based assessment measure.

The Phase 2 IFSP meeting began with team members, including Ms. Lexington and the parents, selecting family outcomes. A family needs assessment form completed by the Johnsons prior to the IFSP meeting helped the family prioritize outcomes. Functional child goals and objectives were developed using family concerns and the curriculum-based assessment information gathered by Ms. Lexington. The goals and objectives were developed collaboratively by considering family priorities and professional evaluation results.

The team ensured that the IFSP was an effective, useful document by writing goals and objectives that were functional, meaningful, generative, and measurable. Team members selected four priority goals to assist in focusing intervention activities and ensure manageable data collection. Ms. Lexington explained that the selected IFSP goals and objectives would be embedded within the Teeter Totter Toddler Program's activities.

Upon completion of the IFSP, Ms. Clark told Mr. and Mrs. Johnson that they could take some time to think about the IFSP before signing the document. Mr. Johnson asked when services could begin and Ms. Lexington agreed to have Marcus start the following week.

Planning

Ms. Lexington called Mr. and Mrs. Johnson and invited them to the next Teeter Totter Toddler Program staff meeting. Ms. Lexington introduced Mrs. Johnson and Marcus and asked her to provide the staff with information about Marcus.

The staff introduced themselves, discussed their program and team philosophy, and explained that they hold weekly planning meetings to discuss weekly activities. Ms. Lexington explained that all the goals and objectives were embedded into the classroom routine and at times related service professionals took on the "activity leader" role. For example, many times the communication specialist leads a snack activity to target specific communication objectives and collect data, whereas the occupational therapist may plan and lead snack on another day to embed adaptive skills and collect data.

The team shared the activity schedule with Mrs. Johnson and explained that most skills could be embedded across the daily activities to allow children to practice their IFSP objectives in functional and meaningful contexts. The Teeter Totter Toddler Program staff reviewed Marcus's IFSP and discussed the selected goals and objectives. Mrs. Johnson reported that she and her husband were comfortable with the objectives on the IFSP and that they were *ready to sign the IFSP, knowing that the IFSP could be revisited after the physical therapist assessed Marcus.*

The team members agreed that the IFSP contained functional goals for Marcus and that the physical therapy assessment could be completed in the Teeter Totter Toddler Program the following week. The team members were delighted to see that the IFSP contained only four goals to help them focus their intervention activities and manage data collection. The following are two of the goals:

Marcus will use his index fingers to activate a variety of objects throughout the day.
During routine and planned activities, when provided with a verbal model, Marcus will imitate a consonant–vowel combination to refer to an object, person, and/or event across 3 consecutive days.

The meeting concluded with the staff and Mrs. Johnson developing an activity schedule for embedding Marcus's objectives into the program's activities. The activity schedule is shown in Figure 2.

Intervention

Mrs. Johnson arrived at the Teeter Totter Toddler Program and began to take off Marcus's jacket. This was Marcus's third week of class and she was delighted to see that he already looked forward to going to the classroom. Upon arrival, Ms. Lexington greeted Mrs. Johnson and showed her how to target an IFSP goal as she removed Marcus's jacket.

Marcus noticed the toys in the center of the room near the other children. He crawled over to the toys and began to play. The instructional aide joined Marcus and assisted him in manipulating the toys. She was aware of the fine motor IFSP objective and used naturally occurring opportunities during free play time to encourage the use of his index finger to activate objects.

Today, the communication specialist was in the classroom. The communication specialist, as well as the other related services personnel, were scheduled to be in the room for 1 hour, 1–2 times a week. Time blocks varied across days, which allowed for the observation of children in a variety of activities and the opportunity to model strategies across activities and children. The communication specialist noticed Marcus was playing with a large toy dump truck. She moved toward Marcus and began to embed a communication goal by labeling objects and providing a consistent consonant–vowel combination model for objects. When Marcus vocalized, he was reinforced by receiving the object. Once the truck was full, he dumped the objects and giggled. The communication specialist wanted to collect data on another child and asked the instructional aide to continue the activity that she just modeled for Marcus.

At 9:20 A.M. the children moved into circle time. Marcus was helped to the circle by Ms. Lexington using one-hand support. This assistance was provided during each classroom transition period. Marcus enjoyed circle time and many of the songs and finger plays were adapted by the circle leader to target his communication goal. After circle time, the children went to the sand table for a planned activity. Again, Marcus was offered one-hand support for his movement to the play area.

Today the occupational therapist led the planned activity that embedded fine motor activities. Marcus pushed the cars around in the sand and used the big spoons to transfer the sand from one object to another. Ms. Lexington collected data on four of the children in the group as they played.

When it was time for the class to go outside, it was raining. As the back-up activity, Ms. Lexington had the children participate in movement activities that included rolling, crawl-

Activity Schedule

	Marcus			
	Uses index finger to activate objects	Walks with one hand support	Brings food to mouth with utensil	Uses consistent consonant–vowel combinations
9 A.M. Arrival Free play	X			X
9:20 A.M. Opening circle		X Transition		X
9:30 A.M. Planned activity	X	X Transition		X
10 A.M. Outside play		X Transition		X
10:20 A.M. Cleanup				
10:30 A.M. Snack			X	X
11 A.M. Story time		X Transition		X
11:20 A.M. Closing circle				X
11:40 A.M. Departure		X Transition		X

Figure 2. An activity schedule developed to embed the objectives of an IFSP into program activities.

ing, stretching, and walking as well as other basic range-of-motion activities. Before starting the movement activities, she asked the children to remove their shoes and socks and place them in their cubbies. After the movement activities, the children were asked to get and put on their shoes and socks. This activity provided many of the children the opportunity to practice adaptive skills and follow one-step directions.

By 10:30 A.M. the children had been in and out of the bathroom in which they had the opportunity to engage in adaptive skills (e.g., washing their hands and faces before snack time). Today, snack included finger foods and foods that required using an eating utensil. Marcus was asked to use his spoon for the applesauce. The instructional aide helped Marcus in transferring the food to his mouth. During snack the children were provided with developmentally appropriate communication models or prompts to request snack items. Opportunities to prac-

tice adaptive, communication, and social skills were provided and encouraged by the staff. Af-
ter snack the children were asked to clean up their snack areas before moving to the book area.

The children completed the day by participating in story time and closing circle activity.
Closing circle allowed Marcus to practice targeted communication skills. Parents who did
not stay for the entire session were encouraged to arrive in time for closing circle activities.
Closing circle time was used for children to share what happened that day. Mrs. Johnson al-
ways enjoyed this part of the day because it allowed her to hear highlights of what Marcus
may have said or done, as well as what the other children achieved or practiced. In closing,
parents assisted the children in getting ready to leave for the day and classroom staff an-
swered questions as the children prepared to leave.

After the children were gone for the day, Ms. Lexington and the instructional aide dis-
cussed the success of the various activities. They noted their observations in order to share
with the other team members during the weekly planning meeting. The children's perfor-
mance data were discussed and transferred to the weekly data collection sheet.

The Analysis

This case study describes the necessary structure of a collaborative team
practice in assessment and intervention services, emphasizes the many opportunities that occur naturally within a child's play, and emphasizes how to take
advantage of the situations that occur while collaboratively assessing and intervening with young children with disabilities and their families.

CONCLUDING REMARKS: FUTURE DIRECTIONS

This chapter began by acknowledging the considerable differences between a traditional multidisciplinary and collaborative approach to assessment, intervention, and evaluation. The differences were emphasized through the presentation
of three case studies in which traditional procedures were contrasted with a collaborative process in two case studies and a collaborative team process illus-
trated in the third case study.

This chapter presents a synthesis of the principles and competencies
thought to be essential to collaborative team building and practice that have
been extracted from other chapters in this book and from other relevant literature. The authors have tried to operationalize the many competencies that, they
believe, underlie in large measure successful teams.

The importance of setting a climate conducive to collaboration has also
been emphasized. For most people making independent decisions, formulating
isolated plans, and then implementing those plans as each person sees fit is difficult to relinquish. Collaboration requires negotiation, compromise, elimination
of barriers, and, most significantly, change. Change is difficult for most people
and moving from traditional approaches to cooperative endeavors requires considerable change. Without a genuine commitment to the development and maintenance of collaborative practice, teams will not succeed over time. Equally
important is the need for an environment or climate that reinforces individual
and group attempts at collaboration. In the beginning stages, teams are likely to
stumble, fall, and even crash and burn—to get over such challenges requires sig-

nificant environmental support for regrouping and continuing toward the goal of effective collaborative practice.

Clearly, the presence of a supportive climate is a necessary but not a sufficient condition for collaboration to occur. In addition, team members require a set of guiding principles and an array of specific competencies if they are to initiate and maintain effective collaborative practice. These principles and competencies have been extracted from the authors' clinical experiences and from the descriptive literature because, so far as they know, there is no empirical basis for the selection of such principles and competencies.

The quality of the assessment, intervention, and evaluation that occurs in early intervention will be largely depend on the professionals' success in learning how to collaborate. Therefore, there are two challenges all the disciplines associated with early intervention programs must begin to face. The first challenge is for professionals to dedicate themselves to the acquisition of knowledge and skills that will lead to increasingly successful collaboration. The second challenge is to study the collaborative process so that in the future early intervention professionals can build training content and process based on what is known to be effective rather than on what is thought to be effective.

REFERENCES

Bayley, N. (1993). *Bayley Scales of Infant Development—Second Edition Manual*. San Antonio, TX: The Psychological Corporation.

Frankenburg, W.K., Dodds, J.B., Fandal, A.W., Kazuk, E., & Cohrs, M. (1975). *Denver Developmental Screening Test manual* (Rev. ed.). Denver: University of Colorado Medical Center.

Fullan, M., & Stiegelbauer, S. (1991). *The new meaning of educational change* (2nd ed.). New York: Teachers College Press.

Hedrick, D.L., Prather, E.M., & Tobin, A.R. (1975). *Sequenced Inventory of Communication Development (SICD)*. Seattle: University of Washington Press.

Kovarsky, D. (1992). Ethnography and language assessment: Toward the contextualized description and interpretation of communication behavior. In W.A. Secord & J.S. Damico (Eds.), *Best practices in speech language pathology* (pp. 115–122). San Antonio, TX: The Psychological Corporation.

Lester, N.B., & Onore, C.S. (1990). *Learning change*. Portsmouth, NH: Heinemann Educational Books.

Pugach, M.C., & Johnson, L.J. (1995). *Collaborative practitioners, collaborative schools*. Denver, CO: Love.

Webster's new universal unabridged dictionary. (1983). New York: Dorset & Baber.

17

INTO THE 21ST CENTURY

Anne Widerstrom
and Diane Bricker

GIVEN THE NUMBER AND VARIETY of disciplines represented among the authors of the preceding chapters, it is noteworthy to find so much agreement in identifying issues of concern related to team training. Nearly all the authors agree that training students and professionals in the field of early intervention to collaborate effectively as team members is challenging. In many cases, the authors also agree about reasons for the difficulty and about possible solutions. In this chapter the major issues of concern raised in the previous chapters are examined as well as specific foundational issues associated with team training as the 21st century approaches.

ISSUES OF CONCERN ACROSS CHAPTERS

The most frequently expressed concern among the authors of this book, regardless of discipline represented, is the need for collaboration in team training. In each chapter, the difficulty in establishing and maintaining effective team collaboration is acknowledged and discussed. A major barrier mentioned by several authors is that most disciplinary training does not prepare students to work collaboratively with professionals from other disciplines. Instead, coursework tends primarily to reflect the discipline awarding the degree or license, with minimal content introduced from related disciplines. In addition, students are given few opportunities to participate in practicum or clinical settings with students from other disciplines. The lack of interdisciplinary course content and field-based settings is matched by the lack of well-functioning, exemplary teams in the field that can serve as models for recommended practice. Consequently, students have little opportunity for exposure to the content and practice of other disciplines or to see effective teams at work. These problems exist in most academic training programs in the United States.

Most disciplines associated with early intervention have fairly extensive licensing requirements. Therefore, training program faculty may see few opportunities to extend their training to encompass the content and fieldwork necessary to train students to become collaborative team members. There is uniform agreement that the professional working in early intervention should use a team approach; however, in 1996, this is not happening, which poses a major question. Is the field of early intervention sufficiently committed to collaborative teams to offer the interdisciplinary training necessary to prepare professionals to successfully participate on teams?

The question of commitment raises another concern mentioned by several authors, including Bricker and LaCroix in reporting the results of a national training survey (see Chapter 3). Training programs vary widely in the amount and quality of training they offer. Some programs call themselves interdisciplinary when in actuality they offer students little interdisciplinary content or field-based practice. There is variation among training programs, for example, in the amount of time students from different disciplines spend together in coursework and internship experiences; yet nearly all programs surveyed by Bricker and LaCroix called themselves interdisciplinary (see Chapter 3). The fact that the need for team collaboration skills was emphasized by all of the authors of this book suggests that the leaders in the early intervention field are fully aware of the limited team training found in many of the training programs and of the lack of collaborative practice in community programs serving young children and their families. The field of early intervention must acknowledge this fact and move toward considering various models and strategies for achieving better collaboration in training and subsequent practice.

Systematic examination is needed to determine what makes training effective—that is, what does and does not work. Serious thought should be given to the kind of professional practitioners needed in early intervention programs. Effective practice should be identified through data-based research methods that measure outcomes, rather than exclusively through opinion surveys as is the current approach (e.g., Gallagher, Shields, & Staples, 1990; Hanson & Lovett, 1992; National Association for the Education of Young Children (NAEYC), 1994). Training programs should then be developed around objectively based tenets of effective team practice. It is unfortunate that the human services disciplines seem more inclined than the scientific fields to accept practice based on opinion rather than on objective data. As a result, early intervention practices are often embraced because intuitively they appear superior to what they replace. Yet, often the data to support these practices are either lacking altogether or the data collection occurs long after the practice has become established. Although all of the authors of this book agree in principle that team training represents recommended practice in early intervention, the data to support such a view are insufficient.

What constitutes effective team practice and how can it be measured? This is a more important question than whether teams should be multi-, inter-, or transdisciplinary in their functioning style. Criteria for effectiveness should be established as functional outcomes that can be measured in team practice. Functional outcomes should be established and measured for parents and family members as well as for the children who are the target of early intervention. In addition, the way resources are used in early intervention should be examined. For example, does team collaboration result in desired outcomes for children? What about for parents? Does it represent a better use of scarce resources? Intuitively, the answers to these questions are affirmative, but data are needed to confirm or reject the authors' intuitions. An associated set of important questions focuses on determining which training practices result in professionals who are collaborative team members and who can produce desired outcomes for children and families and use resources wisely. Systematic observation and data collection are needed to answer these questions. Such outcome data would do much to enrich the ongoing discussion of how to develop effective personnel training systems (Bennett, Watson, & Raab, 1991; Fenichel & Eggbeer, 1990; Kemple, Hartle, Correa, & Fox, 1994; McCollum & Bailey, 1991).

A final issue addressed by many authors is the significant barrier to establishing effective team training across and between disciplines given the climate found in many universities in the mid-1990s. The administrative and funding structures of most universities work against cross-disciplinary teaching. Typically, teaching loads of the university faculty are tied to departmental budgets that are generated by student credit hours, making it difficult to offer interdepartmental courses and practica. Some universities have attempted to create interdepartmental, cross-disciplinary programs only to discontinue them in the face of administrative barriers that seem insurmountable.

Clearly, the authors agree on the need for training students and professionals in the field to become effective team members. They also agree that significant challenges remain before effective team training can be achieved. Training programs often lack the necessary content and supervised practice to assist students in becoming effective team members. Perhaps a more fundamental challenge is the lack of objective data for choosing the content and training practices that should be employed. In addition, the political climate and fight for diminishing resources make the modification of university-based training programs a major challenge.

FOUNDATIONS FOR EFFECTIVE TEAM TRAINING

At the national level there are several broad-based foundational issues that affect the success of team training. These issues include 1) funding, 2) state regulations, 3) comprehensive training plans, 4) collaboration between early intervention and early childhood education (ECE), and 5) federal incentives for collaborative training.

Funding

Many difficulties associated with team training are directly related to economics. Sufficient funds to conduct effective team training are essential. A perusal of the chapters in this book quickly makes apparent the complex and extensive content that early interventionists are required to master. The training necessary to acquire competence in any single discipline represented in this book is considerable. Once having grasped their discipline-specific content and skills, professionals then need to go on to study additional complex material related to team functioning. Because it is not economically feasible to keep students in school for extended periods of time, most training programs are faced with a serious dilemma of developing a balance between team training and discipline-specific training. In addition, there is often significant pressure for professionals to enter the field as soon as possible so they can provide much-needed services to children and families.

The solution is to develop preservice and in-service training programs that integrate team content and strategies directly into the disciplinary training.

Rather than viewing team building as a separate and additional set of content and skills, this content must be seen as integral to the professional training.

State Regulations for a Seamless System

PL 99-457, the Education of the Handicapped Act Amendments of 1986 (reauthorized as PL 102-119, the Individuals with Disabilities Education Act Amendments of 1991), permits states to develop service delivery systems that fit their situations. Unlike PL 94-142, the Education for All Handicapped Children Act of 1975, which mandated special education services for school-age children, PL 99-457 was based on the premise of states' rights. Whereas PL 94-142 mandated the same service delivery system nationwide for children ages 5–21, PL 99-457 gave states flexibility in the type and quantity of services they could provide to young children and their families, including no services for infants and toddlers if they chose.

Consequently, states have adopted different service delivery models. Some states have chosen to develop a seamless system for offering early intervention services to children from birth to 6 years of age (e.g., Colorado, Iowa, Michigan, Oregon, Wisconsin). These states have established early intervention systems based in the state department of education to serve all eligible young children from birth to 6 years of age. California and Illinois, however, are among states that have elected to serve infants and toddlers ages birth to 3 through a designated lead agency different from the state Department of Education, which is responsible for serving 3- to 5-year-olds. Whether a delivery system is seamless is important because it establishes the context in which training takes place and affects a number of important dimensions. For example, it may affect how professionals are prepared to serve on teams. Professionals in programs for children from birth to 3 years old and their teams may function differently from those teams who serve 3- to 5-year-olds. In addition, preparing for transitions in non-seamless systems may take considerably more time and effort than in moving children and their families along in seamless systems.

States also vary in how they defined the children's eligibility for services. Some states serve children considered to be at risk for disability or developmental delay; others serve only those who fully meet the criteria of having a delay or a disability. The lack of continuity in service delivery from state to state makes it difficult to maintain a national standard or accepted model for team training. Therefore, states need to adopt a set of regulatory guidelines that is consistent within and across states so, in turn, training programs can design team content that is appropriate and effective for professionals working in all states.

Comprehensive Training Plans

The need for a coordinated, comprehensive, nationwide training system is acknowledged by nearly all professionals involved in higher education and team training. There are some components that most would agree should be included in a model national training plan. These components include an interdisciplinary focus (Fenichel & Eggbeer, 1990), training divided into levels or stages to allow for career advancement (Hanson & Brekken, 1991), long-range training goals that include both preservice and in-service components (Bruder & Nikitas, 1992), information about community-based service delivery, an emphasis on prevention, attention to issues of cultural and linguistic diversity (Christensen, 1992), and a focus on children who are birth to 6 or 8 years old with sufficient emphasis on including families in partnership roles (Thurman et al., 1990).

Given the economic climate in the United States in the mid-1990s as well as the increasing numbers of young children who are being identified as needing services, service delivery must become increasingly cost effective in the coming decades. A team approach that promotes role sharing among members can be economical if paraprofessionals, parents, and other staff members can receive appropriate training (Widerstrom, Mowder, & Sandall, 1991). Career ladders that offer opportunities for advancement to paraprofessionals and professionals alike should be considered an important component of such a plan (Hanson & Brekken, 1991). In addition to cost-effective practices such as team role release, trends in service delivery include giving the consumer (i.e., the child's family) a greater, more responsible role in the intervention process and moving service delivery into community settings such as public school clinics, Head Start, child care, and the child's home (Widerstrom et al., 1991).

As the 21st century approaches, more children who are medically or environmentally at risk are being identified at birth or during infancy, which makes the possibility of preventing serious disabilities increasingly important (Bricker & Cripe, 1992). Team training should therefore include information about prevention, which should be available to community-based staff (e.g., child care workers). In addition, more use of prevention as a tool of public policy could result in the government eliminating the root causes of risk (i.e., poverty, drug abuse, teen pregnancy, and other social problems) (Widerstrom et al., 1991). One way to address the issue of prevention is to train early interventionists to assume the role of policy advocate. Because early intervention is dependent on public funding, parents and professionals must work together to ensure the continuance of programs. Team training has the potential to effectively bring together people of various disciplines to advocate for quality services for young children at risk and with disabilities.

A comprehensive training model should be coordinated both across and within disciplines. To prepare students to work effectively in situations that call for interagency collaboration and interdisciplinary cooperation, not only should professionals in health, psychology, education, social work, and communication disorders share extensive coursework and internship experiences, but students in early intervention programs should share experiences with those serving older children who are at risk and/or have disabilities (Widerstrom et al., 1991). Related to this is the need for a greater variety of appropriate training materials to reflect the team approach. A serious need exists for up-to-date curriculum guides and instructional materials in film, print, videotape, and interactive computer formats especially designed for training people from diverse disciplines in collaborative team practice. This is a time-consuming and expensive task that has received inadequate attention from the early intervention field (Widerstrom et al., 1991).

Collaboration Between Early Intervention and Early Childhood Education (ECE)

As the fields of early intervention and ECE join to serve all young children in the mainstream, foundational issues for team training emerge that are related to both fields (Division for Early Childhood of the Council for Exceptional Children, NAEYC, & Association of Teacher Educators, 1994). Early childhood educators work primarily in private preschools, Head Start programs, or child care programs. These programs often have less rigorous training requirements for their staff than those found in early intervention. Although many teachers employed in ECE programs have master's degrees, Head Start and child care programs typically require an associate or bachelor's degree. Because early intervention programs typically require both a graduate degree and a special education credential, there is an obvious discrepancy in the levels of training required for each field. Reconciling these varying training needs presents a challenge to programs serving young children.

Collaborative efforts in training are often part of the interagency agreements required by federal law between Head Start programs and school districts to facilitate inclusion of young children with disabilities in general education programs (Hanson & Widerstrom, 1993). Joint and other types of in-service training are difficult to conduct when two groups with disparate needs are combined. Finding a middle ground between the training needs of special educators and of early childhood educators may mean that the staff development needs of neither group are met. Furthermore, efforts to use a collaborative training model may be complicated by the inclusion of therapists and other specialists.

At least two problems need to be addressed in developing a successful collaborative training model. First, the addition of other professionals to the training results in a third set of training needs because therapists and other team members (e.g., physicians, nurses, social workers), although accustomed to working with children individually, generally lack knowledge about how to work with groups of children. Learning how to work with groups of children is usually at the foundation of training programs in the field of education, so early interventionists and early childhood educators generally enter graduate training having already had extensive practice in working with large or small groups of children. They have usually mastered these skills. Second, although the specific discipline-based knowledge that other team members bring to training is valuable for early interventionists and early childhood educators, the problem of role release may inhibit the sharing process. For example, therapists may be trained to provide specific interventions, especially those for children with severe disabilities or medical needs, that they believe should not be carried out by professionals outside their field. Although it may be true that some specialized procedures should not be used by those who lack specialized training, many therapeutic and medical procedures can be used by other team members if they receive adequate training. A commitment to collaborative team training requires that the issue of role release be directly confronted by all participating disciplines.

Federal Incentives for Collaborative Training

As part of the federal policy that encourages the delivery of services to infants and toddlers with disabilities, federal funding has become available to train higher-education faculty for working with children from birth to 3 years old. Four regional institutes have been funded by the U.S. Department of Education to increase the number of higher-education programs that provide training in working with children age birth to 3 to professionals from the various disciplines associated with disabilities. The four institutes, based at Temple University, the University of Colorado, the University of North Carolina, and the University of Minnesota, work closely with state departments of education and health to coordinate in-service training for faculty. Other institutes provide similar training in other regions of the nation. This type of institute represents a first step in the development of a coordinated, comprehensive national training system. Although current institutes are focused on the birth-to-3 population, they could be expanded both horizontally and vertically to include content related to older children and also to expand the number of disciplines represented.

Federal incentives for collaborative training are fundamental to the success of these training efforts. Without federal support and encouragement, neither states, professional organizations, nor universities can or will mount the efforts necessary to build and maintain preservice and in-service programs that will prepare professionals from a broad range of disciplines to appreciate, understand, and engage in effective collaborative practices.

CONCLUDING REMARKS

This book should make it clear the challenges ahead are not only important but difficult. To put it simply, as the 21st century approaches, professionals cannot move forward in early intervention without the general installation of collaborative team practices among professionals and between professionals and family members. Also clear is that the establishment of collaborative practices will not happen without adequate training for the professionals who are assigned this critical task. Finally, it is clear that changes in training programs (both in-service and preservice) will not occur without leadership, advocacy, and the necessary funding and policy.

Will comprehensive team training happen? In a national environment with ever-increasing competition for resources, the answer is not clear. However, it seems certain that without a commitment and effort by most professionals associated with early intervention, comprehensive team training most assuredly will not happen. We hope this book contributes to the building of that effort and that as we move into the 21st century we do so with the firm conviction that collaborative team practice will happen.

REFERENCES

Bennett, T., Watson, A.L., & Raab, M. (1991). Ensuring competence in early intervention personnel through personnel standards and high-quality training. *Infants and Young Children, 3*(3), 49–58.

Bricker, D., & Cripe, J. (1992). *An activity-based approach to early intervention.* Baltimore: Paul H. Brookes Publishing Co.

Bruder, M.B., & Nikitas, T. (1992). Changing the professional practice of early interventionists: An inservice model to meet the service needs of P.L. 99-457. *Journal of Early Intervention, 16,* 173–189.

Christensen, C.M. (1992). Multicultural competencies in early intervention: Training professionals for a pluralistic society. *Infants and Young Children, 4*(3), 49–63.

Division for Early Childhood of the Council for Exceptional Children, National Association for the Education of Young Children (NAEYC), & Association of Teacher Educators. (1994, October). *Personnel standards for early education and early intervention: Guidelines for licensure in early childhood special education.* Washington, DC: Authors.

Education for All Handicapped Children Act of 1975, PL 94-142. (August 23, 1977). Title 20, U.S.C. 1400 et seq: *U.S. Statutes at Large, 89,* 773–796.

Education of the Handicapped Act Amendments of 1986, PL 99-457. (October 8, 1986). Title 20, U.S.C. 1400 et seq: *U.S. Statutes at Large, 100,* 1145–1177.

Fenichel, E., & Eggbeer, L. (1990). *Preparing practitioners to work with infants, toddlers and their families: Issues and recommendations for the professions.* Arlington, VA: National Center for Clinical Infant Programs.

Gallagher, J.J., Shields, M., & Staples, M. (1990, May). *Personnel preparation options: Ideas from a policy options conference.* Chapel Hill: Carolina Policy Studies Program, University of North Carolina. (ERIC Document Reproduction Service No. ED 327 026)

Hanson, M.J., & Brekken, L.J. (1991). Early intervention personnel models and standards: An interdisciplinary field-developed approach. *Infants and Young Children, 4*(1), 54–61.

Hanson, M.J., & Lovett, D. (1992). Personnel preparation for early interventionists: A cross-disciplinary survey. *Journal of Early Intervention, 16*(2), 123–135.

Hanson, M.J., & Widerstrom, A.H. (1993). Consultation and collaboration: Essentials of integration efforts for young children. In C.A. Peck, S.L. Odom, & D.D. Bricker (Eds.), *Integrating young children with disabilities into community programs: Ecological perspectives on research and implementation* (pp. 149–168). Baltimore: Paul H. Brookes Publishing Co.

Individuals with Disabilities Education Act Amendements of 1991, PL 102–119. (October 7, 1991). Title 20, U.S.C. 1400 et seq: *U.S. Statutes at Large, 105,* 587–608.

Kemple, K., Hartle, L., Correa, V., & Fox, L. (1994). Preparing teachers for inclusive education. *Teacher Education and Special Education, 17*(1), 38–51.

McCollum, J.A., & Bailey, D.B. (1991). Developing comprehensive personnel systems: Issues and alternatives. *Journal of Early Intervention, 15,* 51–56.

National Association for the Education of Young Children (NAEYC). (1994). NAEYC position statement: A conceptual framework for early childhood professional development. *Young Children, 49*(3), 68–77.

Thurman, S.K., Brown, C., Bryan, M., Henderson, A., Klein, M.D., Sainato, D.M., & Wiley, T. (1990). *Some perspectives on preparing personnel to work with at risk children birth to five.* Washington, DC: U.S. Department of Education, Office of Educational Research and Improvement. (ERIC Document Reproduction Service No. ED 343 342)

Widerstrom, A.H., Mowder, B.A., & Sandall, S.R. (1991). *At-risk and handicapped newborns and infants.* Englewood Cliffs, NJ: Prentice Hall.

INDEX

Page numbers followed by "f" indicate figures; those followed by "t" indicate tables.